EMERGENCY MEDICINE

the essentials

A Concise, Comprehensive Guide To The
Diagnosis And Treatment
Of Emergency Medical Conditions

Stephen P. McElroy, M.D., FACEP

Health Emergency Publishing

Emergency Medicine The Essentials
Stephen P. McElroy, M.D.
Health Emergency Publishing

ISBN 0-9722470-0-9

Published by
Health Emergency Publishing
43 Whaler Lane, Suite 100, Quincy, MA 02171.

Printed in the United States of America
First Printing

"We are all here to help others; what on earth the others are here for I don't know."- W. H. Auden

This book is dedicated to Lauren, Shannon, and Jake

TABLE OF CONTENTS

Chapter 1: ALLERGY 1
   I.   ALLERGIC REACTIONS 1
      A. Anaphylaxis/Allergic Reaction 1
      B. Angioedema/Urticaria 3

Chapter 2: ANESTHESIA 5
   I.   RAPID SEQUENCE INTUBATION; ALTERNATIVE
       AIRWAY OPTIONS 5

Chapter 3: CARDIOVASCULAR 10
   I.   ACLS- see appendix
   II. ABDOMINAL AORTIC ANEURYSM (AAA) 10
   III. AORTIC DISSECTION (THORACIC) 11
   IV. ARRHYTHMIAS 13
      A. Atrial Fibrillation (AF) 13
      B. Multifocal Atrial Tachycardia 15
      C. Paroxysmal Atrial Tachycardia 16
      D. Paroxysmal Supraventricular Tachycardia (PSVT) ... 16
      E. Ventricular Bigeminy/Trigeminy 17
      F. Ventricular Tachycardia 18
      G. WPW (Wolff-Parkinson-White) Syndrome 20
   V. CARDIOMYOPATHY 21
   VI. CONGESTIVE HEART FAILURE 22
   VII. DEEP VENOUS THROMBOSIS (DVT) 26
   VIII. ECG DIAGNOSIS 29
   IX. HYPERTENSIVE CRISIS 36
   X.   MYOCARDIAL INFARCTION 37
      A. Myocardial Infarction (MI) 37
      B. Specific Acute MI (AMI) Categories 45
      C. Unstable Angina 46
   XI. MYOCARDITIS 47
   XII. PERICARDIAL DISEASE 49
      A. Pericarditis 49
      B. Cardiac Tamponade 50
      C. Constrictive Pericarditis 50
      D. Pericardial Effusion 50

    XIII.   PULMONARY EMBOLUS 51

Chapter 4: DENTAL **55**
    I.   GENERAL DENTAL CONDITIONS 55

Chapter 5: DERMATOLOGY **57**
    I.   ALLERGIC CONTACT DERMATITIS/POISON IVY . 57
    II. ERYTHEMA MULTIFORME/STEVENS-JOHNSON .. 57
    III. LICE/SCABIES 59
    IV. SUNBURN 60

Chapter 6: ENDOCRINE **61**
    I.   ADRENAL INSUFFICIENCY 61
    II. DIABETIC KETOACIDOSIS (DKA) 62
    III. HHNK (Hyperglycemic Hyperosmolar Nonketotic) 64
    IV. HYPERTHYROIDISM 65
    V.   HYPOTHYROIDISM 66

Chapter 7: ENT **68**
    I.   EPISTAXIS 68
    II. PERITONSILLAR ABSCESS 69

Chapter 8: ENVIRONMENTAL **71**
    I.   ANIMAL/HUMAN BITES; RABIES 71
    II. BURNS/INHALATION INJURY 74
    III. COLD ILLNESS 77
         A. Frostbite 77
         B. Hypothermia - see also ACLS section. 78
    IV. DYSBARISM 80
         A. Barotrauma of Descent 80
         B. Barotrauma of Ascent 81
         C. Decompression Sickness 81
    V.   ELECTRICAL INJURY/LIGHTNING 82
    VI. HEAT ILLNESS 85
         A. Heat Cramps 85
         B. Heat Exhaustion 85
         C. Heat Stroke 86
    VII. HIGH ALTITUDE MEDICINE 88

VIII.   NEAR DROWNING 89
IX.   RADIATION INJURIES 90
X.   SNAKEBITES 92
XI.   WARFARE: BIOLOGICAL AND CHEMICAL 94
  A. Biological Warfare Agents 94
  B. Chemical Warfare Agents 99

Chapter 9: FOREIGN BODY (FB) REMOVAL 102

Chapter 10: GASTROINTESTINAL 106

I.   ABDOMINAL PAIN 106
II.   ANORECTAL DISEASE 107
III.   APPENDICITIS 108
IV.   CONSTIPATION 110
V.   DIARRHEA/FOOD POISONING 111
VI.   DIVERTICULAR DISEASE 114
VII.   DYSPHAGIA 116
VIII.   GALLBLADDER DISEASE 117
  A. Cholangitis 117
  B. Cholecystitis 118
  C. Cholelithiasis 119
IX.   GASTROESOPHAGEAL REFLUX 120
X.   GI BLEED 120
XI.   HEPATITIS/JAUNDICE 122
XII.   INFLAMMATORY BOWEL DISEASE 124
  A. Crohn's Disease 124
  B. Ulcerative Colitis 125
  C. Complications 126
XIII.   MESENTERIC ISCHEMIA 126
XIV.   PANCREATITIS 128
XV.   PEPTIC ULCER DISEASE/GASTRITIS 129
XVI.   SMALL BOWEL OBSTRUCTION (SBO) 131
XVII.   VOLVULUS 132
XVIII.   VOMITING 133

Chapter 11: GENITOURINARY 135

I.   THE ACUTE SCROTUM 135

    A. Epididymitis 135
    B. Testicular Torsion 136
    C. Torsion of Appendix Testes 137
II.   NEPHROLITHIASIS 137
III.   URINARY RETENTION 140

Chapter 12: HEMATOLOGY/ONCOLOGY 142

I.   BLOOD PRODUCTS 142
II.   HEMOPHILIA 142
III.   ONCOLOGIC EMERGENCIES 144
    A. Neutropenic Fever 144
    B. Spinal Cord Compression 145
    C. Superior Vena Cava Syndrome 146
IV.   SICKLE CELL DISEASE 146
V.   TTP (Thrombotic Thrombocytopenic Purpura) 149

Chapter 13: INFECTIOUS DISEASE 151

I.   CELLULITIS 151
II.   DIARRHEA- see Chapter 10
III.   ENDOCARDITIS 152
IV.   EPIDIDYMITIS- see Chapter 11
V.   HERPES ZOSTER 153
VI.   HIV- Related Illnesses 154
    A. CNS Disease 154
    B. Ophthalmologic Disease 155
    C. Pulmonary Disease 155
    D. Drug reactions 156
VII. INFLUENZA 156
VIII. MENINGITIS 158
IX.   OTITIS EXTERNA 160
X.   PHARYNGITIS 161
XI.   PNEUMONIA 162
    A. Pneumonia 162
    B. Aspiration Pneumonia 166
    C. Specific Pathogens 166
XII. RHEUMATIC FEVER 168

XIII. SEXUALLY TRANSMITTED DISEASES 169
    A. Pelvic Inflammatory Disease (PID) 169
    B. Other STDs 171
    C. Prophylaxis After Sexual Assault 172
XIV. SINUSITIS 173
XV. TETANUS 174
XVI. TICK-BORNE ILLNESSES 175
    A. Lyme Disease 175
    B. Rocky Mountain Spotted Fever 176
XVII. URINARY TRACT INFECTION (UTI) 177
    A. UTI 177
    B. Pyelonephritis 179

Chapter 14: LEGAL ISSUES 181
  COBRA/EMTALA 181

**Chapter 15: METABOLIC/ELECTROLYTE DISOR-
DERS 183**
  I. ACID-BASE DISORDERS 183
  II. CALCIUM 184
  III. POTASSIUM 185
  IV. SODIUM 188

Chapter 16: NEUROLOGY 190
  I. ALTERED MENTAL STATUS IN THE ELDERLY 190
  II. BELL'S PALSY 191
  III. GUILLAIN-BARRE SYNDROME 192
  IV. HEADACHE 193
  V. MULTIPLE SCLEROSIS 196
  VI. MYASTHENIA GRAVIS 197
  VII. SEIZURES 198
    A. Seizures 198
    B. Status Epilepticus 201
    C. Pseudoseizures 203
  VIII. STROKE/TIA (Transient Ischemic Attack) 203
  IX. SUBARACHNOID HEMORRHAGE 209
  X. SYNCOPE 212

XI.   VERTIGO 215

Chapter 17: OB/GYN 218

  I.   DELIVERY 218
      A. Normal Delivery Procedure 218
      B. Shoulder Dystocia- Delivery Procedure 218
      C. Breech Delivery Procedure 219
      D. Post-Partum Hemorrhage 219
  II.   DYSFUNCTIONAL UTERINE BLEEDING 220
  III. ECTOPIC PREGNANCY 222
  IV. PLACENTAL ABRUPTION; PLACENTA PREVIA 224
  V.   PREECLAMPSIA/ECLAMPSIA 226
  VI. SPONTANEOUS ABORTION 227

Chapter 18: OPHTHALMOLOGY 231

  I.   CELLULITIS 231
      A. Periorbital (Preseptal) Cellulitis 231
      B. Orbital Cellulitis 231
  II.   CONJUNCTIVITIS 232
  III. CORNEAL ABRASION 233
  IV. GENERAL EYE SYMPTOMS/MEDICATIONS 234
  V.   GLAUCOMA- Acute narrow-angle 236
  VI. LID DISORDERS 237
      A. Blepharitis 237
      B. Chalazion 237
      C. Hordeolum (stye) 237
  VII. RETINAL ARTERY OCCLUSION 238
  VIII. RETINAL DETACHMENT 239
  IX. SCLERITIS 240
  X.   TRAUMA 240
      A. Globe Rupture 241
      B. Lid Lacerations 241
      C. Orbital Fractures 242
  XI. UVEITIS (Iritis) 242

Chapter 19: ORTHOPEDICS 244

  I.   ANKLE 244

II.	FOOT	246
III.	FOREARM	248
IV.	HAND	250
V.	HUMERUS/ELBOW	254
VI.	KNEE	256
VII.	LOW BACK PAIN/RADICULOPATHY	259
VIII.	PEDIATRICS	262
IX.	PELVIS/HIP	265
X.	SHOULDER	268
XI.	WRIST	272

Chapter 20: PEDIATRICS 275

I.	Pediatric ALS- see Appendix	
II.	ANESTHESIA	275
	A. Analgesia/Sedation	275
	B. Rapid Sequence Intubation (RSI)	277
III.	ASTHMA- see Chapter 23	
IV.	CARDIOVASCULAR	280
	A. Congenital Heart Disease	280
	B. Congestive Heart Failure	282
	C. Supraventricular Tachyarrhythmias	283
V.	CONSTIPATION	284
VI.	CYANOSIS	285
VII.	DERMATOLOGY	285
	A. Candida Diaper Dermatitis	285
	B. Seborrheic Dermatitis	286
	C. Tinea Capitis	286
	D. Tinea Corporis (ringworm)	287
VIII.	GASTROENTERITIS	287
IX.	HEMOLYTIC-UREMIC SYNDROME	288
X.	HENOCH-SCHONLEIN PURPURA	289
XI.	INFECTIOUS DISEASE	290
	A. The Febrile Child (Without a Source)	290
	B. Bronchiolitis	293
	C. Conjunctivitis (newborn)	294
	D. Croup (laryngotracheobronchitis)	294

    E. Epiglottitis (Supraglottitis) 296
    F. Erythema Infectiosum (Fifth disease) 297
    G. Hand, foot and mouth disease 297
    H. Impetigo 297
    I. Kawasaki Disease 298
    J. Lymphadenitis 298
    K. Measles (Rubeola) 299
    L. Meningitis/Sepsis 299
    M. Mononucleosis 302
    N. Omphalitis 303
    O. Orbital/Periorbital Cellulitis- see Chapter 18
    P. Osteomyelitis 303
    Q. Otitis Media 303
    R. Pharyngitis- see Chapter 13
    S. Pityriasis Rosea 305
    T. Pneumonia 305
    U. Retropharyngeal/Peritonsillar Abscess 307
    V. Roseola 308
    W. Sinusitis- see Chapter 13
    X. Urinary Tract Infection (UTI)/Pyelonephritis 309
    Y. Varicella (Chicken Pox) 310
  XII.   INTUSSUSCEPTION 311
  XIII. JAUNDICE 312
  XIV. METABOLIC 313
  XV. REYE'S SYNDROME 313
  XVI. SEIZURES 314
    A. Seizures 314
    B. Febrile Seizures 318
  XVII. SICKLE CELL DISEASE- see Chapter 12
  XVIII. STRIDOR 319

Chapter 21: PSYCHIATRY 320

  I. PANIC DISORDER 320
  II. PSYCHOSIS 320

Chapter 22: RENAL 322

  I. ACUTE RENAL FAILURE 322

Chapter 23: RESPIRATORY **323**
   I.   ASTHMA 323
   II.   COPD 328

Chapter 24: RHEUMATOLOGY **331**
   I.   ACUTE ARTHRITIS 331
   II.   GOUT 332

Chapter 25: TOXICOLOGY **334**
   I.   GENERAL TOXICOLOGY 334
   II.   ACETAMINOPHEN 338
   III. AMPHETAMINES 340
   IV. ANTICHOLINERGICS 341
   V.   BENZODIAZEPINES 342
   VI. BETA BLOCKERS 343
   VII. CALCIUM CHANNEL BLOCKERS 344
   VIII. CARBON MONOXIDE (CO) 345
   IX. CAUSTIC INGESTIONS 347
   X.   CHOLINERGICS 348
   XI. COCAINE 349
   XII. CYANIDE 351
   XIII. DIGOXIN 353
   XIV. ECSTASY 355
   XV. ETHANOL 356
      A. Alcohol Intoxication 356
      B. Alcohol Withdrawal 356
      C. Alcohol-related Seizures 357
      D. Alcohol-related Complications 358
   XVI. ETHYLENE GLYCOL 359
   XVII. GAMMA-HYDROXY BUTYRATE (GHB) 361
   XVIII. IHHALANTS/OCCUPATIONAL EXPOSURE 362
   XIX. IRON 364
   XX. ISOPROPYL ALCOHOL 366
   XXI. LEAD 367
   XXII. LITHIUM 368
   XXIII. METHANOL 369

XXIV.	METHEMOGLOBINEMIA	371
XXV.	POISONS/ANTIDOTES	372
XXVI.	SALICYLATES	373
XXVII.	SEROTONIN SYNDROME	374
XXVIII.	SULFONYLUREAS	375
XXIX.	THEOPHYLLINE	376
XXX.	TRICYCLIC ANTIDEPRESSANTS	377
XXXI.	WARFARIN (COUMADIN)	379

Chapter 26: TRAUMA **380**

I.	ABDOMINAL TRAUMA	380
	A. Blunt Abdominal Injury	380
	B. Penetrating Abdominal Injury	382
II.	GLASGOW COMA SCALE (GCS)	383
III.	HEAD TRAUMA	383
	A. General Head Injury	383
	B. Concussion	386
	C. Epidural Hematoma (EDH)	386
	D. Subdural Hematoma (SDH)	387
IV.	MAXILLOFACIAL TRAUMA	387
V.	NECK TRAUMA	389
	A. Blunt Neck Injury	389
	B. Penetrating Neck Injury	390
VI.	PEDIATRIC TRAUMA (Blunt)	391
VII.	PELVIS/GENITOURINARY TRAUMA	392
	A. Blunt Pelvic Injury	392
	B. Penetrating Pelvic Injury	394
VIII.	PREGNANCY AND TRAUMA	395
IX.	SPINAL TRAUMA	396
	A. Cervical Spine Trauma	396
	B. Spinal Cord Injury Syndromes	400
	C. Thoracolumbar Trauma	400
X.	THORACIC TRAUMA	402
	A. Blunt Thoracic Injury	402
	B. Penetrating Thoracic Injury	406
XI.	VASCULAR TRAUMA (Penetrating)	407

APPENDICES **409**

   I.   Basic Life Support
      A. CPR/Rescue Breathing 410
      B. Foreign body/Airway Obstruction 411
  II.   ACLS protocols
      A. Ventricular Fibrillation/Pulseless VT 412
      B. PEA 413
      C. Asystole 414
      D. Atrial Fibrillation 415
      E. Narrow Complex Tachycardia 416
      F. Stable Ventricular Tachycardia 417
      G. Bradycardia 418
      H. Pulmonary Edema 419
      I. Hypothermia 420
  III. Pediatric ALS
      A. Bradycardia 421
      B. Asystole/PEA 422
      C. Tachycardia 423
      D. VF/Pulseless VT 424
      E. Pediatric Vital Signs 425
      F. Pediatric Resuscitation Supplies 426
  IV. Neonatal Resuscitation
      A. Protocol 427
      B. Apgar Scoring/ETT/Laryngoscope 428
  V.   Metric Conversions 429
  VI. Normal Lab Values 430

INDEX **431**

CHAPTER 1
ALLERGY

I. ALLERGIC REACTIONS

A. Anaphylaxis/Allergic Reaction

•**General**•
1) Allergic reactions can range from mild local reactions to life-threatening anaphylaxis.
2) In anaphylactic reactions, an antigen binds to IgE on previously sensitized mast cells and basophils. This releases mediators (histamine, leukotrienes, prostaglandins), which cause increased vascular permeability, decreased vascular tone, bronchial smooth muscle contraction, and increased secretions.
3) In anaphylactoid reactions, an inciting substance causes a direct release of mediators (i.e., it is not mediated by IgE).
4) The most common causes of anaphylaxis include parenteral antibiotics, Hymenoptera stings, and certain foods (peanuts, shellfish).

•**Clinical Presentation**•
1) Exposure to an inciting agent may produce symptoms that include flushing, pruritis and urticaria; more severe symptoms include angioedema, bronchospasm, and throat tightness.
2) As symptoms progress, patients may become hypotensive and tachycardic.
3) Some patients have a biphasic reaction with recurrence of symptoms in 6-24h.

•**Treatment**•
1) **If in shock**
   a) Insert 2 large bore IVs. Place patient on monitor. Administer oxygen, lower head. Assess and stabilize the airway.
   b) IVNS bolus 1-2L.
   c) 0.3-0.5 mg of 1:10,000 epinephrine IV (peds: 0.01 mg/kg of 1:10,000) or continuous infusion of aqueous epinephrine (1:1000) 1 ml per 250 ml of 5% dextrose at 1 mcg/min.

    d) Consider glucagon (1-5 mg IV over 5 min) if patient is on beta-blockers (it works independently of beta-receptors as a positive inotrope and chronotrope).

    e) Diphenhydramine 50 mg IV every 6-8h (an antihistamine).

    f) Solumedrol 125 mg IV (glucocorticoids stabilize mast cell membranes and inhibit histamine release).

    g) Cimetidine 300 mg IV (an antihistamine; do not administer cimetidine if patient is on a beta-blocker, as it prolongs the activity of the beta-blocker).

    h) Albuterol nebulizer.

    i) Nebulized epinephrine.

    j) If pregnant, instead of epinephrine, consider ephedrine 25-50 mg IV.

    k) If anaphylaxis was precipitated by an insect sting, consider administering epinephrine at the site of the bite; consider applying a loose tourniquet proximal to the sting and loosen every 10-15 min. Remove the stinger, elevate the affected extremity and apply ice.

    l) If on beta-blocker and no response to epinephrine, consider isoproterenol (1 mg in 500 ml dextrose) at 0.1 ug/kg/min; may double every 15 min.

2) If not in shock, but significant symptoms are present

    a) Consider 0.3-.5 mg 1:1000 epinephrine SC or IM (0.1-0.2 mg in children), max of 3 doses (use caution if elderly or cardiovascular disease).

    b) Diphenhydramine 50 mg IV every 6-8h (an antihistamine).

    c) Solumedrol 125 mg IV (glucocorticoids stabilize mast cell membranes and inhibit histamine release).

    d) Cimetidine 300 mg IV (an antihistamine; do not administer cimetidine if patient is on a beta-blocker, as it prolongs the activity of the beta-blocker).

    e) Albuterol nebulizer.

    f) Nebulized epinephrine.

3) If mild symptoms

    a) Diphenhydramine

    b) Consider prednisone, cimetidine, and albuterol inhaler.

•Disposition•

1) Admit if significant general reaction. Strongly consider admission for any patient on beta-blockers.

2) Consider discharge if patient has no respiratory symptoms and normal vital signs for 4-6h. Discharge on prednisone 40 mg/d (taper the dose), diphenhydramine 25-50 mg every 4-6h, and cimetidine 300 mg qid for 2-5d. Arrange follow-up in 1-2d. Consider prescribing an Epi-pen and allergy referral.

3) If an insect sting causes significant symptoms, the patient should be referred to an allergist for possible immunotherapy and desensitization, which is very effective in preventing future episodes of anaphylaxis.

B. Angioedema/Urticaria

•General•

1) Angioedema and urticaria both result from vascular leakage that is mediated by kinins, histamine, and serotonin; angioedema involves vessels in the layers below the dermis, while urticaria is more superficial. These conditions may occur together or in isolation (although urticaria does not occur with hereditary or acquired angioedema), and may be classified as chronic (lasting longer than 6 weeks) or acute.

2) Angioedema may be classified as idiopathic (secondary to ACE inhibitors and other agents), hereditary (characterized by recurrent episodes of angioedema; patients either have low levels of C1 esterase inhibitor or dysfunctional C1 esterase inhibitor), or allergic (IgE mediated from antigen exposure; often occurs with urticaria). Most cases of angioedema are drug-induced, often secondary to ACE inhibitors; angioedema usually occurs within 1 week of the initiation of ACE inhibitors, although it may be delayed for years.

3) Urticaria has 3 principle etiologies: medications (penicillins, aspirin, NSAIDs, opiates), food (chocolate, shellfish, nuts, eggs, milk), and infection (sinus, gallbladder, GU).

•Clinical Presentation•

1) Angioedema may present with acute onset of edema in the tongue,

uvula, lips, and orbital area; the extremities, face, and genitalia are most commonly involved. The edema is non-pitting, and not erythematous or pruritic. Edema of bowel wall may cause abdominal pain.
2) Urticaria is characterized by erythematous wheals, plaques or papules that blanch under pressure; it is usually pruritic.

•Treatment•
1) Treatment of angioedema involves maintaining a secure airway, which may necessitate nasotracheal fiberoptic intubation or a surgical airway. Medication options are similar to those for an allergic reaction (epinephrine, steroids, and H1/H2 blockers). In hereditary angioedema, these medications are often ineffective, so consider administering stanazol, danazol, and C1 concentrate (or fresh frozen plasma if C1 concentrate is unavailable).
2) Treatment of both acute and chronic urticaria involves antihistamines (H1and H2 blockers). In the acute setting, a short course of oral prednisone may be a reasonable adjuvant therapy (prednisone 40 mg daily for 4 days). If antihistamines are ineffective, oral Doxepin may be useful. In general, the use of systemic corticosteroids should be avoided for the management of chronic urticaria. If the cause is identified, advise patients to avoid that trigger.

CHAPTER 2

ANESTHESIA

I. RAPID SEQUENCE INTUBATION; ALTERNATIVE AIRWAY OPTIONS

A. Rapid Sequence Intubation

•Indications•

Intubation is indicated in patients who are unable to protect their airway, or are unable to maintain adequate oxygenation and ventilation.

•Equipment•

1) Laryngoscope blade, either curved or straight (straight is preferred in infants and small children). Check to ensure a functioning light.
2) Endotracheal tube (ETT) with stylet inserted (distal end of stylet should be 1-2 cm proximal to end of ETT); adult males can accommodate 7.5 mm-8.5 mm tubes, while adult females can accommodate 7.0 mm-8.0 mm ETT. Consider applying a lubricating agent to the end of the ETT, and use a small amount of lubricant on the stylet (to facilitate removal). Have several different sizes of tubes ready.
3) Bag-valve mask attached to high-flow oxygen.
4) Suction.
5) Prepare optional methods for intubation. Options include the laryngeal mask airway (LMA), the esophageal tracheal Combitube, fiberoptic bronchoscope or laryngoscope, use of a lighted stylet, percutaneous transtracheal ventilation, cricothyroidotomy, retrograde tracheal intubation, and the digital method.

•Procedure•

1) **Preoxygenate** with 100% oxygen. Establish IV. Prepare equipment and medications. Have suction ready and place the patient on a cardiac monitor and pulse oximetry. Check laryngoscope light and endotracheal tube (ETT) cuff. Place patient in the sniffing position. To avoid gastric distention, only use bag-valve mask if there is no respiratory effort. Apply cricoid pressure when bagging patients; consider always using a nasal airway when bagging patients. In the trauma patient, one

person performs jaw-thrust, while another bags.

2) Premedicate

a) Consider fentanyl 2 mcg/kg (onset 1 min, lasts 30 minutes) for analgesia in awake patients; opioids have sedative and analgesic effects and blunt increases in heart rate and blood pressure (but may increase intracranial pressure).

b) If heart rate is <120 bpm in children, consider atropine 0.02 mg/kg IV.

c) Consider lidocaine 1.5 mg/kg IV push, especially if head injury (it decreases the cough and gag response and blunts the release of catecholamines and thus blunts the intracranial pressure response to intubation).

d) Consider giving a defasciculating dose of Vecuronium (0.02 mg/kg IV push) or succinylcholine (0.1 mg/kg IV). Defasciculation blocks increased intracranial pressure; *do not defasciculate if patient is younger than 5 years.*

e) Wait 3 minutes after giving medications.

3) Sedate

Sedation options for different clinical situations:

<u>Normotensive</u>: Thiopental or Etomidate or Midazolam.

<u>Hypotension without head injury</u>: Etomidate or Ketamine or 1/2 dose Midazolam.

<u>Head injury without hypotension</u>: Thiopental.

<u>Head injury with hypotension</u>: Etomidate or decreased dose of thiopental.

<u>Status asthmaticus</u>: Ketamine or Midazolam.

<u>Status epilepticus</u>: Thiopental or Midazolam.

Sedative Doses

<u>Diazepam</u> 0.25-0.5 mg/kg- onset 2-4 min, duration 40 min; has minimal effect on intracranial pressure and blood pressure.

<u>Etomidate</u> 0.2-0.4 mg/kg- onset 1 min, duration 2-3 min; minimal effect on intracranial pressure, intraocular pressure, and blood pressure. Repeated use may cause adrenal suppression.

<u>Fentanyl</u> 2-10 ug/kg- onset 1 min, lasts 30 min; little hemodynamic effect; may cause chest wall rigidity and increased ICP.

<u>Ketamine</u> 1-2 mg/kg- onset 1-2 min, duration 10 min; bronchodilates;

increases intracranial pressure, intraocular pressure, and secretions; will not usually cause hypotension. Use with asthma. Premedicate with atropine. Do not give if cardiac disease.

Methohexital 1-1.5 mg/kg- onset 10 sec, duration 15 min; decreases blood pressure.

Midazolam 0.1-0.4 mg/kg- onset 1-2 min, duration 30 min; minimal effect on intracranial pressure and blood pressure.

Thiopental 2-5 mg/kg- onset 30 sec, duration 15 min; decreases intracranial pressure and blood pressure; increases bronchospasm. Use with status epilepticus, but avoid in asthma because it may cause histamine release.

4) Paralyze- short-acting agent (depolarizing agent (succinylcholine) or rocuronium).

Succinylcholine 1-1.5 mg/kg (1-3 mg/kg if <10 kg)- onset 30 sec, duration 5 min; increases intracranial pressure, intraocular pressure; may cause bradycardia or hypokalemia. May be given IM.

Rocuronium 1 mg/kg- onset 60 sec, duration 30 min; may use instead of succinylcholine.

5) Placement. Pass the endotracheal tube; apply cricoid pressure. Placement is best confirmed with direct visualization of the tube passing through the vocal cords. Inflate balloon cuff when tube is in place. If patient becomes bradycardic during placement, administer atropine 0.5 mg IV (in adults).

6) After Intubation- Confirm ETT placement by observing bilateral chest rise with each ventilation and listening for equal breath sounds in the bilateral anterior chest and bilateral mid-axillary line; also, listen over the epigastrium for air entering the stomach. Consider secondary confirmation with an end-tidal CO_2 detector or bulb aspiration device. The depth of ETT insertion should be approximately 23 cm in men and 21 cm in women (from the corner of the mouth). Secure ETT. Obtain CXR to verify correct depth of ETT (it should be approximately 2 cm above the carina). Attach ETT to ventilator with appropriate settings (typically, use a tidal volume of 6-7 ml/kg, a respiratory rate of 12-15, and a FiO2 of 100%).

7) Paralyze- long acting (non-depolarizing agents).

Vecuronium 0.1 mg/kg (or 0.2 mg/kg for RSI, with onset 90 sec)- onset

2-3 min, duration 40 min; few cardiovascular effects; low risk for histamine release.

Pancuronium 0.1 mg/kg- onset 2-5 min, duration 60 min; may cause histamine release.

*Non-depolarizing agents can be reversed with 0.5-1 mg/kg IV edrophonium.

8) Long-term sedation- administer diazepam 0.02-0.03 mg/kg IV if SBP >120 mm Hg; 0.01-0.02 mg/kg IV if SBP 70-120 mm Hg; hold if SBP <70 mm Hg. Consider morphine.

B. Alternative Airway Options

1) Cricothyroidotomy
- **a)** Hyperextend the neck (if no suspicion of cervical spine injury). The cricothyroid membrane is identified between the thyroid cartilage superiorly and the cricoid cartilage inferiorly.
- **b)** If obese or trauma patient, consider first finding the airway with a needle and syringe and keep it in place as a guide.
- **c)** Use left hand to immobilize the larynx and do not let go until procedure is complete.
- **d)** Make a vertical midline incision through skin (vertical incisions minimize bleeding and help to retract the skin).
- **e)** Retract skin and dissect to cricothyroid membrane.
- **f)** Incise the cricothyroid membrane horizontally, and stabilize the proximal trachea by applying traction with a tracheal hook.
- **g)** Dilate the incised cricothyroid membrane with a hemostat, and place a #6-0 endotracheal tube or Shiley tracheostomy tube.
- **h)** Alternatively, there are cricothyroidotomy kits that use the Seldinger technique.

2) Digital Method
- **a)** Approach patient facing the head of the bed.
- **b)** Use nondominant hand and try to place middle finger on epiglottis; bend endotracheal tube to 45 degrees 5cm proximal to the distal end.
- **c)** The middle finger acts as the laryngoscope and lifts the epiglottis anteriorly, while the index finger guides the endotracheal tube under the epiglottis and into the trachea.

3) Nasotracheal Intubation

a) Contraindications for nasotracheal intubation include severe maxillofacial injuries, apnea (if the blind technique is used), and bleeding diathesis.

b) To perform nasotracheal intubation, place the patient sitting up in a sniffing position and use a vasoconstrictor in nares. Also, apply lidocaine to the nasal airway (consider a 4% lidocaine nebulizer).

c) Use a well-lubricated 7.0 endotracheal tube with bevelled edge (long edge) against the septum.

d) With cricoid pressure, advance the tube while listening for breath sounds, and pass the tube on inspiration.

e) If unsuccessful, the ETT is usually lodged laterally in the piriform sinus or posteriorly in the esophagus. If the ETT is lodged in the esophagus, the head should be hyperextended on subsequent attempts.

4) Retrograde Tracheal Intubation

a) Point the needle of a central line kit cephalad through cricothyroid membrane; thread wire through needle, grasping wire in the posterior pharynx with McGill forceps.

b) Thread the wire through the side port of the endotracheal tube; keep tension on the wire and pass the endotracheal tube.

CHAPTER 3
CARDIOVASCULAR

I. ACLS- see appendix

II. ABDOMINAL AORTIC ANEURYSM (AAA)

•**General**•
AAAs most often result from degeneration of the media of the artery, usually associated with atherosclerosis. A mycotic aneurysm or collagen vascular diseases can also cause AAA.

•**Clinical Presentation**•
1) Patients may experience mild abdominal, groin or back pain prior to aneurysm rupture.
2) An expanding or ruptured AAA may cause sudden, constant, severe abdominal, flank, back, or groin pain.
3) Patients may present in shock. If ruptured, an aneurysm may present with syncope, followed by spontaneous recovery, then abdominal or back pain.
4) A hematoma may lead to symptoms of inguinal hernia, testicular pain, or jaundice and RUQ pain (secondary to compression of common bile duct). Also, symptoms may include hematuria and flank pain (and an IVP consistent with obstruction). 10% of patients with AAA present with urologic symptoms.
5) Rupture into the mesentery or left colon may cause LLQ pain and tenesmus; rupture into the right retroperitoneum may cause right hip or RLQ pain.
6) A fistula may present with GI bleed and mid-thoracic pain.
7) An inflammatory aneurysm presents with chronic pain, weight loss, and an increased ESR (CT is 50% sensitive for inflammatory aneurysm).
8) AAA may also be a painless incidental finding.

•**Physical Findings**•
1) Palpate above the umbilicus (where the aorta bifurcates); an aorta

>3 cm is abnormal.

2) Hypotension, tachycardia, and a pulsatile abdominal mass are present in 30-50% of ruptured aneurysms; check for bruit.

3) Check peripheral pulses. Perform complete cardiovascular and neurologic exams.

4) Tenderness to palpation of aneurysm requires urgent evaluation for surgery, even if stable.

•Evaluation•

1) Check ECG, CBC, platelets, PT/PTT, and BUN/Cr. Type and crossmatch for blood (at least 10 units).

2) Ultrasound and abdominal CT are equally sensitive, but CT is better for detection of leaking and extension (if ruptured, most bleed into the retroperitoneum). Unstable patients should not leave the department for imaging studies (if the diagnosis is unclear, ultrasound can be performed at bedside).

3) Plain abdominal films may show a calcified aortic wall.

•Treatment•

1) Insert 2 large bore IVs (avoid placing femoral IV lines). Place patient on monitor. Administer oxygen. Assess and stabilize the airway. Obtain surgical consult.

2) If necessary, resuscitate patient with IVNS 2L and blood transfusion.

3) If hemodynamically unstable, the patient should be taken directly to surgery. If patient is stable, consider imaging study prior to surgery.

III. AORTIC DISSECTION (THORACIC)

•General•

1) Type A thoracic aortic dissections involve the ascending aorta; type B dissections do not.

2) A proximal dissection may involve the right coronary artery, causing an inferior myocardial infarction.

3) Hypertension is the etiology in 90% of patients with aortic dissection.

•Risk Factors•

Risk factors include hypertension, Marfan's disease, Ehlers-Danlos,

11

and pregnancy.

•Clinical Presentation•

1) 90% of patients with aortic dissection have pain.
2) The classic presentation is pain of abrupt onset, most severe at onset, and a ripping quality; pain may also be described as sharp. The location of pain may be substernal, jaw, interscapular, or lumbar and correlates with the location of the dissection (thus, it may migrate).
3) Patients may also present with neurological deficits.

•Evaluation•

1) Check CXR, ECG, CBC, PT/PTT, BUN/Cr, and type and crossmatch (for 10 units).
2) Check for pulse deficits in all extremities (commonly transient from intimal flaps); check blood pressure in both arms. Check for murmur (aortic regurgitation occurs in 50%).
3) If hypotensive, there may be either involvement of the pericardium (tamponade) or aortic rupture. If the patient has refractory hypertension, the aneurysm may involve the renal arteries.
4) Transesophageal echocardiogram is probably the best diagnostic test for aortic dissection, especially if the patient is unstable (it can be performed at the bedside). Alternatively, consider chest CT.
5) The CXR is abnormal in 80-90% of patients with aortic dissection; 75% have mediastinal widening. Other CXR findings suggestive of aortic dissection include calcification separated by >5 mm from the aortic wall, loss of aortic knob, tracheal deviation, depression of left main stem bronchus, deviation of nasogastric tube, left pleural effusion, left apical cap, and loss of the left paratracheal stripe.

•Treatment•

1) Establish 2 large bore IVs. Monitor patient. Administer oxygen.
2) Nitroprusside: start at 0.5-3 mcg/kg/min (after first dose of beta-blocker); keep SBP 100-120 mm Hg. Nitroprusside decreases shear forces acting on the aortic wall.
3) Propranolol 1 mg IV q 5 min (max 10 mg); or metoprolol 2.5 –5mg q 5 min; or esmolol. The goal is to keep the heart rate 60-80 bpm. Consider trimethaphan if beta-blockers are contraindicated. This de-

creases the velocity of left ventricular contraction, thus decreasing shear forces acting on the aortic wall.

4) An alternative to nitroprusside and propranolol is single agent therapy with labetalol 10-20 mg q 2-4 min to achieve effect, then 1-2 mg/min infusion.

5) Transfuse blood as necessary.

6) Consult cardiothoracic surgery.

7) Type A requires surgery; type B may be treated medically.

IV. ARRHYTHMIAS

A. Atrial Fibrillation (AF)

•**General**•

1) Conditions associated with AF include mitral valve disease, hypertensive heart disease, ischemic heart disease, CHF, cardiomyopathy, pericarditis, hyperthyroidism, pulmonary embolus, alcohol, and COPD. AF may be acute (paroxysmal) or chronic. "Lone" AF is AF without underlying structural cardiac disease or hypertension.

2) AF may lead to decreased cardiac output. A large pulse deficit (the difference between the heart rate measured by auscultation and pulse) indicates a significant reduction in cardiac output.

3) AF increases the risk of stroke, and also leads to atrial remodeling.

•**Clinical Presentation**•

Chronic AF may present with lethargy, dyspnea and fatigue, while paroxysmal AF may present with palpitations, chest pain, or lightheadedness.

•**Evaluation**•

1) Check ECG, CXR, electrolytes, and cardiac enzymes. Consider thyroid function tests and toxicology screen.

2) ECG- In atrial fibrillation, multiple re-entry circuits expose the A-V node to 300-600 impulses/minute, producing fibrillatory waves and an irregularly irregular ventricular rhythm. In the absence of intraventricular conduction delay, the QRS complexes are narrow.

•**Treatment**•

Treatment involves controlling rate, and consideration of anticoagulation and restoration of sinus rhythm.

1) Rate Control Options if Patient is Unstable

    a) Cardiovert, start with 200 J; sedate first if SBP >90 mm Hg (if on digoxin, it is acceptable to cardiovert if levels are normal, but use 10-40 J). Cardioversion has a high failure rate, depending on the duration of atrial fibrillation, and even if successful, it is often short-lived. Also, cardioversion may not immediately lead to atrial contraction because of atrial stunning.

    b) Therefore, another option in an unstable patient is chemical rate control (consider esmolol with its half-life of 9 min) combined with vasopressors (dopamine).

2) Other Options for Rate Control

Rate Control with Normal Cardiac Function

    a) Diltiazem (Cardizem) 0.25 mg/kg IV bolus over 2 min; may repeat 0.35 mg/kg in 15 min. Or, consider boluses of 5 mg every 3 min; may start infusion 5-15 mg/h for up to 24h.

    b) Or verapamil 5-10 mg IV, may repeat in 5-10 min (effective for 4-6h). Or propranolol 1-3 mg IV bolus every 2 min (usual total dose is 10-20 mg; effective for 4-10h). Or esmolol loading dose 500 ug/kg IV over 1 min, then 50 ug/kg/min; may repeat loading dose and increase infusion every 5-10 min.

Rate Control with Impaired Cardiac Function

    a) Digoxin, load 0.4-0.6 mg IV, then 0.1-0.3 mg every 4-6h x 2-4 doses. Or diltiazem; or amiodarone.

*To lessen the hypotensive effects of calcium channel blockers, consider giving calcium chloride first.

3) Conversion of Rhythm

If duration of symptoms is less than 48h, consider DC cardioversion, amiodarone, ibutilide (1 mg over 10 min (.01 mg/kg if <60 kg), may repeat in 10 min), flecainide, propafenone, or procainamide. Consider transesophageal echocardiography to evaluate for the presence of atrial thrombi before conversion. Consider delaying cardioversion for anticoagulation.

If duration of symptoms is longer than 48h, conversion is generally delayed until the patient is anticoagulated (to decrease the risk of embolization of atrial thrombi). Or, consider transesophageal echocardiography to evaluate for the presence of atrial thrombi; if absent, cardioversion may be considered (with anticoagulation), and anticoagulation continued for 3-4 weeks.

4) Anticoagulation

a) Patients with atrial fibrillation of greater than 48h duration are generally anticoagulated to decrease the risk of embolization of atrial thrombi. Transesophageal echocardiography may be performed to evaluate for the presence of atrial thrombi; if absent, cardioversion may be considered (with anticoagulation), and anticoagulation continued for 3-4 weeks.

b) Some recommend that all patients with new-onset atrial fibrillation be given anticoagulants on presentation and for 3-4 weeks after conversion, because Holter monitoring has shown that patients in atrial fibrillation may be asymptomatic (and therefore the onset of AF may not be clear), and it often takes 24h for the atrium to begin contracting after cardioversion.

•Disposition•

1) Consider admitting all patients with new onset atrial fibrillation for evaluation, rate control and possible cardioversion. A significant percentage of patients will spontaneously convert to sinus rhythm in the first 24h.

2) Asymptomatic patients with chronic atrial fibrillation with good rate control and no precipitating factors may be considered for discharge.

B. Multifocal Atrial Tachycardia

•Etiology•

Etiologies include decompensated lung disease, CHF, sepsis, acidosis and methylxanthine toxicity. Digoxin toxicity is an unlikely cause.

•Evaluation•

1) Check ECG, CXR, electrolytes, and cardiac enzymes.

2) ECG- Irregular rhythm between 100-180 bpm, with 3 or more distinct P waves and varying PR intervals.

•Treatment•

1) Treat the underlying disease (e.g., consider administering oxygen and bronchodilators, and correct acidosis or any electrolyte abnor-

malities).
2) Antiarrhythmic treatment is rarely indicated (Mg 2 g IV or verapamil 5-10 mg IV or amiodarone may be considered).
3) Cardioversion is ineffective.

C. Paroxysmal Atrial Tachycardia

•General•
1) Paroxysmal atrial tachycardia is secondary to digoxin toxicity in 50-75% of patients. It is often associated with cor pulmonale and CAD.
2) As the arrhythmia is due to re-entry or abnormal automaticity of the atrium, medications or maneuvers that delay AV node conduction will not terminate this rhythm.

•Evaluation•
1) Check ECG, electrolytes and digoxin level. Consider CXR.
2) ECG- Atrial rate is usually 150-200 bpm, often with an unusual P wave morphology; the QRS complexes are usually narrow and regular. There is usually some degree of A-V block (2:1 block or Wenkebach).

•Treatment•
1) If the patient is taking digoxin, stop digoxin.
2) If on digoxin, electrical cardioversion is contraindicated; consider diltiazem or beta-blockers. If on digoxin, consider administering phenytoin.
3) If patient is not on digoxin, use diltiazem, verapamil, beta-blocker, or digoxin to slow conduction. Amiodarone or sotalol may be required for conversion.

D. Paroxysmal Supraventricular Tachycardia (PSVT)

•General•
It is a regular rhythm from either a re-entry or ectopic pacemaker above the bifurcation of the bundle of His.

•Evaluation•
ECG- Junctional (A-V nodal) tachycardia has a narrow complex; the rate is regular without preceding P waves with <10 bpm variation. It may also present as an ectopic atrial pacemaker (PAT). If the heart rate

is >200 bpm, the most likely mechanism is an accessory pathway.

•Treatment•

1) Vagal maneuvers (which include Valsalva and carotid sinus massage; ocular pressure is contraindicated) stimulate the vagus nerve and increase the AV block, slowing and potentially terminating an arrhythmia.

2) Adenosine 6 mg rapid IVP, may repeat twice with 12 mg. Adenosine slows the SA node and A-V node; it will increase A-V nodal block (i.e., slow the ventricular response) in atrial fibrillation/flutter or re-entrant atrial tachycardia. Adenosine terminates SVT of A-V nodal re-entry, sinus node re-entry, and A-V re-entry involving an accessory pathway.

3) **If normal cardiac function**, priority order is: DC cardioversion; calcium channel blocker; beta-blockers; digoxin; procainamide; amiodarone; or sotalol.

4) **If impaired cardiac function**, priority order is: digoxin; amiodarone; diltiazem. Consider DC cardioversion.

•Disposition•

If patient has converted to sinus rhythm and has no comorbid conditions or significant precipitating event, observe for 2-4h and consider discharge.

E. Ventricular Bigeminy/Trigeminy

•Etiology•

It may be secondary to stress, caffeine, cocaine, or underlying cardiac disease. If it occurs with a change in position, consider mitral valve prolapse.

•Evaluation•

1) Check ECG; consider CXR.

2) Consider checking electrolytes and cardiac enzymes. Consider echocardiography, Holter monitor, or stress test to evaluate for possible cardiac disease.

3) ECG- Every second (bigeminy) or third (trigeminy) beat is of ventricular origin.

•Disposition•

If secondary to stress, it should resolve over 6-8h. Consider admission to telemetry if patient is high risk.

F. Ventricular Tachycardia

•General•

1) Ventricular tachycardia (VT) originates from an ectopic ventricular focus (which is usually a consequence of structural heart disease), and may be classified as monomorphic or polymorphic.
2) VT may or may not result in hemodynamic deterioration; it may degenerate into ventricular fibrillation.
3) Electrolyte abnormalities may contribute to VT.

•Evaluation•

Check ECG, electrolytes, cardiac enzymes, CBC, and CXR.

ECG

1) The QRS is > 140 ms and usually regular.
2) P waves are usually lost.
3) A-V dissociation is present; fusion and capture beats are present.
4) The rate is usually >100, <220; QRS axis is between –90 and ±180.
5) An RS in the precordial leads is absent; RS>100 ms; R/S <1 in V6.

Left BBB morphology: QRS >160 ms; notched S downstroke in lead 1 or V2; any q wave in lead V6; right QRS axis; r>30 ms in V1 or V2.

Right BBB morphology: QRS >140 ms; Rsr' in lead V1; monophasic/biphasic QRS in lead V1. A taller left rabbit ear in V1 favors ventricular tachycardia.

Distinguishing VT from SVT with aberrant conduction

1) In general, it is difficult to diagnose aberrancy with certainty; it is safer to assume the patient has VT. If the patient is in CHF or there is a history of CAD, assume VT. Hemodynamic stability does not rule out ventricular tachycardia.
2) Response to adenosine cannot be used to exclude VT, as some patients with VT will convert to sinus rhythm with adenosine.
3) **Indications of likely aberrancy include**: rSR' in V1; R/S > 1 in V6; normal frontal QRS axis; QRS <140 ms; ventricular rate > 170; no A-V dissociation; and it usually has a RBBB pattern.
4) **Ventricular tachycardia is more likely if**: mono or biphasic in V1;

frontal axis < 30; QRS >140 ms; ventricular rate < 170; or A-V dissociation.

Brugada rules for identifying ventricular tachycardia:

1) If there is no RS complex in any precordial lead, it is ventricular tachycardia (100%).

2) If there is an RS, then if interval from onset of R to deepest part of S is >100 ms, then it is ventricular tachycardia.

3) If RS interval <100 ms, then look for A-V dissociation, which is ventricular tachycardia.

4) If no dissociation, look for classic, concordant morphology in V1 and V6.

*One study did not validate the use of these criteria in the ED.

•Treatment•

1) If unstable, cardiovert and administer medications according to ACLS protocols.

2) **If monomorphic VT and normal cardiac function**: Procainamide 20 mg/min, max 17 mg/kg, then drip 1-4 mg/min; or amiodarone 150 mg over 10 min, then 1 mg/min; or lidocaine 1.5 mg/kg IVP, repeat 0.5-.75 mg/kg (max 3 mg/kg), then drip at 2-4 mg/min; or sotalol.

3) **If monomorphic VT and impaired cardiac function**: amiodarone 150 mg over 10 min; or lidocaine 0.5-0.75 mg/kg IVP; then synchronized cardioversion.

4) **If polymorphic VT and normal baseline QT interval**: consider any one of: beta-blockers; or lidocaine; or amiodarone; or procainamide; or sotalol. If impaired heart function, use amiodarone.

5) **If polymorphic VT and prolonged baseline QT interval (suggests Torsades)**: magnesium; overdrive pacing; isoproterenol; phenytoin; lidocaine.

6) **Torsades de Pointes**
   a) Torsades is a polymorphous ventricular tachycardia with a rate between 150 and 250 bpm, with the QRS demonstrating an undulating axis. It is associated with a markedly increased QT interval. It usually occurs in episodes of <20 sec.
   b) Torsades may be precipitated by hypokalemia or hypomagnesemia or antiarrhythmic drugs.

    c) Treatment includes Mg 2 gm IVP, overdrive pacing (100-120 bpm), isoproterenol, or cardioversion; treat any hypokalemia.

•Disposition•
Admit all patients with VT to a monitored unit.

G. WPW (Wolff-Parkinson-White) Syndrome

•General•
1) Kent bundles (which may conduct in an anterograde direction, retrograde direction, or both) are accessory pathways that directly link the atria to the ventricles; they are present in patients with WPW.
2) Concealed bypass tracts account for 20% of all supraventricular tachycardia (SVT).

•Evaluation•
ECG
1) The classic ECG demonstrates a short PR interval, a delta wave (an initial distortion of ventricular activation), and a wide QRS. However, depending on the location of the accessory pathway and the method of conduction, the ECG may appear normal.
2) If the electrical impulse from the atria arrives simultaneously at the ventricle through both the AV node and the accessory pathway, then the ECG will appear normal. If the electrical impulse from the accessory pathway arrives early (pre-excitation), the ventricles are initially activated through the accessory pathway, producing slow initial forces, a delta wave, and a widened QRS interval.
3) In the majority of tachyarrhythmias, the re-entrant SVT occurs with conduction down the normal A-V system and up the bypass tract (thus there is a normal QRS and no delta wave). If atrial fibrillation/flutter, either or both conducting systems may be used (the QRS may have different morphologies), and a very rapid heart rate is possible.

•Clinical Presentation•
There is a high incidence of tachyarrhythmias. Patients may present with syncope or palpitations.

•Treatment•
1) If re-entrant SVT and orthodromic (i.e., <u>narrow QRS</u> without delta

waves, since the A-V node is used for anterograde conduction and the accessory pathway is used for retrograde conduction), treat as other SVTs: adenosine or calcium channel blockers. Beta-blockers are usually ineffective.

2) If antidromic (<u>wide QRS</u> with delta waves and short PR interval, since the accessory pathway is used for the anterograde limb), then it is usually associated with a short refractory period of the bypass tract and thus at risk for rapid heart rate and degeneration into ventricular fibrillation. Treat with adenosine, procainamide (20 mg/min; max 17 mg/kg) and, if unstable, electrical cardioversion. Avoid beta-blockers and calcium channel blockers (they may shorten the refractory period of the bypass tract).

3) **If Atrial fibrillation/flutter with rapid ventricular response**, the best treatment is cardioversion; alternatively, use procainamide (20 mg/min; max 17 mg/kg) or amiodarone or flecainide or propafenone or sotalol. Avoid beta-blockers and calcium channel blockers as they have a variable effect on accessory conduction. Digoxin is contraindicated as it may shorten the refractory period and enhance conduction over the bypass tract.

V. CARDIOMYOPATHY

A. Dilated Cardiomyopathy

1) Dilated cardiomyopathy is characterized by depressed systolic function and cardiomegaly. It is usually idiopathic; consider toxic, metabolic or infectious etiologies.

2) Patients present with symptoms of CHF (fatigue, dyspnea, orthopnea). Patients may develop mural thrombi.

3) CXR usually shows cardiomegaly. The ECG is almost always abnormal (LVH and left atrial enlargement). An echocardiogram is usually diagnostic.

4) Treat with digoxin, diuretics, ACE inhibitors, and consider chronic anticoagulation.

B. Hypertrophic Cardiomyopathy

1) Hypertrophic cardiomyopathy is characterized by increased left ventricle (LV) mass without dilation, and asymmetric septal hypertro-

phy. The ejection fraction is usually normal.

2) Patients present with dyspnea on exertion, chest pain, and palpitations. A systolic ejection murmur increases with decreased LV filling (Valsalva, standing) and decreases with increased LV filling (squatting, hand grip).

3) ECG may demonstrate left ventricular hypertrophy or septal Q waves (upright T waves distinguish these from ischemia). A normal ECG virtually excludes hypertrophic cardiomyopathy. The CXR is usually normal.

4) Treat with propranolol.

C. Restrictive Cardiomyopathy

1) Restrictive cardiomyopathy is characterized by diastolic dysfunction. It may be idiopathic or secondary to intrinsic heart muscle disease. It may be confused with constrictive pericarditis.

2) Patients may present with dyspnea, orthopnea, peripheral edema, and chest pain.

3) CXR usually does not show cardiomegaly.

4) Treat with digoxin and diuretics.

VI. CONGESTIVE HEART FAILURE

•General•

1) Congestive heart failure (CHF) may be secondary to ischemia, MI, valvular disease, cardiomyopathy, or hypertension. If the heart pump cannot maintain adequate circulation, CHF may develop, in which elevated venous pressure causes pulmonary capillaries to leak into the interstitium and alveoli of the lung, resulting in dyspnea; decreased forward flow may cause fatigue and weakness.

2) Heart failure may be described as left ventricular failure, right ventricular failure, or both. Also, pulmonary edema may be secondary to impairment of left atrial outflow.

3) Heart failure may be due to systolic dysfunction (in which there is impaired cardiac contractility, increased filling pressures, and usually an ejection fraction < 40%) or diastolic dysfunction (the ejection fraction and heart size are usually normal, but the ventricular wall is stiff and noncompliant, leading to impaired diastolic filling;

it usually occurs together with systolic dysfunction). Patients with diastolic dysfunction are preload dependent, and aggressive diuresis or venodilation may result in hypotension.

4) In CHF, a decrease in cardiac output activates the renin-angiotensin system (which increases systemic vascular resistance (SVR) and aldosterone levels), increases vasopressin levels, and activates the sympathetic CNS (in which an increase in norepinephrine increases cardiac contractility, heart rate, and SVR). These compensatory mechanisms result in increased sympathetic tone, salt and fluid retention, and ventricular remodelling. These changes initially allow heart failure to remain stable (or compensated), but are ultimately maladaptive and eventually worsen left ventricular output.

5) Also, a counterregulatory process occurs in which a stretch stimulus results in release of B-type natriuretic peptide (BNP) from the myocardium; BNP decreases aldosterone levels and vascular resistance and promotes sodium excretion.

•Clinical Presentation•

1) If left-sided heart failure predominates, dyspnea (especially with exertion) is the primary symptom; the patient may also have orthopnea, paroxysmal nocturnal dyspnea, and fatigue. On exam, the patient may demonstrate tachycardia, tachypnea, pulmonary rales and a third heart sound.

2) Right-sided heart failure presents with increased venous pressures (jugular venous distention) and peripheral edema; hepatic congestion may cause right upper quadrant abdominal pain.

•Evaluation•

1) Check ECG, pulse oximetry, CXR, CBC, electrolytes, BUN/Cr, and cardiac enzymes. Consider echocardiogram. B-type natriuretic peptide (BNP) is secreted from the ventricles in response to pressure overload; if elevated, it may help distinguish CHF from other causes of dyspnea.

2) A normal ECG is strong evidence against LV dysfunction. Look for ischemia, left atrial enlargement, LVH, and a bundle branch block.

3) CXR may demonstrate cephalization of pulmonary vessels, perihilar haze, peribronchial cuffing, Kerley B lines, basilar and perihilar patchy white alveolar infiltrates, and an enlarged cardiac silhouette

(cardiomegaly may not be present with acute cardiac decompensation, such as MI or valve disease). Pleural effusions are nearly always bilateral or right-sided; if only left-sided, consider other possibilities.

4) Non-cardiogenic pulmonary edema typically has a CXR without cardiomegaly, predominantly central distribution of interstitial infiltrates, and lack of pleural effusions. It may result from sepsis, renal failure, fluid overload, PE, near drowning, or smoke inhalation.

5) If there is a new murmur, normal heart on CXR, and the patient is unresponsive to treatment, consider acute valve incompetence.

6) JVD, hypotension without gross pulmonary edema and peripheral edema suggest right ventricle infarct or tamponade.

•Treatment•

1) Establish IV. Place patient on monitor and pulse oximetry. Administer oxygen. Assess and stabilize the airway. Consider non-invasive positive pressure ventilation (e.g., CPAP) as an early intervention; intubate if respiratory failure. Consider urinary catheter to monitor urine output.

2) Nitrates. Administer SL nitroglycerin. Consider IV nitroglycerin 0.125 mcg/kg/min, titrate up to 2 mcg/kg/min by doubling every 15 min. At low doses, nitroglycerin venodilates; at higher doses, it dilates resistance vessels only if the preload is high (which acts as a safeguard against hypotension). Nitroglycerin reduces afterload and preload, and effects coronary vasodilation. Onset is 2-5 min, duration 5-10 min. Nitroglycerin is safer than nitroprusside for most patients, especially if there is concurrent angina/MI (it has anti-ischemic effects). Nitroprusside is a balanced vasodilator but does not protect the myocardium; it is best for acute CHF with severe hypertension.

3) Diuretics. Administer furosemide (Lasix) 20-40 mg IV (or a dose equal to twice the patient's daily usage); it venodilates within 3-4 min and causes diuresis within 15-20 min. Monitor urine output; the dose may be doubled in 20-30 min if there is a poor response. Furosemide reduces preload and antagonizes salt retention. Loop diuretics activate the neurohumoral axis, causing vasoconstriction, which in turn increases left ventricle dysfunction for ~2h; thus it is

important to give it with an ACE inhibitor and nitrates, which support the ventricle (however, ACE inhibitors may cause hypotension after aggressive diuresis). Bumetanide is another loop diuretic; 1 mg of bumetanide equals 40 mg furosemide. If sulfa allergy, administer ethacrynic acid 50 mg.

4) Consider nesiritide (Natrecor) 2 mcg/kg bolus followed by 0.01 mcg/kg/min IV. It is a BNP that venodilates, reduces preload and afterload, antagonizes the sympathetic nervous system and decreases aldosterone levels. It may be added to standard treatment (except NTG).

5) Morphine 2-3 mg IV, may repeat every 10-15 min; avoid if decreased blood pressure. Morphine relieves anxiety and decreases afterload by dilating resistance vessels.

6) If hypotension, consider dobutamine (start 2.5 mcg/kg/min) if signs of poor perfusion with a systolic BP > 90 mm Hg; dobutamine decreases afterload and is a positive inotrope. Or, consider dopamine (start 2-3 mcg/kg/min). If hypotension unresponsive to dobutamine, consider milrinone 50 mcg/kg over 10 min, then 0.375-0.750 mcg/kg/min; it is an inotropic agent. Use norepinephrine only as a temporizing measure. Consider intra-aortic balloon pump.

7) ACE inhibitors. Captopril (if SBP ≥ 110 mm Hg, 25 mg powder placed sublingually; if SBP 90-110 mm Hg, 12.5 mg sublingual) or enalapril 1.25 mg IV. ACE inhibitors improve the cardiac index, lowers end diastolic pressure, promotes vasodilation, generally improves renal blood flow, and reduces aldosterone.

8) Consider hydralazine 10-20 mg IV, may repeat 10 mg every 1h. Hydralazine dilates arterioles and increases cardiac output; combine with IV nitroglycerin to decrease preload.

9) In patients admitted with class III-IV CHF, consider DVT prophylaxis with Lovenox (enoxaparin).

10) Digoxin inhibits Na-K ATPase pump. This increases intracellular sodium, which in turn increases calcium via the Na-Ca exchange pump and results in increased contractility. Digoxin is not a good agent for acute CHF.

11) Beta blockers block deleterious adrenergic stimulation; it is not an acute treatment.

12) Phlebotomy may be necessary in patients with polycythemia.

VII. DEEP VENOUS THROMBOSIS (DVT)

•General•
1) The majority of lower extremity DVTs begin in the deep veins of the calf.
2) Thrombi may propagate and embolize (propagation usually occurs before embolization), resulting in pulmonary emboli.
3) Progression of venous thrombi may produce other long-term sequelae, including valve damage and venous flow obstruction.
4) Most isolated calf thrombi dissolve without therapy.

•Risk Factors•
1) *Hypercoagulability*- from previous thromboembolic disease, malignancy, sepsis, protein S or C deficiency, antithrombin deficiency, Factor V Leiden, prothrombin mutation, lupus anticoagulant, inflammatory conditions or increased estrogen (from pregnancy, recent pregnancy, abortion or oral contraceptive pills).
2) *Stasis*- from immobility, paralysis, or use of cast.
3) *Endothelial injury*- from IV drug use, trauma, or recent surgery.
4) Advancing age.

•Clinical Presentation•
1) Patients may present with lower extremity pain, swelling, or sense of fullness, usually occurring over several days. Involvement is almost always unilateral.
2) Consider DVT in any patient with unexplained unilateral extremity pain or swelling, especially in the presence of risk factors.
3) Patients may also present with symptoms of pulmonary emboli (i.e., chest pain, shortness of breath).

•Physical Exam•
1) In general, the physical exam is insensitive and inaccurate for DVT.
2) Exam may demonstrate unilateral calf swelling, with or without pitting edema. Examine for signs of compartment syndrome. Palpation may elicit tenderness of the calf muscles. Erythema or warmth over the thrombosis may be present.
3) Lack of measurable calf swelling does not rule out DVT.
4) A palpable cord, most often in the popliteal fossa, is specific but not

sensitive for DVT.

5) Although DVT rarely produces a fever > 102 F, it may be difficult to clinically distinguish DVT from cellulitis.

6) Superficial thrombophlebitis (tender, indurated distention of subcutaneous veins) may be associated with DVT.

7) Homan's sign (posterior calf pain with foot dorsiflexion) is an inaccurate test for DVT.

•Diagnosis•

1) Ultrasound is the diagnostic test of choice for suspected DVT; color-flow duplex detects 95% of acute clots above the knee. Duplex scanning detects only 80% of distal clots. Ultrasound is less accurate in advanced pregnancy, due to the gravid uterus compressing the inferior vena cava (consider MRI after 20 weeks gestation if ultrasound is indeterminate). If the patient is at high risk for DVT and has a negative ultrasound, consider repeat clinical evaluation and ultrasound in 1 wk.

2) MRI is an accurate test for DVT, including for thrombus below the knee.

3) D-Dimer by the rapid whole blood agglutination test (SimpliRED), when elevated, is 93% sensitive and 77% specific for proximal DVT. The gold standard is the ELISA method; latex methods are generally not reliable. If a patient has a negative D-dimer and no risk factors, there is a less than 1% chance of proximal DVT.

4) If suspected pulmonary embolism (PE), consider V/Q scan or chest CT (at least 40% of patients with DVT have clinically silent PE, as demonstrated by VQ scan).

5) Obtain blood for future studies.

•Treatment•

1) Most patients with DVT can be managed as outpatients. Consider enoxaparin (Lovenox) 1 mg/kg SC every 12h for inpatient or outpatient treatment (for inpatient treatment, another option is enoxaparin 1.5 mg/kg SC q day). Enoxaparin is a low molecular weight heparin which, when compared to unfractionated heparin (UFH), exerts less of an inhibitory effect on thrombin and a greater inhibitory effect on factor Xa. Therapeutic levels are achieved within 30 min and last

24h (its effect may be prolonged in patients with renal failure). There is less of an incidence of thrombocytopenia than with UFH. Enoxaparin was shown to be at least as effective as UFH for treatment of DVT, with a decreased risk of bleeding. If close follow up can be arranged, and if patients do not meet certain exclusion criteria (pregnancy, hereditary bleeding or thrombotic disorders, active bleeding, significant cardiopulmonary comorbidity, morbid obesity, acute CHF, renal insufficiency, suspected PE, or geographic inaccessibility), then outpatient treatment is acceptable. Enoxaparin should be administered for at least 5d, with warfarin started on the same day or the day after (until the INR is therapeutic).

2) If enoxaparin is not indicated, administer heparin 80 u/kg bolus followed by 18 u/kg/h. Heparin blocks extension of the thrombus and reduces the risk of emboli. Usually, warfarin 10 mg is started concomitantly.

3) If heparin is contraindicated (active internal bleeding, malignant hypertension, recent major trauma or surgery, CNS neoplasm, or history of heparin-induced thrombocytopenia) or if complications develop while patient is anticoagulated, a vena cava filter is indicated.

4) Thrombolytic therapy may be indicated in certain cases (young patients with an acute onset of extensive DVT or patients with massive iliofemoral thrombosis). Thrombolytic therapy may result in improved vessel patency, preservation of valve function, and a decreased incidence of post-phlebitic syndrome.

5) Bed rest; elevate leg; compression stockings.

6) **Calf thrombi**- management is controversial; at least 15-20% of isolated calf thrombi propagate and embolize. Either anticoagulate patient or arrange for serial ultrasounds to document clot regression.

7) **Upper extremity DVT**- clots may cause PE. Diagnosis is usually with duplex ultrasound. Treatment is either anticoagulation or catheter-directed thrombolysis with urokinase or tPA.

8) **Superficial thrombophlebitis**- obtain ultrasound (25% of patients with superficial phlebitis have involvement of the deep venous system), and, if negative, treat with compression bandages and NSAIDs. Patients who do not have co-existing varicose veins, have no other

clear etiology for a superficial thrombophlebitis (IV drug use, trauma, recent IV catheter), or have involvement of the greater saphenous vein above the knee, are at higher risk for DVT.

9) Phlegmasia alba dolens- 'milky-white' leg from extensive iliofemoral thrombosis and complete venous obstruction, which may progress to shock or gangrene. There is usually painful swelling of the entire leg to the groin; the leg may have a doughy consistency. Treat with IV fluids, vasopressors if necessary, heparin, elevation of leg, and consider thrombolysis or thrombectomy.

10) Phlegmasia cerulea dolens- 'blue leg' from massive iliofemoral obstruction; the leg may become tensely swollen, painful and cyanotic. Swelling may cause arterial insufficiency, pallor, coolness of extremity, and diminished pulses; it may progress to shock or gangrene. Treat with IV fluids, vasopressors if necessary, heparin, elevation of leg, and consider thrombolysis or thrombectomy.

VIII. ECG DIAGNOSIS

Hexaxial Reference (for determination of electrical axis)

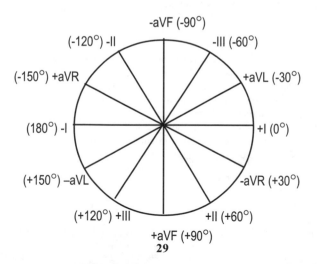

A. The Basics/Normal Values

The septum is depolarized left to right.

Heart rate can be determined by the number of large boxes between 2
QRS segments; if there is a one box separation; the rate is 300 bpm;
if 2 boxes, it is 150; if 3 it is 100; if 4 it is 75; if 5 it is 60 (a small box
is 0.04 sec, a large box is 0.2 sec).

Axis: Normal is -30° to +100°. Left axis deviation is -30° to -90°. Right
axis deviation is 100° to 180°; extreme right axis deviation is 180° to
-90°.

P wave: should be up in leads I, II, V4-V6, aVF; down in aVR; equivocal in leads III, aVL,V1-V3; maximum duration is 0.11 sec.

P-R interval: Duration of 0.12-0.2 sec; decreases at increased rates.

Q wave: may be normal if small (1-2 mm); should be absent in leads I,
aVL, aVF, V5-V6; a deep Q is normal in aVR. It is normally < 0.04
sec, and <25% of the height of the following R wave.

QRS interval: Duration of 0.05-0.10 sec; amplitude >5 mm, <25-30
mm. It is normally up in leads I, II, V5, and V6; it is normally down
in aVR and V1.

ST segment: compare with TP segment (compare with several con-
secutive complexes, averaging the TPs); curves gently into the T
wave.

T wave: Amplitude should be <5 mm in the limb leads, <10 mm in
precordial leads; should be up in leads I, II, V3-V6; down in aVR;
equivocal in leads III, aVL, aVF, V1-V2.

QT Interval: If heart rate is 60-100 bpm, the QT should not exceed 1/2
the RR interval; with other rates, the interval is corrected: QTc =
QT/square root of RR

U wave: same polarity as T; increases with decreased potassium; inverted with ischemia or left ventricular overload.

B. AtrioVentricular Block

1st degree: PR interval is >0.2 sec.

2nd degree

Mobitz I (Wenkebach): progressive PR interval prolongation until a P
wave fails to conduct to the ventricle. Grouped beating is present. The
block is usually in the AV node (which is more likely if the QRS is

narrow), and may be secondary to acute myocardial infarction, beta-blockers, calcium channel blockers, digoxin, or increased vagal tone. Mobitz I usually requires no specific therapy, except to withhold medications that may increase the AV nodal block.

<u>Mobitz II</u>: sudden dropped QRS without prolongation of the PR interval. The site of the block is in the infranodal His-Purkinje system (which is lower than the site of the block in Mobitz I and has a worse prognosis), and therefore the QRS is usually wide. The ECG may demonstrate 2:1 or 3:1 conduction. Atropine may worsen the conduction ratio by increasing the number of atrial impulses without improving conduction. Mobitz II is usually the result of myocardial infarction. Patients with Mobitz II require a pacemaker.

3rd degree

<u>Complete Heart Block</u>: No P waves conduct to the ventricle; there is no relationship between the P waves and the QRS (the QRS rate is slower than the P wave rate). The QRS may be junctional or idioventricular; there is a fixed P-P interval. Not all A-V dissociation is complete heart block- if the underlying supraventricular or junctional rhythm rate is not fast enough to overcome any infranodal pacemakers, then A-V dissociation is present, but not complete heart block. Complete heart block may result from acute myocardial infarction, digoxin, calcium channel blockers, or beta-blockers. Treat with atropine, pacer, isoproterenol.

<u>A-V dissociation</u>: no relationship between P and QRS; the QRS rate is faster than the P rate.

C. Conduction Delays

Bundle Branch Blocks (BBB)

* To determine the site of the block, examine Lead I. In this lead, the terminal QRS forces point to the side of the bundle block; i.e. if the terminal forces are negative (pointing to the right, away from the positive pole of lead I), then it is a RBBB. In other words, in lead I, RBBB has a terminal S wave, and LBBB has a terminal R wave. Also, in lead V1, a RBBB has a terminal R wave, and LBBB has a terminal S wave.

Left BBB

1) QRS >0.12 sec and has normal general orientation.
2) Ventricles are activated right to left (opposite from norm); septum is

depolarized right to left, just after right ventricle depolarization.

3) The ECG has many variations, including: deep S in V1-V3 (monophasic QS or rS complexes) or tall R wave in leads I, AVL, V5-V6; left axis deviation; very small R wave in leads V1-V3 (Qs complex); less steep upstroke of initial QRS; no septal Q in leads I, AVL, V5-V6.

4) ST depression and T wave inversion are discordant (i.e. opposite to main deflection of the QRS); T wave should be opposite to the terminal QRS (if not, consider ischemia).

5) The block is incomplete if the duration is 0.10-0.12 sec.

Right BBB

1) QRS >0.12 sec and has late rightward and anteriorly directed forces in leads V5-6.

2) Lead I has a broad (>0.04 sec) terminal S.

3) AVR has a terminal broad R; V1 has an rSR' complex.

4) There is a normal first 1/2 of QRS, but then no opposing right to left forces. The T wave is usually opposite in direction to the terminal deflection of the QRS (if not, consider ischemia).

5) The block is incomplete if the QRS is 0.1-0.12 sec.

6) If an anteroseptal infarct is present, the initial septal forces disappear, and V1 may just have a Q and late R wave.

Intraventricular Conduction Delay

Definition: QRS $\geq$ 0.108 sec with a pattern nonspecific for LBB or RBB.

Left anterior hemiblock: normal or slightly prolonged QRS duration; left axis deviation (-30 to -90); S>R (rS) in leads II, III, AVF; qR or R in leads I, AVL; AVR with terminal positivity.

Left posterior hemiblock: normal QRS; right axis deviation; R, small q in leads II, III, AVF; small R, deep S in leads I, AVL; no RVH. It is difficult to diagnose on a single ECG.

D. Hypertrophy

Right Atrial Enlargement

1) P wave is tall and peaked in leads II, III, and AVF; amplitude is > 2.5 mm.

2) It is seen with congenital heart disease, pulmonary disease, and

RVH.

Left Atrial Enlargement
1) Wide P wave >0.11 sec.
2) Notch in P wave with two peaks >0.04 sec apart.
3) Negative deflection in terminal P wave in V1 $\geq$ 1 mm deep and 1 mm wide.
4) Seen with mitral valve disease.

Right Ventricular Hypertrophy
1) Tall R in V1 (R/S >1.0).
2) Right axis deviation.
3) Taller R in right precordium and deeper S in left precordium.
4) Negative QRS in lead I.
5) Right ventricular strain with T wave inversions in leads V1-V3.
6) A tall R in V1 may also be seen with MI (but there is usually evidence of inferior MI and T wave inversion) or benign cardiac rotation (in which there are no other ECG abnormalities).

Left Ventricular Hypertrophy
1) R in I + S in III $\geq$25 mm.
2) S in V1 + R in V5 or 6 $\geq$ 35 mm.
3) R in AVL >11 mm.
4) Left axis deviation; left atrial enlargement; poor R wave progression with loss of septal R waves (may have a QS complex in V1-V3 with ST segment discordance showing ST elevation that may mimic an acute MI).
5) QRS >.1 sec; strain with downsloping ST depression and asymmetric biphasic or inverted T wave inversion in leads with prominent R waves (I, AVL, V5-V6).

E. Extrasystoles

Most premature atrial complexes (PACs) depolarize the sinus node, resetting the intrinsic sinus rate and causing a noncompensatory pause. Some PACs may not be conducted to the ventricles. Premature ventricular complexes (PVCs) usually have a fully compensatory pause; the impulse is blocked at the A-V node, so the sinus node is not reset.

F. Early Repolarization

Characteristics of early repolarization include: diffuse J-Point elevation; no T wave inversion; and PR depression in either limb or precordial leads, but not both (unlike pericarditis). It occurs in 20% of young black men. The patient should be asymptomatic.

G. ECG Evidence of Ischemia

General: Acute ischemia may be subendocardial (with ST depression) or transmural (ST elevation). In an acute MI, ST changes appear rapidly, Q waves may not appear for several hours, and T wave inversions are variable.

Ischemia: symmetrical inverted T waves and horizontal or downsloping ST depression ≥ 1 mm.

Nonspecific ST-T Changes: <1 mm ST depression or elevation; blunted, flattened, or biphasic T waves without obvious inversion or hyperacuity.

Acute MI: ST elevation with or without abnormal Q waves and hyperacute T waves.

<u>Anterior MI</u>: ST elevation in leads I, AVL, V1-V4; these leads may have pathologic q waves. ECG may only show poor R wave progression, with reciprocal changes in leads II, III, AVF, and the posterior chest. If A-V block is present, it is usually below the His bundle trifurcation and is more permanent and may progress to complete heart block. It is usually from LAD or LCA obstruction.

<u>Anterolateral MI</u>: ST elevation in leads V1-V6; tall R in leads V1-2.

<u>Anteroseptal MI</u>: ST elevation in leads V1-V3.

<u>Inferior MI</u>: ST elevation and possible pathologic q waves in leads II, III, AVF with reciprocal changes in leads I, AVL and anteriorly. If A-V block is present, it is usually above the trifurcation of His and is partly due to increased vagal activity and normal conduction is usually reestablished. It is usually from RCA obstruction.

<u>Lateral MI</u>: ST elevation in leads I, AVL, V4-V6. It is usually from left circumflex obstruction.

<u>Posterior MI</u>: ST depression V1-V2 with tall, broad R waves (which represent reciprocal changes); R/S > 1 in V1 or V2. May have coexisting acute inferior or lateral MI. Posterior MI usually occurs with RCA or left circumflex obstruction.

RV infarction: ST elevation ≥ 1 mm V4R-V6R; may also have elevation in leads II, III, and AVF. RV infarction occurs with RCA obstruction and is usually associated with inferior MI.

Wellens' Syndrome- Biphasic or deep, symmetrically inverted T waves
in leads V2 and V3, often in V1 and V4, and occasionally in V5 and
V6. If these ECG changes are associated with chest pain, no pathologic precordial Q waves, little or no ST segment elevation and no loss
of precordial R waves, Wellens' criteria indicate left anterior descending artery disease.

Coronary Vessel Distribution

Right Coronary Artery: supplies the inferior and posterior myocardium,
S-A node, most A-V nodes, right atria, right ventricle, and right bundle
branch.

Left Anterior Descending: supplies the anterior myocardium, and the
superior 2/3 of the septum.

Left Circumflex: supplies the anterolateral myocardium.

Posterior Descending: supplies the inferior 1/3 of the septum.

H. Specific ECG Definitions

Pathologic q wave: 0.04 sec wide or 1/3 the height of the QRS in two or
more contiguous leads.

ST Depression: ≥1 mm depression at 0.8 mm from the J-point; a
downsloping ST segment is most specific for ischemia.

Coronary Insufficiency: ST depression; horizontality of ST segment
with sharp angle with T wave; inverted U wave.

Poor R wave Progression: R wave is not positive by lead V4; R/S < 1 in
V5; R wave not progressively larger from V4-6.

I. ECG Manifestations of Metabolic Abnormalities

Hypokalemia: ST depression; flat T wave; U wave is present.

Hyperkalemia: Tall peaked T wave; prolonged PR interval; wide QRS
interval.

Hypercalcemia: Short QT interval, prolonged PR and QRS intervals.

Hypocalcemia: Prolonged QT interval.

Digoxin: Sloped ST depression; atrial tachycardia, paint brush or fist-
like ST depression, and various arrhythmias.

IX. HYPERTENSIVE CRISIS

•General•
1) Severe hypertension is defined as diastolic blood pressure >120 mm Hg or mean arterial pressure (MAP) >130 mm Hg. MAP = DBP + 1/3 (SBP-DBP).
2) Hypertensive emergency is hypertension associated with evidence of end-organ damage (usually CNS, cardiovascular, or renal).
3) Hypertensive urgency is hypertension (>115 mm Hg diastolic) without evidence of end-organ dysfunction.
4) Hypertensive crisis may occur at lower blood pressures with acute eclampsia or renal disease.

•Etiology•
Etiologies include an abrupt increase in essential hypertension; renovascular disease; aortic dissection; eclampsia; acute glomerulonephritis; pheochromocytoma; withdrawal or discontinuation of meds; and drugs (cocaine).

•Clinical Presentation•
1) In a hypertensive crisis, the patient may present with shortness of breath, chest pain, visual changes, or neurological deficits. Intracranial hemorrhage, aortic dissection, eclampsia, oliguria, CHF or ischemic chest pain also indicate hypertensive emergency.
2) Headache and dizziness are nonspecific symptoms unless they occur with fundoscopic changes or other CNS dysfunction.
3) Hypertensive encephalopathy presents with severe headache, nausea and vomiting and altered mental status.

•Evaluation•
1) Check CXR (evaluate for pulmonary edema), ECG (evaluate for ischemia and hypertrophy), CBC, electrolytes, BUN/Cr, and urinalysis. Lab evidence of organ dysfunction includes hemolysis, increased BUN or creatine, hematuria, or proteinuria.
2) Obtain head CT if severe headache or focal CNS signs.
3) Perform fundoscopic exam (papilledema indicates hypertensive emergency) and complete neurologic and cardiovascular exams.
4) Check blood pressure in both arms.

•Treatment•

1) If hypertensive emergency, the initial guideline is a 30% reduction in blood pressure in 30 min. Options include:

  a) Nitroprusside (0.1-10 mcg/kg/min, start with <0.25 mcg/kg/min if renal insufficiency); it has an immediate onset and lasts 1-5 min.

  b) Nitroglycerin: start 10 mcg/min, onset 2-5 min; nitroglycerin is the agent of choice in ischemia.

  c) Labetalol: bolus 20-80 mg IV every 10 min or 2 mg/min; onset 5-10 min.

  d) Furosemide 20-80 mg IV.

  e) Esmolol.

2) Alternatively, the appropriate antihypertensive agent can be determined by the clinical circumstances:

  a) Myocardial ischemia: nitroglycerin or beta-blockers.

  b) Aortic dissection: nitroprusside and propranolol.

  c) Congestive heart failure: nitroglycerin, furosemide, and morphine.

  d) Hypertensive encephalopathy with DBP > 130 mm Hg: nitroprusside or labetalol.

  e) Stroke: labetalol.

  f) Eclampsia/Preeclampsia: magnesium plus either hydralazine or labetalol.

  g) Pheochromocytoma: phentolamine, nitroprusside or labetalol.

3) If the hypertension is long-standing and the work-up is negative and the patient is asymptomatic, consider re-starting previous oral medications and observe until blood pressure decreases. **Clonidine** is a safe and effective oral treatment (onset 30 min, peak effect 2-4h, duration 6-8h; may cause sedation); other options include loop diuretics, ACE inhibitors, or beta-blockers. If only hypertensive urgency is diagnosed, the goal is a gradual reduction in blood pressure over 1-2d.

X. MYOCARDIAL INFARCTION/ACUTE CORONARY SYNDROMES

A. Myocardial Infarction (MI)

•Pathophysiology•

1) Coronary thrombosis is triggered when a fibrous cap overlying a vulnerable plaque ruptures; this leads to the deposition of platelets and fibrin and the formation of a platelet plug at the subendothelial disruption site.

2) Coronary thrombi vary in composition. Thrombi from acute MI are more likely to have older thrombin within the clot, and stasis within the vessel allows fibrin and RBCs to add to the platelet rich thrombus; this gives the appearance of a 'red thrombus'. In contrast, thrombi in unstable angina are more likely to be newer and smaller, and consist primarily of platelets with little fibrin, and appear as a 'white thrombus'. The varying content of thrombi may explain the varied efficacy of anti-platelet and anti-thrombin therapy in different acute coronary syndromes.

•Clinical Presentation•

1) The Chest Pain (CP) Study Group showed that the character of pain cannot reliably determine which patients are having a cardiac event. The group found that if CP lasts <2 min or >2 d, it is unlikely due to MI; 23% with burning pain had MI; 20% with sharp pain had ischemia; 15% of patients with MI had chest wall tenderness; 15% of patients with MI had pain radiation to the right arm.

2) Dyspnea is the most frequent anginal equivalent.

3) CNS injury (CVA, multiple sclerosis, ALS) may lead to silent MI.

4) Isolated emesis or diaphoresis are rare presentations of MI.

5) The elderly often present atypically. Many patients over age 85 who have an MI present atypically, with acute weakness, syncope, or mental status change. The elderly often present with complications from MI rather than symptoms (CHF, bradycardia, A-V block) and should be ruled out for MI.

•Evaluation•

1) Check ECG, CXR, CBC, and cardiac enzymes (CPK, CPK-MB, and troponin). Consider PT/PTT, electrolytes, and BUN/Cr.

2) Repeat ECGs as necessary.

3) Echocardiogram or radionuclide scanning may be helpful in evaluating patients with chest pain.

ECG

Changes seen with left ventricle infarct may include:

1) Pathologic q waves (q waves may be normal in lead III).

2) ST-T elevation ≥ 1 mm or depression >1 mm.

3) T wave inversion (inversion may be normal in leads III, AVR and V1); or peaked hyperacute T waves ($>50\%$ as high as the preceding R wave in 2 or more leads).

4) 13% of MIs have a normal ECG; the ECG is diagnostic in 25-50% of MIs.

5) Acute ischemia may be subendocardial (with ST depression) or transmural (ST elevation). In an acute MI, ST segment changes appear rapidly, q waves may not appear for several hours, and T wave inversion is variable.

6) Always obtain a right-sided ECG in patients with an inferior MI.

7) The negative predictive value of a normal ECG does not improve with increased time from symptom onset.

ECG Correlation with Location of Injury

Ischemia: symmetrical inverted T waves and horizontal or downsloping ST depression ≥ 1 mm.

Nonspecific ST-T Changes: <1 mm ST depression or elevation; blunted, flattened, or biphasic T waves without obvious inversion or hyperacuity.

Acute MI: ST elevation with or without abnormal Q waves and hyperacute T waves.

Anterior MI: ST elevation in leads I, AVL, V1-V4; these leads may have pathologic q waves. ECG may only show poor R wave progression, with reciprocal changes in leads II, III, AVF, and the posterior chest. If A-V block is present, it is usually below the His bundle trifurcation and is more permanent and may progress to complete heart block. It is usually from LCA obstruction.

Anterolateral MI: ST elevation in leads V1-V6; tall R in leads V1-2.

Anteroseptal MI: ST elevation in leads V1-V3.

Inferior MI: ST elevation and possible pathologic q waves in leads II, III, AVF with reciprocal changes in leads I, AVL and anteriorly. If A-V block is present, it is usually above the trifurcation of His and is partly due to increased vagal activity and normal conduction is usually reestablished. It is usually from RCA obstruction.

Lateral MI: ST elevation in leads I, AVL, V4-V6. It is usually from left circumflex obstruction.

RV infarction: ST elevation ≥ 1 mm V4R-V6R; may also have elevation in leads II, III, and AVF. RV infarction occurs with RCA obstruction and is usually associated with inferior MI.

Posterior MI: Horizontal ST depression in leads V1-V2 with tall, broad R waves (which represent reciprocal changes); R/S > 1 in lead V1 or V2; and upright T waves in leads V1-V3. May have coexisting acute inferior or lateral MI. Posterior MI usually occurs with RCA or left circumflex obstruction.

Wellens' Syndrome- Biphasic or deep, symmetrically inverted T waves in leads V2 and V3, often in V1 and V4, and occasionally in V5 and V6. If these ECG changes are associated with chest pain, no pathologic precordial Q waves, little or no ST segment elevation and no loss of precordial R waves, Wellens' criteria indicate left anterior descending artery disease.

Lab Findings

CK-MB: rises in 2-6h, peaks at 10-24h, returns to normal in 36-72h. The sensitivity in the first 24h is 94-100% (90% in 5-6h), specificity 96-98%. CK is not elevated in ischemia.

Myoglobin rises within 2-4h (as early as 1h), peaks at 4-12h, and is less specific than other cardiac enzymes. If carbonic anhydrase is not elevated, then myoglobin is more likely cardiac. Myoglobin is the most sensitive marker in the early hours; it is detected in 2/3 of MI within 3h, and in nearly all by 6h. Myoglobin may rise with just ischemia. One study showed a repeat myoglobin that doubled within 1-2h (even if still in the normal range) is highly specific for acute MI. Patients with chronic renal failure do not clear myoglobin well.

Troponin I, T rises in 2-6h, peaks at 10-24h. Its sensitivity for ischemia is 100% at 6-10h. Troponin persists for 7-10d, and is specific for infarction. A positive Troponin T is associated with a 40% increased risk of adverse outcome.

•Treatment•

1) Establish IV access. Place patient on monitor. Administer oxygen.

2) **Consider PCI (Percutaneous Coronary Intervention) or fibrinolytic therapy (see below).**

3) Aspirin 160-325 mg chewed (onset is within 60 min; lasts 9d). Aspirin permanently inactivates the platelet enzyme cyclooxygenase; the ISIS-2 trial demonstrated a 23% reduction in mortality with aspirin use. If patient is aspirin allergic, administer clopidogrel (Plavix) 300 mg po loading dose, then 75 mg/d. Clopidogrel is an ADP inhibitor and may take several days for peak effect. (Another option, ticlopidine, is associated with neutropenia and thrombocytopenia).

4) Nitroglycerin (NTG). Initially, administer sublingual NTG (0.4 mg/dose for 3 doses as needed). If the patient has persistent pain, start IV NTG, bolus with 12.5-25 mcg, then 10-20 mcg/min, may increase by 5-10 mcg every 5-10 min. IV NTG is recommended for the first 24-48h in patients with CHF, hypertension, large anterior MIs or persistent ischemia. Avoid NTG if hypotension, bradycardia or tachycardia, as it may worsen ischemia. NTG reduces preload, afterload, myocardial oxygen consumption and dilates coronary vessels; there is a 20-30% reduction in mortality in acute MI. Titrate to pain.

5) Low molecular weight heparin (enoxaparin) or unfractionated heparin. Antithrombin therapy with heparin prevents extension of thrombosis and allows clot dissolution by the fibrinolytic system. Always start heparin or enoxaparin if the patient is undergoing PCI or CABG; strongly consider heparin if large or anterior MI, or if atrial fibrillation. Fully anticoagulate patients even if therapeutic on Coumadin.

a) Enoxaparin (Lovenox) 1 mg/kg SC as been shown to be superior to unfractionated heparin in the treatment of non-ST segment elevation acute coronary syndromes (non-Q-wave MI and unstable angina), unless CABG is planned within 24h. Enoxaparin may be given to patients undergoing PCI. Enoxaparin (30 mg IV bolus followed immediately by 1 mg/kg SC q12h) may also be superior to unfractionated heparin in the treatment of ST segment elevation MI.

b) If enoxaparin is not given, consider IV heparin. If given with fibrinolytic therapy, the recommended dose of IV heparin is 60 u/kg bolus, then 12 u/kg/h infusion, max 4000 u bolus, 1000 u/h infusion (this dose may decrease the incidence of bleeding). If the patient has ST-segment elevation and fibrinolytic therapy or glycoprotein inhibitors are not given, consider IV heparin 60-70 u/kg bolus (max 5000 units) then 12-15 u/kg infusion.

6) Metoprolol 5 mg IV every 5 min x 3, followed in 15 minutes by 25-50 mg po q6h x 24h; or administer atenolol 5 mg IV every 10 min x 2 or esmolol drip at 50 ug/kg/min. Contraindications include asthma, high A-V block, heart rate<50 bpm, PR >240 ms, SBP <90 mm Hg, CHF, severe COPD, or moderate to severe left ventricle dysfunction. Beta-blockers decrease myocardial oxygen consumption, reduce mortality and non-fatal reinfarction, and decrease the incidence of primary ventricular fibrillation.

7) Morphine 2-4 mg IV if persistent or recurrent pain. Hypotension is an uncommon side effect if the patient is not volume depleted. Morphine reduces anxiety; it also decreases preload and afterload.

8) Consider glycoprotein inhibitors, which block platelet aggregation (aspirin only inhibits 30% of platelet activity, and heparin does not interfere with platelet aggregation; also, fibrinolysis activates platelets, sometimes causing reocclusion). It has established benefits for non- ST segment elevation acute coronary syndromes (unstable angina and non-Q wave MI) when patients undergo percutaneous coronary intervention; it should also be considered in patients with ongoing ischemia who are not undergoing interventions.

9) ACE inhibitors reduce mortality and the incidence of CHF associated with MI; ACE inhibitors also decrease reperfusion arrhythmias and help maintain cardiac function. ACE inhibitors are especially beneficial in patients with anterior infarction, CHF, or LV dysfunction. Do not give in the first 6h. Start at low dose within 24h with captopril 6.25 mg.

10) MgSO4 1-2 gm if high-risk for hypomagnesemia (alcoholic, on diuretics, or poor diet) then 15 g over 24h (Mg acts as an antiarrhythmic, inhibits platelets, may decrease afterload and acts as a calcium channel blocker; consider holding Mg if shock, hypotension, or complete heart block).

11) Lidocaine if frequent (>5/min) PVCs, multifocal PVCs, ventricular tachycardia or ventricular fibrillation.

12) <u>Pacemaker Indications</u>: Indications include asystole, complete heart block, RBBB with developing hemiblock, developing LBBB, type II second degree A-V block, or symptomatic bradycardia unresponsive to atropine. Also, consider pacemaker for overdrive pacing with PAT, atrial flutter, ventricular tachycardia, and Torsades.

13) <u>Intra-Aortic Balloon Pump Indications</u>: Indications include cardiogenic shock, acute mitral regurgitation or ventricular septal defect, incessant ventricular arrhythmias with hemodynamic instability, unstable angina, and as a bridge to bypass operation.

14) **PCI (Percutaneous Coronary Intervention)**

a) In multiple studies, PCI appears to be superior to fibrinolytic therapy, if experienced facilities are available within 90 minutes (door to balloon time). PCI offers the greatest benefit for the elderly (who are at increased risk of hemorrhage with fibrinolytic therapy) and those with extensive or anterior MIs.

b) PCI is the best option for patients in cardiogenic shock (but consider administering fibrinolytic therapy while waiting for PCI). Patients who have had a previous CABG may not respond to fibrinolytic therapy; consider PCI in these patients.

c) Indications for transfer to a facility with PCI capabilities include patients with contraindications to fibrinolytic therapy, post-infarction or post-reperfusion ischemia, persistent ventricular dysrhythmias, or persistent hemodynamic instability.

15) **Fibrinolytic Therapy**

a) Fibrinolytics activate plasminogen to plasmin, which then dissolves the fibrin component of the occluding coronary artery thrombus. Different fibrinolytics exhibit different degrees of fibrin specificity and intrinsic thrombogenic potential (fibrinolytics can result in a paradoxical activation of the coagulation cascade: thrombin is exposed during fibrinolysis, which then results in platelet activation and aggregation).

b) **Doses for Different Fibrinolytic Agents**

1) <u>TNK-tPA</u>: single weight-adjusted IV bolus over 5-10 sec:

> If < 60 kg, give 30 mg bolus;
> If ≥ 60 kg but < 70 kg, give 35 mg bolus;
> If ≥ 70 kg but < 80 kg, give 40 mg bolus;

If ≥ 80 kg but < 90 kg, give 45 mg bolus;

If ≥ 90 kg, give 50 mg bolus.

The optimal antithrombin regimen with TNK-tPA is probably enoxaparin 30 mg IV bolus followed immediately by 1 mg/kg SC. Alternatively, administer unfractionated heparin: for patients weighing < 67 kg, give 4000 unit IV bolus, then 800 u/h infusion; for patients weighing >67 kg, give 5000 unit IV bolus, then 1000 u/h infusion.

2) t-PA (alteplase): 15 mg bolus, then 0.75 mg/kg up to 50 mg over 30 min, then 0.5 mg/kg up to 35 mg over 60 min. Heparin is given with tPA: 60 u/kg bolus, then 12 u/kg/h infusion (max 4000 u bolus, 1000 u/h infusion).

3) r-PA (reteplase): double bolus infusion of 10 U, 30 minutes apart. Heparin is given with rPA: 60 u/kg bolus, then 12 u/kg/h infusion (max 4000 u bolus, 1000 u/h infusion).

c) Indications for Fibrinolytics

1) Chest pain or its equivalent suggesting MI, with time to therapy <12h from symptom onset; and an ECG that demonstrates ≥ 1 mm ST elevation in ≥ 2 contiguous leads or new or presumed new left bundle branch block (LBBB).

2) If clinical presentation suggests acute MI, consider fibrinolytic therapy in any type of BBB (RBBB, LBBB, paced rhythm, and new or old BBB).

3) Also, consider fibrinolytic therapy if ST depression ≥ 1mm with upright T waves in 2 or more contiguous anterior precordial leads (suggesting posterior MI).

4) Also, consider fibrinolytic therapy in patients with atypical presentation of acute MI and any BBB with concordant ST segment elevations ≥ 1 mm toward the major QRS deflection or discordant ST segment elevation ≥5mm in 2 or more contiguous leads.

d) Contraindications to Administering Fibrinolytics

Altered mental status, recent head trauma, previous hemorrhagic CVA, intracranial or intraspinal surgery within 2 months, major surgery within 2 weeks, blood pressure > 200/120 mm Hg despite treatment, active internal bleeding, intracranial neoplasm, arteriovenous malformation, aneurysm, bleeding diathesis, or suspected aortic dissection.

*Age alone is not a contraindication to fibrinolysis; however, the risk for hemorrhage increases with age (as do post-MI complications).

e) Relative Contraindications to Fibrinolytics

Active PUD, previous ischemic CVA, major surgery within 2 months, subclavian line, prolonged CPR.

f) After Administering Fibrinolytic Therapy

1) If massive bleed with cardiovascular compromise, give 10 u of cryoprecipitate and stop fibrinolytic therapy.

2) After fibrinolytic therapy, markers for reperfusion are inaccurate, but consider rescue PCI or post-MI ischemia if worsening hemodynamics or persistent severe symptoms after 90 min. However, complete ST resolution (i.e. >70%) within 3h has a low mortality risk and lack of resolution (<30%) indicates persistent ischemia and is associated with high mortality.

3) If there is no recurrence of angina or documented ischemia, elective PCI following fibrinolytic therapy has no proven benefit.

B. Specific Acute MI (AMI) Categories

1) AMI Diagnosis in Patients with LBBB (or with pacer)

a) There have been many proposed ECG signs of ischemia in patients with LBBB. The most reliable method of determining ischemia in LBBB appears to be a point system proposed by Sgarbossa:

1) Concordant (in the same direction as the QRS complex) ST elevation ≥ 1 mm in any lead (5 points); or,

2) ST depression ≥ 1 mm in leads V1-3 (3 points); or

3) Discordant (opposite QRS) ST elevation ≥ 5 mm (2 points).

A total score of 3 or more points suggests acute MI; the Sgarbossa criteria are specific but not sensitive for AMI.

b) Other proposed ECG signs of AMI in LBBB include elevation or depression of ST segment of 7-8 mm in the opposite direction of the major QRS complex or more than 1/2 the height of T wave; Q waves in at least 2 of leads I, AVL, V5-6; and R wave regression in leads V1-4.

c) The T wave is not useful in diagnosing acute MI with LBBB.

d) RBBB does not hinder ECG diagnosis of AMI (ST elevation is reliable, depression is not).

2) Right Ventricle Infarction

<u>Clinical Presentation</u>- Patients may present with shock, jugular venous distention, clear lungs, a holosystolic murmur of tricuspid regurgitation, or a right-sided gallop. Right ventricular infarction occurs in 40% of patients who have an inferior MI.

<u>ECG</u>- ST elevation of 0.5-1 mm in V4R is 90% sensitive, 80% specific for right ventricular infarction; there may be ST elevation in right-sided leads III, V1, V4-6, AVR.

On the standard ECG there is prominent ST depression in leads V1-3.

<u>Treatment</u> (in addition to usual acute MI interventions)

1) IV fluids.

2) Consider RV afterload reduction with nitroprusside.

3) If patient is hypotensive, use dobutamine; avoid diuretics, opiates, and nitrates.

4) The RCA supplies the sinoatrial and A-V nodes; thus consider cardioversion if atrial fibrillation.

3) Posterior MI

<u>ECG</u>- It may show coexisting acute inferior or lateral MI; tall, broad R wave with increased voltage in leads V1-3; R/S > 1 in V1 or V2; horizontal ST depression in leads V1-3; and a prominent positive T wave in leads V1-V3. (When the ECG is held upside down and backwards, the R wave indicates a Q wave, and ST-T changes represent ST elevation with T wave inversion).

4) Anterior; Lateral; Inferior MI- see above ECG Correlation with Location of Injury.

C. Unstable Angina

•Definition•

It is defined as rest angina (anginal symptoms lasting > 20 min); new onset angina (angina with onset within 2 months that occurs with mild exertion); or accelerating angina. ECG has no evidence of acute MI.

•Pathophysiology•

1) If myocardial oxygen demand exceeds supply (usually because a fixed obstruction in a coronary artery limits blood flow during exercise), chest pain results.

2) The development of unstable angina may result from non-occlusive thrombosis on a preexisting plaque, coronary vasoconstriction, progressive coronary obstruction, or coronary inflammation.

•Treatment•

1) Treatment options include with aspirin (or clopidogrel), oxygen, nitroglycerin, beta-blockers, enoxaparin (Lovenox), glycoprotein receptor inhibitors, and morphine; perform repeat ECGs.

2) If low-risk (1 or fewer cardiac risk factors; normal/unchanged ECG; flat T waves): administer aspirin, nitroglycerin; consider enoxaparin.

3) If intermediate-risk (rest or nocturnal angina, diabetes, ST depression 0.5-1 mm, age > 65 years, two or more cardiac risk factors): administer aspirin; IV nitroglycerin and enoxaparin if pain returns.

4) If high-risk (history of CAD, PCI within 6 months, CHF, ongoing rest pain, symmetrical T wave inversion, ST elevation or depression): administer aspirin, IV nitroglycerin and enoxaparin. Consider IV beta-blocker, morphine, platelet glycoprotein receptor inhibitors, and urgent catheterization.

5) Enoxaparin 1 mg/kg SC is slightly better than heparin; PCI appears safe in patients who have received enoxaparin for unstable angina or non ST-elevation MI.

6) If pain persists or recurs, consider platelet glycoprotein receptor inhibitors. It has established benefits for non- ST segment elevation acute coronary syndromes (unstable angina and non-Q wave MI) when patients undergo percutaneous coronary intervention; it should also be considered in patients with ongoing ischemia who are not undergoing interventions.

7) If recurrent angina, CHF, sustained ventricular tachycardia, or hemodynamic instability, consider PCI.

XI. MYOCARDITIS

•General•

1) Myocarditis is an inflammation of the heart muscle, which may lead to a dilated cardiomyopathy.

2) The most common etiologies are viral (Coxsackie B, echovirus), parasitic, Lyme disease, and idiopathic. Also, there are medication-induced, connective tissue disorder, and bacterial etiologies.

3) In Central and South America, Chagas disease is the most common cause of myocarditis.

•Clinical Presentation•

1) Patients may present with fatigue, dyspnea, fever, and precordial chest pain.

2) There is often an antecedent viral syndrome; the majority of cases are subclinical.

3) Myocarditis is frequently accompanied by pericarditis.

4) In children, consider myocarditis if child presents with a low-grade fever, dull substernal chest pain that is present for days, and resting tachycardia.

5) Tachycardia (often out of proportion to the temperature), and tachypnea are common.

6) Acutely ill patients may have signs of heart failure.

•Evaluation•

1) Check ECG, CXR, cardiac enzymes, ESR, and CBC. Patients may have elevated CK-MB, SGOT, LDH; ESR and WBC may be elevated.

2) The ECG usually shows sinus tachycardia, but may demonstrate conduction delays or ST elevation without reciprocal depression.

3) The CXR is usually normal, but may show cardiomegaly.

4) The diagnosis is confirmed with a radionuclide study, echocardiogram, and biopsy.

•Treatment•

1) Establish IV access. Administer oxygen. Admit to monitored setting.

2) Patient should be on bed rest.

3) Treatment is generally supportive.

4) Consider heparin to decrease risk of thromboembolism.

5) Initiate standard treatment for heart failure and arrhythmias as indicated.

6) Do not give NSAIDS or immunosuppressive drugs.

XII. PERICARDIAL DISEASE

A. Pericarditis

•Etiology•

1) Etiologies include viral/idiopathic, malignant, uremia, trauma, radiation, collagen vascular, bacterial, acute MI, and drugs (procainamide, hydralazine, isoniazid, doxorubicin).
2) Dresslers' pericarditis is post-MI pericarditis (usually 2-3 weeks after MI).

•Clinical Presentation•

1) There is often a viral prodrome.
2) Patients may present with substernal chest pain relieved with sitting forward; the pain may be present for days. The pain is usually sharp, and worse with inspiration.
3) Patients may have dyspnea and a low grade intermittent fever.

•Evaluation•

1) Check ECG, CBC, electrolytes, BUN/Cr, and ESR; consider cardiac enzymes (CK-MB may be elevated, as it is often myopericarditis).
2) Check CXR for enlarged cardiac silhouette.
3) Check echocardiogram for effusion (uremic pericarditis has a high association with tamponade; malignant effusions progress to tamponade in 50-85%).
4) A transient pericardial friction rub (superficial grating or scratching sound) may be present and is best heard at the lower left sternal border with the patient leaning forward; it may have presystolic, systolic, and diastolic components.

ECG

These changes are typically seen with infectious causes, and occasionally with other causes:

Stage 1 Concave up ST elevation (elevation seldom exceeds 2 mm) in leads I, II, III, AVL, AVF, V2-6; may have reciprocal ST depression in leads AVR and V1 without T wave abnormality or distinct J point. Most have PR depression in leads II, AVF, or V4-6. In general there is a diffuse, nonanatomic distribution of ECG changes, usually without reciprocal changes; T waves are usually up, as opposed to MI. PR elevation is often seen in AVR.

Stage 2 ST and PR segments normalize.

Stage 3 Diffuse T wave inversions. No Q waves.

Stage 4 ECG normalizes (or T wave inversions become permanent) .

•Treatment•

1) Indomethacin 25-50 mg every 6h; steroids if NSAIDs fail.

2) Dialysis for uremic pericarditis.

3) Treat the underlying disorder.

•Disposition•

Patients with effusions or possible myocardial infarction should be hospitalized. Stable patients with presumptive viral pericarditis without effusions may be discharged.

B. Cardiac Tamponade

1) Patients present with Beck's triad (hypotension, jugular venous distention, muffled heart sounds) and pulsus paradoxus.

2) The ECG may demonstrate electrical alternans. The echocardiogram shows right ventricle diastolic collapse, right atrial compression, and bowing of the septum into the left ventricle with inspiration.

3) Treat with drainage, fluids and dobutamine (afterload reduction with nitroglycerin has not been shown to be beneficial).

C. Constrictive Pericarditis

1) The patient presents with symptoms of right heart failure, usually without chest pain. An early diastolic knock may be heard on cardiac exam. There is usually no pulsus paradoxus and heart sounds are not distant.

2) Diagnosis can be difficult. Distinguish from CHF by the absence of pulmonary edema and the presence of a normal heart size on CXR, no murmurs, and the absence of a bundle branch block or LVH on ECG.

3) Do not treat with diuretics. Treatment is surgery.

D. Pericardial Effusion

1) A pericardial effusion is excess fluid in the pericardial sac. It may be secondary to pericarditis, CHF (from increased hydrostatic pressure),

decreased plasma oncotic pressure, or increased capillary permeability. The exam may demonstrate muffled distant heart sounds. CXR may sow a globular enlarged heart.

2) ECG may show generalized low voltage or electrical alternans (the QRS axis varies beat to beat secondary to movement of the heart within the pericardial sac). CXR may show an enlarged cardiac silhouette. Diagnosis is with echocardiogram.

3) Treatment depends on underlying etiology and hemodynamic status.

XIII. PULMONARY EMBOLUS

•General•

1) Pulmonary embolus (PE) is a complication of underlying deep venous thrombosis (DVT). Over 90% of PEs result from DVTs of the lower extremities, although only 1/3 of patients with PE have clinical signs of DVT.

2) At least 50% of patients with proximal DVTs have asymptomatic PEs at presentation. Consider tumor embolism as the etiology for PE.

•Risk Factors•

1) Age > 40, obesity, immobility, surgery, trauma, malignancy, ulcerative colitis, CHF, vasculitis, IV drug abuse, and nephrotic syndrome.

2) For women, risk factors include hypertension, smoking, therapeutic abortion, exogenous estrogen, and pregnancy.

3) Inherited risk factors include activated protein C resistance, protein C and S deficiency, lupus anticoagulant, and antithrombin deficiency.

4) 12% of patients with PE have no risk factors.

•Clinical Presentation•

1) Symptoms of PE may include pleuritic chest pain (seen in 66%), dyspnea (73%), tachypnea (70%), and tachycardia (30%). The most reliable symptom is dyspnea of acute onset (which may be transient).

2) Many patients are asymptomatic, or have atypical symptoms.

3) The physical exam is often normal in patients with submassive PE.

4) Patients with massive PE may have hypotension secondary to acute

cor pulmonale.

5) Temperature is rarely >102°F.

6) Many patients have rales on lung exam.

7) Less than 1/3 of patients with PE have clinical signs of DVT.

•Diagnosis•

1) **ABG**- An elevated A-a gradient is found in 90-92% of patients with PE. The calculation for the A-a gradient is150-1.2 (pCO2) - pO2; the normal is (age/4) + 4. A normal gradient and pCO2 > 36 have a negative predictive value of 98%. However, in most clinical situations, the A-a gradient and pO2 are not predictive of PE, as many other disease processes may lower the pO2. In patients with preexisting cardiopulmonary disorders, there is no difference in the A-a gradient between those with and without PEs.

2) **Angiogram**- Pulmonary angiogram is the gold standard for the diagnosis of PE. If the V/Q scan is intermediate or low probability, and the clinical suspicion is intermediate or high, consider angiogram, which has a mortality rate of 0.2-0.5%; there is a greater morbidity with unnecessary anticoagulation than with angiogram.

3) **CXR**- The initial CXR is often abnormal. CXR abnormalities may include Hampton's hump (a triangular pleural-based infarction with apex toward hilum), Westermark's sign (dilated pulmonary vessels proximal to embolus with sharp cutoff), atelectasis, effusion (seen in up to 50%; usually small and unilateral), or infiltrate. A normal CXR increases the suspicion of PE.

4) **D-dimer**- It is a fibrin split-product released during fibrinolysis. There are different assays available; the ELISA method is the gold standard, while latex agglutination methods are generally unreliable. In general, D-dimer is not sensitive or specific enough for the evaluation of PE. However, some use D-dimer to decrease the suspicion of PE in patients with no risk factors (as D-dimer is often elevated in patients with many risk factors). If the patient is hemodynamically stable with minimal risk factors, a normal A-a gradient, and a negative D-dimer by the ELISA or SimpliRed method, then PE/DVT is unlikely.

5) **ECG**- The most common ECG abnormalities are tachycardia and

nonspecific ST changes. The ECG may show right heart strain abnormalities, which include right bundle branch block, right axis deviation, peaked P waves in lead II, or the S1Q3T3 pattern (seen in about 12%). The ECG is normal in 20-30% of patients with PE.

6) **Echocardiogram**- Consider obtaining an echocardiogram if there is evidence of right ventricle dysfunction; results may demonstrate acute right ventricular dilation, acute pulmonary hypertension, and tricuspid regurgitation. If the patient is unstable, consider bedside transesophageal echocardiogram, which may detect right ventricular dysfunction and central PE.

7) **Spiral or helical CT**- It is 100% sensitive, 96% specific in detecting lesions within central pulmonary vessels (it is less reliable for subsegmental branches). Therefore, especially in patients with chronic cardiopulmonary disorders (in whom a V/Q scan may be difficult to interpret), consider obtaining a spiral CT instead of V/Q scan. If CT shows PE, start treatment; if CT is normal, obtain a duplex ultrasound of the lower extremities to rule out DVT. If the ultrasound is abnormal, begin treatment (the patient may have subsegmental pulmonary lesions in addition to DVT). If both CT and duplex are normal but there is a high clinical suspicion, a thrombus may be in the subsegmental branches (consider angiogram); or, a thrombus may be in the ileac veins or inferior vena cava.

8) **Ultrasound**- Consider duplex ultrasound of lower extremities to evaluate for possible DVT if the V/Q scan is nondiagnostic (a scan positive for DVT would mandate treatment and be presumptive evidence of PE).

9) **V/Q Scan**- The PIOPED study showed that a high clinical suspicion and high probability V/Q has a 96% positive predictive value for PE; low clinical suspicion and low probability V/Q has a 96% negative predictive value for PE. A V/Q scan is more reliable in patients without underlying cardiopulmonary disorders. If the V/Q scan is indeterminate, a more definitive test must be done to establish a diagnosis. Consider pulmonary angiogram or spiral CT scan of the chest. Or, consider lower extremity Doppler ultrasound (a scan positive for DVT would mandate treatment and be presumptive evidence of PE).

•Treatment•

1) Administer oxygen and establish IV access. Place patient on monitor.

2) If the patient is hypotensive, there is likely right ventricle dysfunction. Consider IV fluids to maintain SBP > 90 mm Hg (be careful not to precipitate pulmonary edema); consider norepinephrine and dobutamine 2.5 mcg/kg/min, max 20 mcg/kg/min (which decreases systemic and pulmonary vascular resistance).

3) Low molecular weight heparins are safer and more effective than unfractionated heparin for the prevention and treatment of PE and DVT. Consider enoxaparin (Lovenox) 1 mg/kg SC q 12h. There should be an overlap period of 5 days with warfarin.

4) If enoxaparin is not given, administer heparin 80 u/kg bolus then 18 u/kg/hr drip (fully heparinize patients who are therapeutic on Coumadin). There should be an overlap period of 5d with warfarin.

5) Consider fibrinolytic therapy if massive PE, hemodynamic instability (even if hypotension is transient or resolves with IV fluids), significant hypoxemia, evidence of acute right heart strain, or obstruction of flow to an entire lobe or multiple segments. Administer tPA (Alteplase) 100 mg over 2h; or, rPA (Retavase) two 10 unit IV boluses 30 minutes apart. (Heparin inhibits clot extension, but does not dissolve existing clot; fibrinolytic therapy dissolves existing clot, and may be beneficial in unstable patients). Fibrinolytics should be started within 24h of symptom onset; heparin is not administered with fibrinolytics.

6) Consider surgical consult for thrombectomy if failed fibrinolysis or if there is a contraindication to fibrinolytic therapy; of if patient remains hypotensive despite heparin and vasopressors.

7) Consider inferior vena caval filters if patient has contraindications to anticoagulation or complications develop while patient is on anticoagulants.

8) Obtain blood for future studies.

9) Admit patient.

CHAPTER 4
DENTAL

I. GENERAL DENTAL CONDITIONS

1) Anatomy

Dentin surrounds the pulp (the neurovascular supply); the coronal portion is covered with enamel. Beginning with midline and counting back, on each upper and lower side there are: 1 medial incisor, 1 lateral incisor, 1 canine, 2 premolars, and 3 molars.

2) Fractures
- **a)** Ellis class I fractures involve only enamel (look for sharp piece causing trauma). Treat by smoothing sharp edges.
- **b)** Ellis class II fractures involve exposure of dentin and may be sensitive to heat/cold. Treat with a calcium hydroxide dressing and cover with gauze or dental foil with adhesive backing (treatment may not be necessary if minor damage and patient is older than 12 years).
- **c)** Ellis class III fractures involve exposure of dentin (pinkish tinge) and pulp (drop of blood); the patient may have exquisite or no pain. Treat with calcium hydroxide dressing and cover with gauze or dental foil with adhesive backing and arrange immediate dental referral.

3) Infection
- **a)** A periapical abscess may have a grossly decayed tooth or no apparent pathology; if abscessed, sharp pain is elicited with percussion.
- **b)** The patient may have associated oral/facial swelling.
- **c)** Consider I & D (if fluctuant), antibiotics, warm saline rinses every 2h, and follow-up within 1d.

4) Post-extraction
- **a)** If the patient has severe pain with foul odor/taste 2-3d post-extraction, the patient may have a dry socket. Treatment includes irrigation, application of medicated dental packing or iodoform gauze slightly dampened with eugenol or Camphophenique, and close follow-up.

  b) After endodontic treatment, some patients may experience buildup of gas in the tooth after it has been sealed; a dentist must reopen it.

5) Subluxation/Avulsion

  a) Minimally mobile teeth heal well with soft diet x 1-2 weeks; grossly mobile teeth require stabilization.

  b) A completely avulsed tooth is an emergency; look for tooth (check x-ray to see if tooth was forced beneath gingiva).

  c) If the avulsed tooth is a primary tooth (6 months to 5 years old), it is not replaced (replaced primary teeth have a high likelihood of fusing to the underlying bone).

  d) Permanent teeth should be replaced as soon as possible (or rinse in normal saline, hold by crown, and place in Hank's solution or milk). The primary goal of reimplantation is to preserve the periodontal ligament, as this decreases ankylosis and improves subsequent repair attempts. Provide immediate referral or stabilization kit.

CHAPTER 5

DERMATOLOGY

I. ALLERGIC CONTACT DERMATITIS/POISON IVY

•General•

1) Allergic contact dermatitis is a T-cell mediated, type IV hypersensitivity reaction.
2) In poison ivy, the plant must be damaged to release resin, which may be carried on shoes or pets. Blister fluid contains no antigen, so scratching cannot spread the rash (unless the antigen remains under a person's fingernails).

•Diagnosis•

1) A linear rash is common. Other characteristics include marked pruritis, and a weeping, oozing, red vesicular rash; there may be occasional large bullae.
2) The rash usually manifests within 2-3 days of contact.
3) Acute (not chronic) dermatitis usually spares palms, soles and scalp.

•Treatment•

1) In poison ivy, the resin quickly penetrates skin; washing has some benefit if done within minutes.
2) Except if very mild symptoms, start oral corticosteroids (prednisone 40-60 mg tapered over 2-3 weeks; less duration may allow symptoms to recur).
3) Potent topical steroids such as clobetasol propionate (Temovate) 3x/d are the only topical medications of any benefit, and are most effective if given early.
4) Symptomatic treatment with diphenhydramine, tap water or Burrow's solution compresses, oatmeal (Aveeno) baths, and Calamine lotion.
5) Poison ivy rarely becomes infected, so topical antibiotics are not indicated. Neomycin, benzocaine spray and topical antihistamines may cause dermatitis.

II. ERYTHEMA MULTIFORME/STEVENS-JOHNSON SYNDROME

•General•

1) Erythema multiforme (EM) and Stevens-Johnsons Syndrome (SJS) are inflammatory reactions to antigenic stimuli, manifesting varying degrees of clinical severity.

2) EM is typically caused by herpes simplex infection. The incidence of EM increases between 20-30 years of age.

3) SJS has a more severe presentation than EM, and is usually caused by medications, including sulfonamides, penicillin, allopurinol, anticonvulsants, and NSAIDs; it has also been associated with Mycoplasma pneumonia. SJS can present at any age. Toxic epidermal necrolysis (TEN) is a more severe form of SJS, characterized by more than 30% of epidermal detachment.

•Clinical Presentation•

EM

1) EM is a self-limited and recurrent disease of young adults that occurs seasonally in the spring and fall. Patients either have no prodrome, or have very mild symptoms of fever and malaise.

2) The rash is often symmetrical and acrally distributed. The typical target lesions have 3 zones: central dusky purpura, an elevated edematous pale ring, and surrounding macular erythema. The central area may blister. Unlike urticaria, the lesions are usually not pruritic. The lesions are found on the extremities, especially the palms and soles; there may be mild mucous membrane blistering. The rash usually resolves in 7-10 days. There is no epidermal detachment.

SJS

1) There is usually a prodrome of fever, malaise, headache, vomiting, and diarrhea. Skin and mucous membrane lesions are more severe than with EM.

2) Skin lesions are typically flat, erythematous, or purpuric, forming incomplete targets that may blister centrally. The lesions are widely distributed, but concentrated on the trunk; SJS is characterized by epidermal detachment and mucous membrane involvement.

3) Eye involvement often occurs. The Nikolsky sign (lesions detach with slight pressure) is often positive.

•Treatment•

1) Determine the cause.

2) **EM**: treatment is symptomatic as most cases are self-limited. Consider antihistamines, NSAIDs, analgesics, and topical steroids. If recurrent HSV is the trigger, chronic suppressive doses of oral valacyclovir or acyclovir are indicated. Topical antivirals and intermittent antiviral therapy have no role in the management. If patients fail to respond to chronic antiviral suppression, dapsone and antimalarial agents may be helpful. As a last resort, azathioprine will control the disease, although recurrences are typical upon discontinuation.

3) **SJS**: treatment is primarily supportive. IV fluid resuscitation as necessary. Consider admission to ICU if the extent of cutaneous involvement exceeds 10 to 30% of total body surface area. Steroid use is controversial (if steroids are used, aggressive dosing and prompt discontinuation within 5-7 days is required). Avoid silvadene use, as it contains sulfa. Obtain an ophthalmology consult if ocular involvement is present. Stomatitis is treated with diphenhydramine and viscous lidocaine mouth rinses.

III. LICE/SCABIES

•General•

1) Lice infestations may be head lice (pediculosis capitis), body lice (pediculosis corporis), or pubic lice (pediculosis pubis, also known as crabs). Head lice are most common, and spread by close physical contact. The adult female lays 3-6 small white eggs (nits) each day at the base of the hair shaft. Patients present with pruritis and excoriations. Diagnosis is based on the observation of eggs or lice; the white ova of head lice are attached to hair, and lice and eggs are often found in seams of clothing.

2) Scabies infections resemble those of lice, but scabies are concentrated around hands and feet, areolae, umbilicus and in web spaces; also, scabies have burrows.

•Clinical Presentation•

Lice- Pediculosis capitis presents with pruritis of scalp and neck, with the presence of nits (whitish eggs firmly attached to hair shafts about

1 cm from scalp). Pediculosis pubis presents with pruritis and nits in the pubic area.

Scabies- There may be burrows up to 1 cm connected to a minute vesicle or papule; secondary changes include excoriations, crusting, and nodules. Patients often have intractable pruritis, which is worse at night. Usual sites include web spaces, wrists, buttocks, abdomen, genitalia, and breasts. In adults, the head and neck are typically spared.

•Treatment•

1) Head lice: over-the-counter permethrin (Nix) 1% for a single 30-60 minute application is effective. Repeated treatment in 1 week is recommended. (Lindane is more toxic and not as effective). For pediculosis pubis, use Nix or 5% permethrin (Elimite) for a single 10 minute application and repeat in 1 week.

2) Scabies: for total body application (not head) in treatment of scabies, use Elimite. Apply once at bedtime and leave on for 8-12h, then wash (a single treatment is usually effective).

3) Use a fine comb to remove nits. Wash all clothing, linen, etc., in hot water.

IV. SUNBURN

•Clinical Presentation•

1) Patients present with skin erythema, blistering, and pain.

2) Severe cases may present with fever.

3) Assess for exposure to photosensitizing medications.

4) Infection, even of severely blistered sunburn, is extremely rare.

•Treatment•

1) Aspirin or other NSAIDs are useful for pain and inflammation; the burn is mediated by histamines (although antihistamines are not effective) and prostaglandins.

2) Topical aloe vera.

3) Cool soaks. Simple elevation should control edema. Consider narcotics if severe pain.

4) If significant systemic reaction (chills, fever, nausea and vomiting, weakness, headache), consider prednisone 50-100 mg/d x 3-5d.

5) Topical steroids are not indicated or effective.

CHAPTER 6

ENDOCRINE

I. ADRENAL INSUFFICIENCY

•General•

1) Primary adrenal insufficiency (Addison's disease) is due to disease of the adrenal cortex; it may be idiopathic, autoimmune, infiltrative, hemorrhagic or drug-induced.

2) Secondary adrenal insufficiency is due to pituitary failure or is iatrogenic from withdrawal of exogenous steroids.

3) The adrenal medulla produces epinephrine and norepinephrine; the cortex produces cortisol, androgens, and aldosterone

•Clinical Presentation•

1) Patients may present with weakness, fatigue, nausea and vomiting, weight loss, abdominal pain, hypotension, hypoglycemia, hyponatremia, or hyperkalemia.

2) Hyperkalemic paralysis is a rare emergent complication.

3) Patients may exhibit hyperpigmentation.

•Evaluation•

1) Check CBC, electrolytes, glucose, BUN/CR, calcium, cortisol level, thyroid function tests, and ECG. Consider evaluation for sepsis.

2) To confirm the diagnosis, measure baseline cortisol and ACTH levels and then administer synthetic ACTH (cosyntropin) 0.25 mg IV/IM. Recheck cortisol levels every 30-60 min. In adrenal insufficiency, serum cortisol levels do not rise; in normal individuals, the cortisol levels should double within 6-8h. If the patient is in adrenal crisis, treatment should not be delayed for diagnostic testing; treatment with dexamethasone will not interfere with serum cortisol measurements.

•Treatment•

1) If the diagnosis is suspected but unconfirmed, administer dexamethasone 4 mg IV every 6-8h (it won't interfere with the cosyntropin test).

2) If the condition is known, administer 100 mg hydrocortisone IV ev-

ery 6-8h (it repletes glucocorticoids and acts to correct hypotension, hyponatremia, hyperkalemia, and hypoglycemia). Florinef 0.1 mg may be added for mineralocorticoid therapy (although high doses of hydrocortisone provide sufficient mineralocorticoid effect). Administer aggressive D5 normal saline.

3) Treat underlying precipitants (sepsis, hypothermia, MI). Correct any metabolic abnormalities. Consider broad spectrum antibiotics if sepsis is suspected.

II. DIABETIC KETOACIDOSIS (DKA)

•General•

1) Hyperglycemia, hyperketonemia, and metabolic acidosis are the hallmarks of DKA.

2) Inadequate insulin effect leads to gluconeogenesis, in which adipose tissue releases fatty acids and the liver in turn releases the acid byproducts (ketones).

3) Lack of insulin prevents tissues from using glucose and ketones, with the subsequent development of hyperglycemia and ketonemia; counter-regulatory hormones (catecholamines, glucagon, cortisol, and growth hormone) worsen ketoacidosis.

4) Glucose in the kidney tubules draws water and electrolytes into the urine, resulting in dehydration and total body depletion of electrolytes.

5) DKA may be caused by infection, medication noncompliance, MI, or stroke, among other precipitants.

•Clinical Presentation•

Patients may present with polyuria, polydypsia, weakness, weight loss, nausea and vomiting, abdominal pain, and altered mental status.

•Evaluation•

1) Check glucose, electrolytes, BUN/Cr, CBC, ABG, serum ketones, amylase, and urinalysis. Consider evaluation for infection. Repeat labs frequently.

2) DKA is usually confirmed by a serum glucose > 250 mg/dL (or a history of diabetes), metabolic acidosis (corrected pH <7.3 or bicarbonate <15), and positive serum ketones.

3) DKA patients often have potassium abnormalities. Potassium is increased by 0.6 mEq/L for every 0.1 decrease in pH (because of acidemia, potassium shifts out of cells). DKA patients are always total body potassium depleted, but because of the acidosis they may initially have a normal or elevated potassium (which resolves after potassium moves back into cells with insulin administration and resolution of the acidemia).

4) Labs may also demonstrate an increased anion gap, increased WBC, and decreased sodium (there is a 1.6 mEq/L decrease in sodium for every 100 mg/dL increase in glucose over 100 mg/dL).

5) Almost all DKA has ketonuria. A urine dip positive for ketones and glucose can rapidly confirm DKA; if negative for glucose, consider alcoholic or starvation ketoacidosis.

6) The glucose may be near normal if the patient was fasting.

7) The nitroprusside reagent test is unreliable, as it doesn't measure beta-hydroxybutyrate, the predominant ketone in serum and urine.

8) Acidemia is not invariably present, especially with prolonged vomiting and severe dehydration (consider alcoholic ketoacidosis). Venous pH probably provides an adequate determination of the acid-base status.

9) Search for the underlying cause of DKA: consider ECG, CXR, urinalysis, LP.

•Treatment•

1) Establish IV. Place patient on monitor. Administer IVNS (500-1000 cc/h x 1-2h); do not over hydrate as it may precipitously lower glucose and cause cerebral fluid shifts (which usually does not develop unless glucose is below 250 mg/dL and insulin is used; however, fatal cerebral edema in adults is rare, so do not under hydrate). Children are more prone to cerebral edema, so reduce glucose more slowly in children.

2) Consider Mg 2 gm IV.

3) When blood glucose decreases to < 250 mg/dL, change fluid to D5NS to keep glucose 200-300 mg/dL while insulin therapy continues to clear ketonemia.

4) If patient is hypotensive, hold insulin initially (it may cause vascular collapse from water moving into cells).

5) Insulin

<u>If patient is admitted to ICU</u>- consider bolus regular insulin 0.1 u/kg IV (although an insulin bolus has not shown to be helpful), then 0.1 u/kg/h IV.

<u>If patient is not admitted to ICU</u>, administer 0.4 u/kg regular (half IV, half SC/IM), then 5-7 u/h SC/IM.

6) Bicarbonate

If pH <6.9, consider 88 mEq HCO3 with 15 mEq KCl every 2h until pH $\geq$ 7. If pH 6.9-7, give 44 mEq HCO3 with 15 mEq KCl. If pH > 7, do not give HCO3.

7) Potassium

If K < 3.4 mEq/L, hold insulin (risk of arrhythmia) and give KCl 10-20 mEq/l x 1-2h; If K <5.5 mEq/L, give 20-30 mEq/l; if K > 5.5 mEq/L, do not give KCl.

*Before potassium replacement, ensure kidney function and urine output are adequate.

•Disposition•

Patients in severe DKA should be admitted to the ICU.

> ## III. HHNK (Hyperglycemic Hyperosmolar Nonketotic Coma)

•Clinical Presentation•

1) HHNK usually occurs in elderly patients with adult onset diabetes (who have a decreased renal clearance of glucose) who present with a several day history of thirst, polyuria or oliguria, polydipsia, and possible fever.

2) Most patients have mental status changes (depending on their osmolality); patients may have seizures or focal CNS deficits.

3) There is usually a precipitating factor.

•Evaluation•

1) Check CBC, glucose, electrolytes, BUN/Cr, serum osmolarity, PT/PTT (as a screen for DIC), and ABG; consider head CT and LP.

2) Look for evidence of infection (CXR, urinalysis, blood/urine cultures) or myocardial infarction (ECG, cardiac enzymes).

3) The hallmarks of HHNK are hyperglycemia and hyperosmolarity

without significant ketosis. Ketoacidosis does not develop perhaps because there is enough insulin to inhibit lipolysis but not enough to prevent hyperglycemia.

4) Glucose is usually greater than 600 mg/dL, and serum osmolarity is usually greater than 320 mOsm/dL. BUN is usually increased.

5) Total body potassium is decreased, as osmotic diuresis leads to severe potassium depletion.

•Treatment•

1) Establish IV. Place patient on monitor. Administer IV fluids, initially with normal saline, then, since fluid loss is hypotonic, change to 1/2 normal saline. Fluid deficit may be as high as 6-10 L. Monitor urine output. When glucose decreases to 250 mg/dL, use solutions that contain 5% glucose.

2) Administer insulin 0.1 u/kg/h IV to gradually lower glucose to 200 mg/dL, and then switch to subcutaneous therapy.

3) Replace potassium (first ensure adequate kidney function and urine output).

4) Dilantin is contraindicated with seizures, as it may impair insulin release.

5) Admit patient.

IV. HYPERTHYROIDISM

•General•

1) Etiologies include Graves's disease, toxic multinodular goiter, and Hashimoto's disease.

2) Thyroid storm is a severe form of hyperthyroidism. There is often a precipitating cause for thyroid storm (consider infection, DKA, MI, stroke, surgery, amiodarone, or antithyroid medication withdrawal).

•Clinical Presentation•

1) Patients may present with weight loss, fever, palpitations, HTN, atrial fibrillation, mental status changes, goiter, exophthalmos, or myopathy.

2) Patients with thyroid storm may present with fever, marked tachycardia, diaphoresis, CNS dysfunction, cardiovascular abnormalities (arrhythmias, CHF) or GI dysfunction. Patients may have eye signs of Graves (exophthalmos) and a palpable goiter. Patients often have a widened pulse pressure.

•Evaluation•

1) Check TSH, free T4 and T3, CBC, electrolytes, BUN/CR, CXR, ECG, cultures, and urinalysis.

2) In hyperthyroidism, TSH is decreased, and free T4 is elevated; CBC often shows leukocytosis and a normocytic anemia. Hypokalemia may be present.

3) Thyroid storm is a clinical diagnosis (thyroid hormone levels are not significantly different than in patients with uncomplicated hyperthyroidism; no lab tests reliably confirm the diagnosis). In thyroid storm, evaluate for possible infection.

•Treatment• (for thyroid storm)

1) Block synthesis of thyroid hormone with propylthiouracil (PTU) 900-1200 mg po loading dose, then 150 mg po every 6h. Alternatively, consider methimazole 20 mg po every 8h.

2) Block release of thyroid hormone with SSKI (iodine) 3-5 drops po every 8h or Lugol's solution 30 drops/d divided tid or qid; it should be given 1h after PTU to avoid increasing intrathyroidal hormone stores. If iodine cannot be used, lithium carbonate may be administered.

3) Block peripheral effects with dexamethasone 2 mg IV every 6h (which blocks conversion of T4 to T3) and propranolol (if no heart block or CHF) 1-2 mg IV every 15 min prn.

4) Supportive treatment includes hydrocortisone 100 mg IV (to replace adrenocortical reserves). Treat hyperpyrexia with acetaminophen and cooling measures (salicylates decrease protein binding and increase free T3 and T4). Provide hydration. Treat CHF with digoxin and diuretics. Treat any precipitating event.

V. HYPOTHYROIDISM

•General•

1) Hypothyroidism may be primary or secondary. Primary hypothyroidism is due to an intrinsic failure of the thyroid (which may be from autoimmune causes or iatrogenic failure after surgery); secondary

hypothyroidism is caused by disease or destruction of the pituitary.
2) There is usually a precipitating factor (often a cold environment).
3) Myxedema coma is a severe form of hypothyroidism.

•Clinical Presentation•

Patients may present with fatigue, cold intolerance, constipation, weight gain, paresthesias, psuedomyotonic DTRs, hypothermia, decreased mental status, or rheumatic symptoms.

•Evaluation•

1) Check thyroid function tests, CBC, electrolytes, glucose, BUN/Cr, calcium, CXR, and ECG. Consider evaluation for infection.
2) Hypothyroidism is demonstrated by an increased TSH (in primary hypothyroidism); free T4 levels are low.
3) ECG may demonstrate a sinus bradycardia, prolonged PR interval, and T wave abnormalities.
4) Labs may demonstrate decreased sodium, increased pCO2, and a decreased pO2.
5) CHF is rare; pericardial effusion is often present, but tamponade is rare.
6) Many patients have an ileus.

•Treatment•- (for myxedema coma)

1) Establish IV access. Monitor patient. Administer oxygen.
2) Administer T4 300-500 mcg IV.
3) Administer stress dose steroids: hydrocortisone 100-300 mg IV.
4) Antibiotics as indicated.
5) Passively rewarm hypothermic patients (active rewarming may be dangerous).
6) Do not treat psychosis with phenothiazines.
7) Admit to a monitored setting.

CHAPTER 7
ENT

I. EPISTAXIS

•Etiology•
Local- Local etiologies include trauma (nose-picking), inflammation, septal deviation, and foreign bodies.
Systemic- Systemic etiologies include atherosclerosis/hypertension, hemophilia, coagulopathy, and Osler-Weber-Rondu.

•General•
1) Epistaxis may be classified as either anterior or posterior nasal bleeding.
2) Anterior bleeding most commonly occurs in Kiesselbach's plexus in the nasal septum; bleeding is often a result of desiccation from dry weather, anatomic abnormalities, or nose picking.
3) Posterior bleeding usually arises from a branch of the sphenopalatine artery; it often occurs spontaneously in the elderly.

•Evaluation•
If significant bleeding is present, check CBC, platelets, INR, type and crossmatch.

•Treatment•
1) If significant bleeding is present, establish IV and place patient on monitor and pulse oximeter. Severe bleeding may require blood transfusion and airway management with intubation.
*Procedure for managing epistaxis:
2) First have patient blow nose to dislodge clots.
3) Use proper lighting and suction.
4) After suctioning, insert gauze moistened with vasoconstrictor (oxymetazoline, phenylephrine 0.5-1.0%, or cocaine 4%) and anesthetic agents (lidocaine 4% or tetracaine 2%) and have patient apply pressure for 10 min. Remove gauze and inspect; if bleeding has stopped, consider scraping mucosa to provoke bleeding, to ensure bleed was anterior.

5) If a bleeding site is identified, consider chemical cautery with a silver nitrate stick (cautery is most effective after bleeding has been controlled; only one side of the septum should be cauterized at a time) followed by application of bacitracin and a hemostatic agent. If bleeding persists, consider Surgicell/gelfoam or a Merecel sponge tampon (consider coating sponge with bacitracin ± surgicell). If bleeding still persists, use petroleum gauze packing or anterior epistaxis balloon. Patients with nasal packs should receive antibiotics (cephalexin, Augmentin, or clindamycin).

6) If unable to visualize bleeding, or if bleeding down pharynx persists, consider posterior epistaxis (10% of all bleeds). Posterior epistaxis requires a posterior packing (a commercial device or Foley catheter), antibiotics, and admission to a monitored setting (the nasopulmonary reflex may cause oxygen desaturation). Posterior packs require anterior packing for effective tamponade. Arrange an urgent ENT evaluation.

7) <u>Home treatment</u>
  a) If bleeding recurs, apply direct pressure and ice (return if bleeding persists after 3 attempts of direct pressure of 10 min each). Nasal packs should be removed in 2d, and patient instructed to return immediately if bleeding recurs.
  b) Advise the use of prophylactic Vaseline/bacitracin applied to the septum, saline nasal spray, and oxymetazoline (Afrin) spray.

II. PERITONSILLAR ABSCESS

•Etiology•
1) Bacterial infection of the tonsils can spread to the peritonsillar space between the tonsillar capsule and the superior constrictor muscle of the pharynx. This may progress to an abscess (presumably preceded by a cellulitis). It is primarily a disease of young adults.
2) Bacteria include Group A beta hemolytic streptococci, S. viridans, and anaerobes.

•Clinical Presentation•
1) Patients present with unilateral pain, and may have trismus and a "hot potato" voice.

2) The abscess may displace the uvula.
3) Patients usually have a coexistent bilateral exudative tonsillitis, with fever, odynophagia, and tender adenopathy.
4) Severe complications include airway compromise, deep space infections of the neck, and mediastinitis.

•Treatment/Disposition•

1) If the abscess is not aspirated, consider admission for IV antibiotics and ENT consult. In general, the approach to children is more conservative; they are usually admitted and treated by ENT. If the patient is not toxic or immunocompromised, consider aspiration of the abscess:
2) Have patient seated and have suction available.
3) Cetacaine spray to pharynx (local lidocaine does not work in an acidic abscess and painfully distends the mucosa).
4) Use a 2-inch 16-gauge needle (catheter removed; a needle guard can prevent deep penetration) and aspirate, in order, superolaterally, inferolaterally, and superomedially. If no pus is aspirated, it may be cellulitis. Avoid the carotid artery (which is 1 cm lateral to tonsil, and usually pushed more laterally by the abscess) by not pointing the needle laterally. Aspiration of pus into the lungs is usually not a problem, as the gag reflex is elicited.
5) Start on antibiotics (cefaclor 250-500 mg tid; Augmentin; clindamycin; erythromycin).
6) Arrange close follow-up.

CHAPTER 8
ENVIRONMENTAL

I. ANIMAL/HUMAN BITES; RABIES

A. Animal Bites

•Etiology• (bacterial)

Dogs- E. coli, Pasteurella, Streptococcus, Staphylococcus, Bacteroides.

Cats- Pasteurella (occurs in 50-80% of bites, with an infection rate up to 50%, usually within 24-48h); Streptococcus and Staphylococcus are the usual pathogens 24h after the bite.

*C. canimorsus is a bacteria carried by dogs and cats; it may cause severe infection in immunocompromised patients, who may rapidly develop a local wound infection, followed by a petechial rash and sepsis.

•Evaluation•

1) Document the neurovascular exam, any bony injury, and any tendon or joint involvement.

2) Consider x-ray of injured part (evaluate for bony injury and foreign body).

•Treatment•

1) Provide local wound care with debridement and extensive irrigation.

2) Leave puncture wounds open, to decrease risk of infection. Consider closing non-punctures with wound tape or, if not infected and <8h old, with suture. Leave hand and foot wounds and crush injuries open. Tissue adhesive is contraindicated.

2) Immobilize and elevate any affected extremity.

3) Administer tetanus vaccine.

4) Provide antibiotic prophylaxis to all face and hand or foot injuries, all cat bites, immunocompromised hosts, if penetration of bone, joint, or tendon, crush injury, and consider prophylaxis in other bites. Consider Augmentin or penicillin. If penicillin allergy, administer azithromycin or doxycycline. Dicloxacillin has poor Pasteurella coverage.

5) Arrange close follow-up.

B. Cat Scratch Disease

1) Cat scratch disease is characterized by persistent lymphadenitis, which is usually unilateral involving arms or legs. The etiologic organism is Bartonella henselae.

2) 3-10d after exposure, a lesion appears at the inoculation site; a week after the appearance of the initial lesion, regional lymphadenopathy develops, and nodes enlarge for 2-3 weeks before starting to resolve. Patients may also have an atypical presentation with high fever, malaise and abdominal pain.

3) Reserve antibiotics for severe disease or immunocompromised patients, as most cases resolve spontaneously over weeks to months.

C. Human Bites

•Etiology• (bacterial)
S. viridans, Staphylococcus, Eikenella, E. coli, Proteus, Bacteroides.

•Evaluation•

1) Document the neurovascular exam, any bony injury, and any tendon or joint involvement.

2) Consider x-ray of injured part (evaluate for bony injury and foreign body).

•Treatment•

1) Provide aggressive local wound care with irrigation and debridement.

2) Leave puncture wounds open, to decrease risk of infection. If less than 24h old, noninfected facial lacerations can generally be closed primarily, as the face has an excellent blood supply. Leave hand and foot bites and crush injuries open. Tissue adhesive is contraindicated.

3) Any invasion of joint space, marked erythema, drainage or late presenting (>24h) infected hand bite requires consult and possible surgical irrigation. Patients with recent bites (within 8h) may only require ED debridement, irrigation, and oral antibiotics. Presentation 8-24h after bite may require surgical evaluation.

4) Immobilize and elevate the affected extremity.

5) Administer tetanus vaccine. Consider hepatitis B vaccine and HIV testing/prophylaxis.

6) Consider antibiotic prophylaxis, especially if patient is high risk, which

is defined as a bite to hand or foot, a deep puncture wound, immunocompromised host, penetration of bone, joint, or tendon, crush injury, if the wound cannot be adequately debrided, or if the age of the wound is >6h. Options include Augmentin or second generation cephalosporin, or penicillin plus dicloxacillin; if penicillin allergic, consider azithromycin or doxycycline. Eikenella is susceptible to penicillin, but not to penicillinase-resistant penicillins. Consider IV antibiotics if hand bite.

7) Arrange close follow-up.

D. Rabies

•**General**•

1) Rabies is a viral infection transmitted in the saliva of infected mammals; it is usually found in skunks, raccoons, bats, and foxes. Rabies is uncommon in rodents (except the woodchuck) and rabbits.

2) In the US, cases due to non-bite exposures (e.g., scratched or licked over an open wound) are more common than bite exposures. Bats may transmit rabies via respiratory exposure.

3) The incubation period is 12d to 12 months; average is 20-90 days.

4) Susceptibility to infection appears to be related to the size and depth of the bite, the size of the inoculum, and proximity to the CNS.

5) After inoculation, the virus enters the nervous system and spreads via retrograde flow.

6) Diagnosis is made by isolation of the virus from saliva, CSF, or CNS tissue; or, by detecting antibodies in brain or nerves.

•**Clinical Presentation**•

1) In patients with rabies, there is usually a prodrome (1-4d) of nonspecific constitutional symptoms; the patient may have pain or paresthesias at the site of the bite.

2) The prodrome is followed by excitement, agitation, confusion, hallucination, fever, CNS symptoms, hypersalivation, and hydrophobia.

3) Rabies progresses over 7-14d. Once symptoms develop, rabies is fatal.

•**Prophylaxis**•

1) Indications for prophylaxis include head or neck bites in children,

immunocompromised patients, and any routine contact with at-risk animals (skunks, raccoons, bats, woodchucks, foxes, and non-domestic dogs). In most areas, if the bite/mucous membrane exposure was from a healthy domesticated animal with known vaccination status, and the animal can be observed for 10d, then prophylaxis is not required (if signs of rabies occur in the animal, it should be sacrificed and sent for testing). If the dog/cat is unknown, consult public health. Unprovoked attacks from domestic animals are more likely to be rabid. Any incidental exposure to bats (even without a bite or scratch) should be prophylaxed. Exposures from lagomorphs and small rodents do not require prophylaxis.

2) Thoroughly clean wound.

3) Administer rabies immune globulin 20 IU/kg (1/2 around wound, 1/2 IM gluteal). Then administer the rabies vaccine intramuscularly in the deltoid on days 0,3,7,14, and 28. The immune globulin provides immediate protection; the vaccine takes 7-10 days for induction of an active immune response, and provides immunity for approximately 2 years. Rabies vaccine is safe for pregnant patients.

4) Consider tetanus vaccine.

II. BURNS/INHALATION INJURY

A. Burns

•Classification•
Superficial burn is a 1st degree burn. Only the epidermis is involved; it is characterized by painful erythema that blanches. Sunburn is an example.

Partial thickness burn is a superficial 2nd degree burn. Part of the dermis is involved; intact skin is red, and bullae are present.

Deep partial thickness burn is a deep 2nd degree burn. Skin is pale, waxy, mottled, and hypesthetic, but pressure sensation is intact.

Full thickness burn is a 3rd degree burn, and characterized by pale yellow or black or waxy insensitive skin.

Estimation of Burn Size- The percent of body surface burned can be calculated by the "rule of nines": head is 9%; anterior trunk 18%; posterior trunk 18%; each upper extremity 9%; each lower extremity 18%;

and perineum is 1%. Or, the surface area of the patient's palm is equal to 1% of his body surface area.

•Evaluation•

1) Consider ABG with COHgb and metHgb. Consider ECG, CXR, CBC, PT/PTT, electrolytes, BUN/Cr, CPK, and urinalysis.

2) Consider checking a cyanide level if patient was exposed to burned plastics, polyurethane, wool, silk, nylon or rubber.

•Treatment•

1) Treatment for Severe Burns

a) Establish IV. Monitor patient and place on pulse oximeter. Monitor urine output.

b) Provide hydration with lactated ringers without glucose, as stress causes hyperglycemia (however, children should receive dextrose, as they have limited glycogen stores). The formula for hydration during the first 24h is 2-4 ml/kg/% body surface area burned; half of this amount is given in the first 8h. Unless the patient is hypotensive, boluses are usually not recommended, since fluid is rapidly lost to the interstitium; instead, titrate IV fluids up or down 25-50% based on the clinical response. Ensure urine output of 30-50 cc/h.

c) No debridement or creams before transfer to burn center.

d) Elevate burned limbs and encourage exercise to prevent edema.

e) Provide analgesia with morphine.

f) Maintain normothermia (avoid wet linens in large burns).

g) NG tube (ileus usually develops with burns >20% body surface area).

h) Cimetidine 300mg IV for stress ulcer prophylaxis.

i) Consider tetanus vaccine.

j) Prophylactic antibiotics are not indicated.

k) If necessary, do escharotomy in mid-lateral or mid-medial line of extremity.

2) Treatment for 2ⁿᵈ Degree Burns

a) Debride draining blisters, as necrotic skin is an excellent culture medium. Some recommend debriding blisters over joints and blisters larger than 2 cm.

    b) Treat with topical Silvadene or bacitracin. Cover with gauze.

    c) Elevate burned extremity and encourage exercise to prevent edema.

    d) Provide analgesia and consider tetanus vaccine. Prophylactic antibiotics are not indicated.

    e) Arrange close follow-up.

3) Treatment for 1ˢᵗ Degree Burns

    Treat 1st degree burns with ibuprofen orally and aloe vera topically.

4) Referral- Criteria for referral to a burn center include:

    a) Partial thickness burns >10% total body surface area (TBSA) in patients younger than 10 years or older than 50 years; or partial thickness burns >20 % in other age groups.

    b) Full thickness burns > 5% TBSA in any age group.

    c) Significant chemical or electrical burns.

    d) Inhalational injuries.

    e) Burns involving face, hands, feet, major joints, or genitalia.

    f) Burns in high risk patients with significant comorbidities.

B. Inhalation Injury

•General•

Most thermal injury is limited to the supraglottic airway; exceptions are steam, explosive gases, and aspiration of hot liquids. Steam burns have much more energy and are more likely to cause edema and lower airway injury.

•Clinical Presentation•

Patients may present with facial burns, hoarseness, rales, rhonchi, wheezes, or carbonaceous sputum.

•Evaluation•

1) Check CXR (although CXR is an unreliable means of diagnosing inhalation injury), ECG, and ABG with COHgb and metHgb.

2) If there is a high suspicion for inhalation injury, consider bronchoscopy or lung scanning with xenon.

•Treatment•

1) Establish IV. Place patient on monitor and pulse oximeter. Administer humidified oxygen.

2) Consider early intubation if decreased level of consciousness, posterior pharyngeal edema, full thickness nasolabial burns, or circumferential neck burns.

3) Bronchodilators and antihistamines may be of benefit.

4) Steroids are not indicated (but consider using steroids if patient has coexisting asthma or COPD and there are no large surface burns).

5) Prophylactic antibiotics are not indicated.

6) Head up position may decrease airway edema.

7) Hyperbaric oxygen in carbon monoxide poisoned patients with inhalation injury is controversial, as it is associated with aspiration, seizure, and shock. However, consider hyperbaric oxygen if altered mental status, carboxyHgb >25%, CNS findings, cardiovascular dysfunction or loss of consciousness.

8) Combustion of plastics, polyurethane, wool, silk, nylon, rubber and paper products can lead to the production of cyanide gas. Consider empiric therapy for cyanide poisoning if the patient has profound CNS and cardiovascular findings and a metabolic acidosis (lactate >10 mmol/L is a sensitive indication), and there is no other explanation for the acidosis. In smoke inhalation patients with possible cyanide poisoning, sodium thiosulfate alone avoids the hypotensive and methemoglobin effects of nitrates (induction of methemoglobinemia is contraindicated in smoke inhalation patients who already have carboxyhemoglobinemia).

•Disposition•

1) Monitor for at least 4h.

2) Consider admission for closed space exposure >10 min, pO2 <60, HCO3 <15, carboxyHgb >15%, carbonaceous sputum, comorbidity, or bronchospasm.

3) Respiratory failure may develop 6-24h after inhalation of poorly soluble gases.

III. COLD ILLNESS

A. Frostbite

•Clinical Presentation•

1) First degree frostbite presents with erythema, edema, and sensory deficits.

2) Second degree frostbite has clear blisters.

3) Third degree frostbite has hemorrhagic blisters.

4) Fourth degree frostbite has involvement of muscles, tendons, or bone.

5) The affected area may have numbness, a "chunk of wood sensation," and pain with reperfusion.

•Treatment•

1) Do not rewarm in the field if there is a potential for incomplete thawing (refreezing is disastrous).

2) Protect the injured part; do not perform friction massage.

3) Stabilize the core temperature.

4) Perform rapid rewarming of the affected part in 38-41°C circulating water (dry heat desiccates tissue); this requires 10-30 min with active motion of the part. Thawing is complete when flushing is observed in the distal tip of the affected part.

5) Provide analgesia.

6) Administer tetanus vaccine if necessary.

7) Administer IV fluids (to decrease viscosity).

8) Debride clear blisters, as they contain mediators of ischemia; leave hemorrhagic blisters intact.

9) Ibuprofen and topical aloe vera inhibit thromboxane production, which mediates ischemia. Apply silvadene to ruptured blebs. Cover with gauze. Elevate affected extremity.

10) Provide streptococcus prophylaxis x 2-3d (cephalexin, dicloxacillin, or erythromycin).

11) Amputation, if necessary, is usually delayed as long as possible; demarcation of viable tissue requires 6-8 weeks.

•Disposition•

Admit all but the most superficial and isolated cases.

B. Hypothermia - see also ACLS section.

•Definition•

Mild hypothermia is defined as 32-35°C. Moderate hypothermia is defined as 30-32°C (86-90°F). Severe hypothermia is defined as less than 30°C.

•Clinical Presentation•

1) Clinical presentation depends on the degree of hypothermia.

2) Hypothermia causes progressive CNS depression, and may result in atrial or ventricular arrhythmias. The patient may be volume depleted secondary to "cold" diuresis (impaired renal concentrating ability).

3) Patients may have cold, mottled skin. There may be evidence of trauma or frostbite.

•Evaluation•

1) Check core temp with low-reading rectal, esophageal, or bladder probe.

2) Check ECG, CBC, electrolytes, glucose, and BUN/Cr; consider checking amylase and DIC panel. There may be wide fluctuations in electrolytes, and the hematocrit increases 2% for each 1°C drop in the core temperature; amylase is often elevated. The ECG may have Osborn (J) waves (a slow, positive deflection at the end of the QRS).

3) Consider evaluation for sepsis. Evaluate for possible trauma.

•Differential Diagnosis•

The differential includes Addison's disease, panhypopituitarism, myxedema coma, and sepsis. Consider alcoholism, opiate overdose, stroke, hypoglycemia, and spinal cord injury.

•Treatment •

1) Establish IV. Place patient on monitor and pulse oximeter. Administer oxygen. Consider administering glucose, thiamine, and naloxone. Consider hydrocortisone for possible adrenal insufficiency.

2) <u>If pulse or breathing are absent</u>: **If temp < 30°C** : perform CPR; do not administer IV medications; limit defibrillations to 3; provide active internal rewarming. **If temp > 30°C**: perform CPR; administer IV medications at longer intervals; provide active internal rewarming.

3) <u>If pulse and breathing are present</u>: **If temp 34-36°C**: provide passive rewarming and active external rewarming. **If temp 30-34°C**: provide passive rewarming; actively rewarm truncal areas only. **If temp <30°C**: provide active internal rewarming.

4) Passive rewarming requires intact thermoregulatory mechanisms and that the patient be capable of metabolic heat production. Remove cold or wet clothes; give blankets.

5) Active rewarming techniques include:

<u>External</u>- heated blankets/warmers (it may result in peripheral vasodila-

tion, returning cold blood to the core, causing "rewarming acidosis").

<u>Internal</u>- warm humidified oxygen; warmed IV fluids (use D5 normal saline or normal saline, not lactated Ringer's, as the liver's ability to metabolize lactate may be impaired); lavage of stomach, bladder, peritoneum, or pleural cavity; and extracorporeal bypass.

6) Most arrhythmias revert with rewarming, and the activity of cardioactive drugs is unpredictable in hypothermia. In general, only treat life-threatening dysrhythmias. Bradydysrhythmias are unresponsive to atropine (they result from decreased depolarization of pacemaker cells). Vasoactive agents induce dysrhythmias and have little effect on already constricted vessels.

7) Treat all neonates with antibiotics if sepsis cannot be ruled out.

8) Consider NG tube as there often is decreased gastric motility.

9) Disposition depends on the clinical status, any underlying etiology, and the degree of hypothermia.

IV. DYSBARISM

A. Barotrauma of Descent

•General•
Gas compresses in enclosed spaces as ambient pressure increases with descent. If there is obstruction to gas exchange, then pressure equalization is precluded; if the space is not collapsible, the pressure imbalance will cause tissue distortion and damage.

•Clinical Presentation•
1) Barotrauma occurs most commonly in ears and paranasal sinuses.

2) If the external canal is occluded, external ear squeeze occurs, which is manifested by petechiae and outward bulging or rupture of the tympanic membrane.

3) If the eustachian tube is occluded, middle ear pressures do not equalize with the environment, and middle ear squeeze occurs; patients present with pain, edema, hemorrhage, and inward bulging of the tympanic membrane (which may rupture).

•Treatment•
Treat with decongestants and avoidance of flying/diving.

B. Barotrauma of Ascent

•General•

1) Barotrauma of ascent is the reverse of the "squeeze" injury that occurs in barotrauma of descent.

2) Ear and sinus trauma is unusual, because impediment of pressure equalization is unlikely if it was achieved with descent.

3) Tooth squeeze may occur; aerogastralgia occurs in novices who swallow air.

4) The most significant injury is pulmonary barotrauma, which occurs when expanding gas in the lungs, if not allowed to escape, dissects into the surrounding tissue. This may result in a pneumothorax or subcutaneous emphysema, or an air embolus may cause cerebral or coronary artery occlusion (air emboli always occur within 10 minutes of surfacing).

•Evaluation•

1) If pulmonary barotrauma is suspected, check CXR, ECG, ABG, and consider CBC, platelets, electrolytes, and BUN/Cr.

2) Consider head CT if neurologic symptoms are present.

•Treatment• (for pulmonary barotrauma or air embolism)

1) Establish IV. Place patient on monitor and pulse oximetry. Administer high flow oxygen. Assess and stabilize the airway.

2) Arrange for treatment with hyperbaric oxygen (call 919-684-8111 or www.diversalertnetwork.org for the nearest facility).

3) Aspirin 325 mg (if there is no suspicion of hemorrhage).

4) Do not place patient in Trendelenburg.

5) Exclude treatable injuries.

C. Decompression Sickness

•General•

Inert nitrogen equilibrates from alveoli to blood, and then with tissue. When ambient pressure is decreased too rapidly, nitrogen does not have time to diffuse out of the tissues; this results in the formation of bubbles and vascular occlusion (the bends).

•Clinical Presentation•

1) Symptoms depend on the location of the gas bubbles, which may form in joints, soft tissue, CNS, or the pulmonary or circulatory systems. Symptoms typically occur 10 min-6h after ascent (symptoms are rarely delayed 24-48h).

2) Type I decompression sickness involves lymphatics and skin; patients may also have periarticular pain.

3) Type II decompression sickness presents with spinal cord involvement (paraplegia or bladder dysfunction), cardiopulmonary involvement, or hypovolemic shock.

4) Arterial gas embolization (AGE) may result in an MI or stroke, and occurs when gas emboli in the arterial blood supply occlude coronary, cerebral, or other systemic arterioles. Cerebral AGE may be differentiated from Type II neurologic decompression sickness by the more rapid onset of symptoms (within 10-20 min) in AGE.

•Evaluation•

1) Consider CXR, ECG, ABG; also, consider CBC, platelets, electrolytes, and BUN/Cr.

2) Consider head CT if neurologic symptoms are present.

•Treatment•

1) Establish IV. Place patient on monitor and pulse oximeter. Administer high flow oxygen. Assess and stabilize the airway.

2) Arrange for treatment with hyperbaric oxygen (call 919-684-8111 or www.diversalertnetwork.org for the nearest facility).

3) Aspirin 325 mg (if there is no suspicion of hemorrhage).

4) Do not place patient in Trendelenburg.

5) Exclude treatable injuries.

V. ELECTRICAL INJURY/LIGHTNING

A. Electrical Injury

•General•

1) High voltage is defined as greater than 600V.

2) Nerves and muscles have the least resistance and thus are the best conductors; bone has the highest resistance.

3) Current passing through the brain produces unconsciousness; alternating current through the chest may produce ventricular fibrillation.

4) Electrical injuries may produce myonecrosis and significant amounts of tissue destruction (sometimes requiring an eventual amputation).

5) Alternating current (household current) produces explosive exit wounds, and generally causes worse damage than direct current. Direct current (batteries and electrical train circuits) causes discrete exit wounds.

•Evaluation•

1) Check ECG, CBC, electrolytes, PT/PTT, and CPK (elevated CK-MB is common without other evidence of myocardial injury, as skeletal muscle injured by current releases high levels of MB; thus CK-MB is unwarranted as a screening test unless chest pain is present). Check urine myoglobin; check LFTs if abdominal injury is suspected.

2) Document the location and extent of any entrance or exit wounds.

3) High voltage electrical burns are typically more extensive than they initially appear.

4) Document the neurovascular status of any injured extremity.

5) Perform a complete neurological and cardiovascular exam.

6) Evaluate for any musculoskeletal injuries secondary to trauma.

•Treatment•

1) Establish IV and place patient on monitor. Hydrate patient with normal saline or Ringer's lactate.

2) Evaluate for the possible development of rhabdomyolysis. If the patient develops rhabdomyolysis, keep urine output >1-1.5 cc/kg/h; add one ampule of bicarbonate/liter of normal saline. Consider 25 gm mannitol bolus then 12.5 g/h to maintain urine output. Consider furosemide. The goal is to prevent acute tubular necrosis secondary to myoglobinuria.

3) Administer tetanus vaccine if necessary.

4) Silvadene for wound.

5) Splint injured extremities in functional position.

6) High voltage electrical burns may require an early fasciotomy to maintain circulation.

7) Consider NG tube, as there is a high risk of ileus.

8) Consult general/burn surgery.

•Disposition•

1) Admit any high voltage injuries (observe for rhabdomyolysis and compartment syndrome).
2) Admit low voltage injuries if accompanied by symptoms of systemic involvement, underlying medical problems, arrhythmia, abnormal CNS exam, or exposure while immersed in water.
3) Admit for 24h monitoring if loss of consciousness, cardiac arrest, abnormal ECG, chest pain or coronary disease.
4) Consider transferring all patients with significant electrical burns to a burn center.
5) If >24 weeks pregnant, admit for 24h fetal monitoring.
6) If pediatric oral burns, consider admitting until scars separate as the labial artery may rupture at that time.

B. Lightning

•General•
1) A lightning strike is a massive current impulse that lasts for microseconds.
2) Lightning usually does not cause significant burns, as there is a very brief duration of contact with the skin; also, there usually are no entrance or exit wounds. Internal burns and rhabdomyolysis are rare.
3) Lightning may result in respiratory arrest, arrhythmias, neurologic damage, vascular spasm, and autonomic disorders.
4) Lightning is associated with intraventricular hemorrhage, subdural/epidural hematomas, and cataracts.
5) Death results from respiratory arrest or arrhythmia (therefore, lightning victims who appear dead should be treated first).

•Clinical Presentation•
1) The patient may have superficial evanescent skin burns that resemble a fern. Large burns are unusual; internal burns are not a concern (current travels around outside of victim and is of short duration).
2) Transient paralysis or mottling (usually of the lower extremities) is common; it is often secondary to vascular spasm, but a possible spinal cord injury should be investigated.
3) Many lightning victims sustain a ruptured tympanic membrane (which does not heal well on its own).
4) The patient may have long-term cognitive deficits.

•Evaluation•

1) Check ECG, cardiac enzymes (although MI is rare), urinalysis, urine myoglobin, CBC, glucose, electrolytes, and BUN/Cr.
2) Obtain head CT if loss of consciousness or focal CNS signs.
3) Perform a complete neurologic and cardiac exam.
4) Evaluate for secondary trauma.

•Treatment•

1) Establish IV. Monitor patient.
2) Fluid loading is unnecessary, as renal involvement (rhabdomyolysis) is rare.
3) Consider admission to telemetry for observation.
4) Arrange ophthalmology and ENT follow-up.

VI. HEAT ILLNESS

A. Heat Cramps

•General•

1) Heat cramps occur in the muscles that are used most, usually after exertion.
2) There is usually copious sweating and hypotonic fluid replacement.
3) Patients may have decreased sodium and chloride.

•Treatment•

1) If mild symptoms, treat with 0.1-0.2% oral salt solution (salt pills are gastric irritants).
2) If symptoms are more severe, administer IV normal saline.

B. Heat Exhaustion

•General•

1) Heat exhaustion occurs when the body can no longer adequately dissipate heat; it occurs in the setting of extreme environmental heat or increased endogenous heat production.
2) If thermoregulatory mechanisms become overwhelmed, heat exhaustion may progress to heat stroke.

•Clinical Presentation•

1) Patients may present with malaise, fatigue, nausea, or headache, usu-

ally after exposure to a hot environment. The patient may have been exercising. The patient may not have had access to hydration or a cool environment (e.g., elderly, disabled, or immobile patients).

2) The core temperature is usually <40°C (often normal).

3) Tachycardia, orthostatic hypotension, and clinical dehydration are often present. There is usually profuse sweating. Mental status is essentially intact.

•Evaluation•

Check core temperature. Assess volume status (check BUN/Cr, Hgb, and sodium).

•Treatment•

1) Rest, cool environment.

2) Replace volume losses with normal saline; correct electrolyte abnormalities.

3) Apply ice packs to the great vessels (neck, axilla, and groin).

4) If the diagnosis is in doubt, treat as heat stroke.

C. Heat Stroke

•General•

1) Under conditions of heat stress, renal/splanchnic vasoconstriction and peripheral vasodilation shunt blood away from the core to the skin; heat is then dissipated mostly through radiation and evaporation.

2) In heat stroke, thermoregulatory mechanisms fail and end-organ damage occurs. Hyperthermia leads to cerebral edema and increased intracranial pressure; CNS dysfunction is universal in heat stroke. Neonates and the elderly are at increased risk for heat stroke. Heat stroke is traditionally classified as classic or exertional.

3) **Classic Heat Stroke**- It occurs in the elderly who may use anticholinergics, diuretics, or antipsychotics. There is usually no sweating, lactic acidosis, rhabdomyolysis or acute renal failure. CPK is usually slightly elevated. It is caused by poor dissipation of environmental heat.

4) **Exertional Heat Stroke**- It typically occurs in healthy men 15-45 years old with excessive heat production from strenuous exercise. Sweating is often present; lactic acidosis, rhabdomyolysis and acute

renal failure are often present. CPK is often markedly elevated.

•Clinical Presentation•

1) Patients present with all of the symptoms of heat exhaustion; however, all patients also have CNS dysfunction (seizures, coma, delirium). CNS dysfunction often has a sudden onset; ataxia is an early finding.
2) The temperature is usually >40°C. Patients often have hot, dry skin (however, cessation of sweating is often a late phenomenon of heat stroke). Patients usually have tachycardia and decreased cardiac output. Patients may have coagulation disorders, hematuria, or oliguria.
3) Unlike malignant hyperthermia and neuroleptic malignant syndrome, heat stroke generally does not present with muscle rigidity.

•Evaluation•

1) Check CBC, electrolytes, glucose, BUN/Cr, LFTs, CPK, toxicology screen, PT/PTT, and urine myoglobin; consider head CT and LP. Check CXR.
2) Hepatic transaminases are almost always elevated. The patient may have DIC. CPK may demonstrate rhabdomyolysis. BUN/Cr may demonstrate acute renal failure.

•Differential Diagnosis•

The differential includes thyroid storm, anticholinergic overdose (in which the patient should have mydriasis), DKA, meningitis, neuroleptic malignant syndrome, and sepsis.

•Treatment•

1) Establish IV. Place patient on monitor. Administer oxygen. Assess and stabilize the airway. Judiciously administer IVNS. Place catheter to monitor urine output.
2) Apply ice packs to great vessels (neck, axilla, and groin).
3) Provide evaporative cooling by undressing the patient, spraying the skin with tepid water and exposing the skin to large fans (this requires intact circulation to take cooled blood to the core, so consider ice water cooling if the patient is in shock).
4) Consider ice water immersion (however, it is generally not recommended because of increased complications and difficulties in monitoring the patient). Consider peritoneal, rectal or gastric ice water lavage. Consider cardiopulmonary bypass.

5) Do not give antipyretics; heat stroke is not caused by an increased hypothalamic thermoregulatory set point. Do not give aspirin (it uncouples oxidative phosphorylation) or acetaminophen (it may cause liver dysfunction). Avoid anticholinergics (which decrease sweating) and alpha-adrenergics (which increase peripheral resistance).

6) Administer lorazepam 2 mg IV or chlorpromazine 25 mg IV for shivering.

7) Admit to ICU.

VII. HIGH ALTITUDE MEDICINE

•General•

1) High altitude is defined as 1500-3500 m above sea level; very high altitude is 3500-5500 m above sea level.

2) Hyperventilation is the initial adaptation to high altitude, and is attenuated by respiratory alkalosis. Renal excretion of bicarbonate then compensates for the alkalosis, pH returns to normal, and ventilation continues to increase. Acetazolamide, which forces a bicarbonate diuresis, facilitates this process.

3) Illness occurs when a rapid ascent overwhelms compensatory mechanisms. Vasogenic brain edema probably results from hypoxia-induced changes in the blood-brain barrier, causing the cerebral forms of altitude illness. Pulmonary edema may be the result of increased pulmonary capillary permeability secondary to hypoxia.

Acute Mountain Sickness

1) Symptoms include lightheadedness, shortness of breath, headache, weakness, and nausea and vomiting. Fluid retention results in peripheral edema.

2) Treat with descent, oxygen, and acetazolamide 125-250 mg. If symptoms are severe, consider hyperbaric therapy and dexamethasone (4 mg every 6h).

High Altitude Cerebral Edema

1) Vasogenic brain edema probably results from hypoxia-induced changes in the blood-brain barrier.

2) Patients may present with altered mental status, ataxia, or coma.

3) Treat with descent, oxygen, and acetazolamide 125-250 mg. If symp-

toms are severe, consider hyperbaric therapy and dexamethasone (4 mg every 6h).

High Altitude Pulmonary Edema

1) High altitude pulmonary edema is a non-cardiogenic pulmonary edema from an exaggerated pulmonary pressor response to hypoxia.

2) Symptoms include cough, poor exercise tolerance, dyspnea, and tachypnea; the patient may have rales on lung exam.

3) Treat with descent, oxygen, and hyperbaric therapy. Consider CPAP and nifedipine 10 mg po (it reduces pulmonary artery pressure and increases O2 saturation). Consider morphine and furosemide (although many discourage the use of furosemide, as patients may already be intravascularly depleted). Acetazolamide has no role in high altitude pulmonary edema, and dexamethasone should only be used if there is associated high altitude cerebral edema.

VIII. NEAR DROWNING

•General•

1) Aspiration induces vagal-mediated pulmonary vasoconstriction/hypertension, surfactant destruction, and endothelial damage. This results in V/Q mismatch, edema, and reduced compliance.

2) Aspiration of 22 ml/kg is required for electrolyte changes (which occur in 15% of near drownings). Freshwater aspiration produces hypervolemia, electrolyte dilution, and red cell lysis; seawater aspiration causes hypovolemia (hypertonicity pulls fluid into alveoli) and increased electrolyte concentrations. 10% of drownings are dry (from laryngospasm).

•Evaluation•

1) Check pulse oximetry, ABG, CXR, CBC, glucose, electrolytes, PT/PTT, and BUN/Cr.

2) Evaluate for associated injuries.

•Treatment•

1) Establish IV. Place patient on monitor and pulse oximeter.

2) If necessary, intubate and add 5-10 PEEP. Maintain cervical spine precautions.

3) Administer high flow oxygen and albuterol nebulizer (if

bronchoconstriction).

4) Steroids are not indicated.

•Disposition•

1) If patient is symptomatic or there is a history of significant immersion, admit for observation.

2) If patient is asymptomatic, has a normal evaluation, a reliable history of a minor immersion, and no signs of respiratory distress, then observe the patient for 4-6h and consider discharge (1 study showed all patients who became symptomatic did so within 4h). Otherwise, admit for observation.

IX. RADIATION INJURIES

•General•

1) Radiation may be classified as ionizing (produced by nuclear weapons and reactors, x-rays, and radioactive material; it causes atoms to convert to ions) or nonionizing (light, radio waves, or microwaves). Radioactive substances emit ionizing radiation.

2) Apart from x-rays, ionizing radiation is usually produced when unstable atomic nuclei decay to more stable forms, giving off energy in the form of photons or particles. Alpha particles, beta particles, and gamma rays are the common types of radiation emitted from the nuclei of radioactive atoms during radioactive decay.

3) Ionization produces free radicals, which can damage DNA and RNA; those cells with the highest turnover (embryo, bone marrow, GI tract epithelium) are most susceptible.

4) Radiation is either electromagnetic or particulate.

5) Electromagnetic radiation occurs in waveform, and includes, in order of decreasing energy, gamma rays, x-rays, ultraviolet rays, visible rays, microwaves, and radio waves. Gamma rays and x-rays easily penetrate tissues and may cause ionization.

6) Particulate radiation includes the alpha and beta particles. The alpha particle consists of 2 protons and 2 neutrons emitted from the nucleus of a radioactive atom; the beta particle is an electron emitted from the nucleus of a radioactive atom. Alpha and beta particles have minimal penetration, but can be harmful if ingested or inhaled, or if an open wound is contaminated.

7) The dose of radiation absorbed is measured in rads or Gray (1 gray = 100 rad). The rem is the absorbed dose in rads multiplied by a biological quality factor (which accounts for the effectiveness of different types of radiation; for most beta and gamma radiation, the quality factor is 1, but alpha particles may have factors of 20). The SI unit for rem is the Sievert; 1 Sievert = 100 rem.

8) With the exception of high-dose neutron radiation, a person or object exposed to ionizing radiation (i.e., gamma or x-rays) does not become radioactive, and thus presents no risk to health care providers. However, unsealed radiation sources or radioactive fallout may contaminate the patient and remain radioactive.

•Clinical Presentation•

1) High dose (>100 rem) whole body radiation exposure may initially cause erythema of skin, nausea and vomiting, and malaise. Later, bleeding, anemia, and infection may occur.

2) The amount of exposure can be estimated by the timing of symptoms. Nausea and vomiting within 2h of exposure suggests exposure to > 400 rem. Nausea and vomiting that occurs more than 2h after exposure suggests exposure to <200 rem. If there are no symptoms after 6h, the exposure is likely <50 rem.

3) Erythema indicates exposure to >300 rem; diarrhea suggests >400 rem exposure.

4) Lower levels of exposure may not cause symptoms.

•Evaluation•

1) Check baseline CBC and platelets. Perform a radiation survey.

2) Lymphocyte counts 48h after exposure can be used prognostically. If >1200/uL, there is a good prognosis. If 300-1200/uL, there is a fair prognosis. If <300/uL, there is a poor prognosis.

•Treatment•

1) If there was a significant exposure, place patient in a reverse isolation atmosphere. Use universal precautions.

2) Perform rapid external and internal body decontamination. Cover open wounds. Remove clothing and deposit in closed receptacles. Wash patient with soap and water, and collect contaminated water. If there was ingestion or inhalation of radioactive particles (transuranics and certain heavy metals), then decorporation is indicated with chelating agents (DTPA). Treatment of critical patients takes precedence over decontamination.

3) Check patient with a GM counter for surface contamination.

4) Administer potassium iodide, which prevents uptake of radioactive iodine by the thyroid. If there was an exposure to 10-30 rem or more, administer 130 mg potassium iodide qd x 14d if older than 13 years old; administer 65 mg if patient is pregnant or 3-12 years old; administer 32.5 mg if patient is younger than 1 year old.

5) Administer IV fluids.

6) Symptomatic treatment.

•**Disposition**•

Disposition depends on symptoms and level of exposure.

X. SNAKEBITES

•**General**•

North American venomous species include:

Coral Snakes (Elapidae family), represented by eastern, Texas, and Arizona coral snakes. They are all brightly colored with black, red, and yellow rings, with the red and yellow rings bordering each other ("red on yellow, kill a fellow; red on black, venom lack"). Coral snakes have round pupils and short, immobile fangs.

Pit Vipers (Crotalidae family), represented by rattlesnakes, pygmy rattlesnakes, massasauga, copperheads, and water moccasins. They are identified by bilateral depressions (pits) between the eye and nostril, 2 long mobile fangs, a triangular-shaped head, and elliptic pupils. Rattlesnakes do not always rattle before striking.

•**Pathophysiology**•

Coral Snakes- Venom does not cause significant local injury; venom contains neurotoxic components.

Pit Vipers- Venom causes local and systemic effects, including local tissue injury, hemolysis, neuromuscular dysfunction, and systemic vascular damage.

•**Clinical Presentation**•

Coral Snakes- Neurologic manifestations include tremors, seizures, fixed pupils, dysphagia, and paralysis (including of respiratory muscles); signs may be delayed up to 12h. Coral snake bites do not cause significant local injury.

Pit Vipers- The severity of the bite is variable, and an initially minimal bite may progress to a severe bite. Patients present with fang marks, localized pain, and progressive edema (edema usually begins within 30 min, but may not start for hours). Other symptoms include vomiting, paresthesias, tachycardia, and hematuria.

Classification of Pit Viper Snakebites:

Minimal Envenomation- swelling/erythema limited to area of bite, minimal systemic symptoms, and normal lab evaluation.

Moderate Envenomation- swelling/erythema may involve most of an extremity, and moderate systemic symptoms (vomiting, mild tachycardia) are present. PT/PTT may be abnormal, but there is no significant bleeding.

Severe Envenomation- rapidly spreading swelling or ecchymosis, and systemic symptoms including mental status change, hypotension, tachycardia, and tachypnea. There is significant bleeding, with severe abnormalities in PT/PTT and other labs.

•Evaluation•

Check CBC, platelets, PT/PTT, fibrinogen, electrolytes, BUN/Cr, and urinalysis. Consider type and crossmatch, ECG, and ABG. Consider CPK to check for rhabdomyolysis.

•Treatment•

1) Pre-hospital: immobilize bitten extremity in neutral position below the heart and maintain strict bed rest. Consider use of constriction bands, especially if there is a prolonged transport. Other devices (suction, electric shock, ice) have not been proven to be of benefit.

2) Call regional poison center or zoo for information on snake identification, toxicity, and where to locate antivenin.

Coral Snakes-Treatment

1) Establish IV. Place patient on monitor.

2) Consider 3 vials of Antivenin, an antivenom, if definite bite. Reserve further Antivenin after symptoms of envenomation occur. Arizona coral snakebites are mild and probably do not require Antivenin. Consider

a test dose, and pretreatment with steroids and H1 blockers.

3) Supportive measures; observe closely for respiratory deterioration.

Pit Vipers- Treatment

1) Establish IV. Place patient on monitor.

2) All crotalid bites with progressive symptoms (worsening swelling, lab abnormalities, or unstable vital signs) should receive antivenom.

3) Antivenin Polyvalent is an antivenom derived from horse serum, and may cause an allergic reaction. Therefore, an intradermal test dose should be given before antivenom is administered.

4) Use at least 10 vials of Antivenin in rattlesnake bites; if rapidly progressing symptoms or unstable vital signs, use at least 20 vials. Water moccasin bites usually require lesser amounts of antivenom; copperhead bites often do not require antivenom. Consider pretreatment with steroids and H1 blockers.

5) A newer antivenom, CroFab, is derived from sheep and is more potent than equine antivenom with less risk of allergy. The initial dose is 4-6 vials.

6) Provide aggressive supportive care, including IV fluids and vasopressors as indicated. Consider blood component replacement if there is active bleeding; consider fasciotomy if compartment syndrome is suspected. Routine fasciotomy and local wound excision are not recommended.

7) There is no proven benefit of prophylactic antibiotics or steroids.

•Disposition•

Coral Snakes- Observe all for 24-48h.

Pit Vipers- Admit all patients receiving Antivenin to ICU. Observe other patients at least 8h; a normal initial physical exam and labs do not exclude significant envenomation.

XI. WARFARE: BIOLOGICAL AND CHEMICAL

A. Biological Warfare Agents

•General•

1) Biological warfare agents may be disseminated by sprays, explosion, or food/water contamination.

2) A small amount of biologic agents may be enough to kill hundreds of thousands of people in urban areas; their efficacy depends upon the size and stability of the agent, and atmospheric conditions.

3) If there is a suspicion of biological warfare agents, protective measures include high efficiency masks, removal of clothes, and thorough showering after aerosol attack. Also, patients should be placed in negative pressure rooms.

4) Of the potential biological warfare agents, only smallpox, plague, and viral hemorrhagic fever are readily spread from person to person.

5) Broad spectrum antibiotic coverage is recommended initially for all victims of biological warfare.

1) Anthrax

a) Anthrax is an aerobic gram-positive bacillus that typically produces disease in goats, sheep, and cattle. Infection occurs primarily through cutaneous exposure, but may occur through respiratory or GI routes. Person to person airborne transmission of anthrax does not occur.

b) 95% of cases are cutaneous, which has an incubation period of 1-5 days and first appears as a small papule that progresses to a vesicle, which ruptures and leaves a necrotic ulcer with varying degrees of edema. Patients also have headache, malaise, and edema; septicemia is rare. If treated with antibiotics, cutaneous anthrax has a 1% mortality.

c) Inhalation anthrax is the most likely form to be used in a terrorist attack. Inhalation anthrax has an incubation period of 1-6 days (but a possible latent period of 60 days), and presents with fever, headache, nonproductive cough, and malaise, followed 2-3 days later with increasing respiratory distress. The CXR classically shows a widened mediastinum (from lymphadenopathy and hemorrhagic mediastinitis) and pleural effusions (but usually no infiltrates). This is followed by septic shock and death (mortality is near 100%). Patients may also develop hemorrhagic meningitis. Diagnosis is through blood cultures.

d) For all presumed cases of inhalational anthrax, ciprofloxacin 400 mg IV q12h (in children, 20-30 mg/kg/d IV divided bid, max 1 gm/d) is recommended. Another option is doxycycline 100 mg IV bid. Consider multiple drug regimens, adding rifampin, vancomycin, ampicillin, imipenim, or clindamycin. Following exposure, administer ciprofloxacin 500 mg bid or doxycycline 100 mg bid x 4 weeks (60 days for inhalational exposure); initiate the vaccine.

2) Botulinum Toxin

a) Clostridium botulinum is a spore-forming, anaerobic, gram-positive bacillus that produces toxins; there are 7 distinct antigenic types of botulinum toxin. There are 3 forms of naturally occurring human botulism: food borne, wound, and intestinal (infant and adult). Inhalational botulism results from a man-made form of toxin that is aerosolized. Food borne botulism has an incubation period of 2h-8 days; inhalational botulism has an approximate incubation period of 72h. Botulism is not spread person to person, and isolation is not required.

b) In botulism, a preformed toxin irreversibly binds to the presynaptic membrane and prevents release of acetylcholine, thus blocking neurotransmission. Botulism is an acute afebrile illness in which patients initially present with neurologic complaints related to ocular and bulbar muscles (diplopia, ptosis, difficulty speaking or swallowing); symptoms then progress to a symmetric, descending flaccid paralysis. There are also autonomic symptoms and respiratory involvement. The toxin does not affect the brain, so patients have a normal mental status.

c) Diagnosis is usually made clinically; confirmation requires specialized tests. Routine labs are usually unremarkable.

d) Admit to ICU for supportive care; consider administering antitoxin (which should be given early, as it will prevent progression of paralysis, but not reverse existing paralysis).

3) Plague

a) Plague (yersinia pestis), a gram-negative coccobacillis, is characterized by abrupt onset of high fever, painful lymphadenopathy, and bacteremia.

b) When plague develops after a flea bite, the bacteria usually spread to regional lymph nodes, and result in the characteristic bubo of bubonic plague and associated constitutional symptoms (there is a 1-8d incubation period before the appearance of bubos). Untreated, septicemia may then develop, with spread to other organs.

c) Inhalation of aerosolized plague is the most likely route of infection during a terrorist attack. Inhalation may cause primary pneumonic plague, which is rapidly fatal and can be spread human to human via the respiratory route. Pneumonic plague has a 1-6 day incubation period, and usually presents with high fever, headache, cough productive of bloody sputum, and sepsis; prominent gastrointestinal symptoms may be present. CXR may reveal patchy or consolidated pneumonia.

d) Diagnosis is made clinically in the appropriate setting; also, blood, sputum, and bubo aspirate should be cultured. A gram stain of sputum or blood may reveal the characteristic gram-negative "safety pin" organism.

e) Once diagnosis is suspected, patients should be isolated, and treated with streptomycin 30 mg/kg/d IM divided bid (add chloramphenicol 50-75 mg/kg/d if hemodynamic instability or meningitis); gentamicin is an alternative. In mass casualty situations or for postexposure prophylaxis of individuals exposed to aerosols or who have had contact with patients who have pneumonic plague, administer doxycycline 100 mg bid or ciprofloxacin 500 mg bid.

4) Ricin

a) Ricin is a toxin derived from the castor plant. Toxicity varies with the route of administration.

b) After inhalation (the most likely route during a terrorist attack), severe respiratory distress may occur within 12-24h if there was a significant exposure.

c) Ingestion of ricin is usually less toxic, but may result in vomiting, hematochezia, fever, and vascular collapse.

d) Diagnosis is generally made on clinical and epidemiological factors.

e) Treatment is supportive.

5) Smallpox

a) Smallpox is caused by the virus variola, which is highly infectious, easily spread, and has a high mortality. Smallpox was eradicated by 1980, and routine vaccination was halted in 1972.

b) Variola is spread by aerosol, and has an incubation period of 7-17d. It is then spread hematogenously to lymph nodes, and then to dermal blood vessels, causing the characteristic skin lesions.

c) Symptoms include fever and constitutional symptoms, followed by a maculopapular rash that progresses in 1-2 days to vesicular lesions and then pustular lesions, with more lesions on the face and extremities than on the trunk. The rash spreads centrifugally, sparing palms, soles, and axillae; also, lesions are in the same stage of progression (as opposed to chickenpox). Patients are most infectious from the onset of rash through the first 7-10 days of rash, until scabs form (although patients should be considered infectious until all scabs are shed).

d) Diagnosis is clinical, and may be confirmed with electron microscopy of vesicular or pustular fluid.

e) In a possible terrorist or warfare situation, it is important to recognize any vesicular exanthem as possible smallpox. All patients and contacts should be quarantined with respiratory isolation. All exposed individuals should be vaccinated. Treatment is supportive; consider vaccinia immune globulin. There is a 30% mortality for variola major in unvaccinated individuals.

6) Tularemia

a) Tularemia is caused by a gram-negative aerobic intracellular bacterium, and is characterized by the abrupt onset of fever, lymphadenopathy, pharyngitis, skin or mucous membrane ulcerations, and sometimes pneumonia. It is not spread person to person.

b) Tularemia is usually acquired via mucous membranes or breaks in the skin. There is an incubation period of 3-6d, after which constitutional symptoms develop, often followed by the appearance of a cutaneous ulcer; enlarged lymph nodes also frequently develop.

c) Diagnosis is usually made by sputum culture or serology.

d) Treatment is with streptomycin 30 mg/kg/d IM divided bid for 10-14d; or gentamicin 5 mg/kg qd IM/IV x10 d or ciprofloxacin IV. Antibiotics for post-exposure prophylaxis or in mass casualty situations include doxycycline 100 mg bid or ciprofloxacin 500 mg bid x 14d.

7) Viral Hemorrhagic Fevers

a) Four different families of viruses exist; the best known agent is the Ebola virus. All agents (except dengue fever) are highly infectious as an aerosol; Ebola is easily spread by body fluids. Patients should be placed in isolation.

b) Infection with these viruses causes an acute generalized illness with circulatory regulatory disorders and increased vascular permeability. Patients may present with fever, bleeding (mucosal and GI), hypotension, vomiting, and malaise.

c) Diagnosis is made through serology.

d) Treatment is supportive.

8) Other potential biological warfare agents include Cholera; Brucellosis; Q Fever; Viral Encephalitides; Dengue; Staphylococcal Enterotoxin B; and Botulinum Toxin.

B. Chemical Warfare Agents

•General•

1) Chemical warfare agents are generally stored as liquids and deployed as aerosols or vapors, and exposure occurs through the skin, eyes or respiratory tract.

2) The first responsibility in the treatment of victims is for the providers to protect themselves, specifically by using the appropriate level of personal protective equipment.

3) Decontamination involves removing the individual from the contaminated environment, removal of clothing, irrigation with water, and rinsing with soap water or 0.5% hypochlorite solution (which neutralizes most nerve agents and mustards). Vapor exposure alone does not require decontamination. Decontamination should ideally occur outside the hospital.

4) There are several categories of chemical warfare agents. These include: **Anticholinergics, Cyanides, Lung Irritants** (Chlorine, phosgene, diphosgene), **Nerve Agents** (VX, sarin, cyclosarin, soman, tabun), and **Vesicating Agents** (Mustards; Lewisite).

1) Mustards

  a) Mustard is a vesicating agent that causes blistering of exposed surfaces. Mustards may damage skin, eyes, respiratory tract, the hematopoietic system, and GI mucosa. The toxicity partly depends upon the route of exposure; symptoms are usually delayed 4-6h.

  b) Skin exposure results in partial or full thickness burns; eye exposure may result in chemosis, corneal abrasions, and ulcers; inhalation may result in airway inflammation and erosion. Mustards may also cause bone marrow suppression.

  c) Rapid decontamination after dermal exposure is essential: remove clothing and wash with soap and water.

  d) Treatment is generally supportive.

2) Nerve Agents

  a) Nerve agents are classified into the G-series and the V-series. The G-series (G stands for German) consist of the organophosphates tabun (GA), sarin (GB), soman (GD), and cyclosarin (GF). The V-series include VE, VG, VM, and VX. The G-series agents are volatile liquids at room temperature; vapors are denser than air. V-series agents are persistent and can remain on clothes and other surfaces for extended periods of time; V agents are less volatile than G agents, and dermal toxicity is more common than inhalational toxicity.

  b) Nerve agents irreversibly inactivate acetylcholinesterase, which results in the accumulation of acetylcholine at nerve terminals, eventually paralyzing cholinergic transmission (resulting in muscular paralysis). Exposure may be dermal or inhalational.

  c) Dermal exposure produces local effects, and, if the dose is large enough, generalized effects (symptoms may be delayed for up to 18 hours). Vapor inhalation may cause toxicity within seconds. Exposure may result in nicotinic or muscarinic manifestations. Victims may experience cholinergic toxidrome symptoms, including copious bronchial secretions, lacrimation, defecation, urination, tachy or bradydysrhythmias, hypertension, miosis, decreasing level of consciousness, seizures, fasciculations, paralysis, and apnea. Mild vapor exposure may result only in miosis and rhinorrhea.

d) Check basic labs. Before treatment, draw blood for RBC cholinesterase activity; severe toxicity may be seen with a 20-25% reduction in activity.

e) Treatment involves decontamination, maintaining an adequate airway, providing adequate ventilation and circulatory support, and treatment with atropine and pralidoxime.

> **1)** Maintain high levels of precaution, and decontaminate skin with soap and water or 0.5% hypochlorite solution; exposure to nerve agent vapor alone does not require decontamination.

> **2)** Mild vapor exposure usually does not mandate treatment with atropine or pralidoxime; observe patients for at least 1 hour for development of worsening toxicity. Eye pain from vapor exposure can be treated with topical homatropine.

> **3)** Mild liquid exposure may require treatment with atropine and pralidoxime. Patients with mild liquid exposures or asymptomatic patients with possible liquid exposures should be observed for 18h.

> **4)** If severe toxicity, consider early intubation (avoid succinylcholine, as it is metabolized by cholinesterase and may result in prolonged paralysis).

> **5)** Atropine 2 mg IV q2-5 min (pediatric dose is 0.02 mg/kg IV) will reverse the muscarinic effects (bronchoconstriction, secretions, and bradycardia) of nerve agents, but has no effect on the nicotinic effects (paralysis). Atropine should be titrated to relieving bronchoconstriction and secretions.

> **6)** Pralidoxime (2- PAM) 1-2 g IV (pediatric dose is 25-25 mg/kg IV) should be given to reactivate acetylcholinesterase (prompt administration of pralidoxime may disrupt the bond between the nerve agent and acetylcholinesterase before it becomes permanent).

> **7)** Treat seizures with benzodiazepines.

CHAPTER 9

FOREIGN BODY (FB) REMOVAL

•General•

If a wound heals poorly or is particularly painful, suspect a foreign body. Virtually all glass is radiopaque, regardless of lead content.

1) Cutaneous Foreign Body

Fishhooks

    a) If barb is superficial, enlarge entry wound and pull out.

    b) Alternatively, grasp hook with needle holder and push through skin, cut hook behind barb and remove the rest of hook in retrograde fashion.

    c) Or, insert 18-gauge needle along wound track, sheathe barb of hook and then back out needle and hook as one.

    d) Or, attempt the string technique, in which an assistant applies downward pressure on the barb of the hook, which releases the barb. Then, a piece of 0 silk suture is passed around the hook at the bend; a quick pull on the string will remove the hook.

Puncture Wounds

    a) Explore puncture wounds for possible FB. Consider x-rays. Irrigate.

    b) Prophylactic antibiotics are not indicated for puncture wounds. Arrange close follow up, as it is often impossible to adequately explore puncture wounds, since the tract closes quickly.

    c) If a wound is infected, suspect FB (consider CT or MRI) or osteomyelitis. (Pseudomonas is the most common infection in puncture wounds to the foot).

Rings

    a) Apply lubricant, elevate and cool digit, then apply traction with circular motion.

    b) Or, perform a digital block, then exsanguinate digit by wrapping tourniquet around digit, distal to proximal and elevate for 5-10 min. Then, remove tourniquet (if digit immediately becomes swollen again, use blood pressure cuff to stop arterial flow), and use a hemostat to pull umbilical tape or a full skin of # 2-0 silk sutures under ring and, beginning at distal edge of ring, wrap around finger to DIP without allowing skin to bulge through. Then, pulling on proximal end of string, unwrap in same direction that it was wrapped.

c) If neurovascular compromise, use ring cutter.

Splinters

a) Wood is very reactive, fragments easily and is radiolucent (consider MRI, ultrasound or CT for diagnosis); any retained wood will cause infection.

b) Irrigation/exploration cannot reliably exclude FB; get three views on x-ray.

c) Consider making an incision along axis of splinter rather than dragging splinter through entrance wound. Do not simply pull out with longitudinal traction, as it will splinter; cutdown over entire length of FB, fillet open subcutaneous tissue and identify and remove all fragments. However, if near tendons and nerves, consider traction only and prompt referral. If splinter is perpendicular to skin, excise an ellipse around wound, excise tissue over tract until FB is visualized, then excise FB and surrounding tissue as a block.

d) If wound is recent and clean, it is usually safe to suture.

Stingers

Remove stinger as soon as possible (method of removal probably does not matter).

Zippers

Clip zipper diamond or median bar, and zipper will fall apart.

2) Ear Foreign Body

a) Emergency removal is only necessary with infection, disc batteries, or insects.

b) Immobilize insects with mineral (or baby/vegetable) oil or lidocaine.

c) Remove FB with irrigation (do not irrigate if FB is vegetable matter, as it will swell), suction with funnel tip, forceps, or right angle hook.

3) Gastrointestinal Foreign Body

a) The majority of foreign bodies pass on their own without complication. Children may present with dysphagia, drooling, or refusing to eat. The physical exam is usually non-specific. Objects in the stomach (including disc batteries) usually pass on their own; however, if the objects are longer than 5 cm and wider than 2 cm, they are unlikely to pass. A FB in the proximal to middle third of the esophagus requires urgent removal, as it may be aspirated. A FB in the lower third of the esophagus may be observed to see if it passes. Indications for prompt endoscopy (which may be diagnostic and therapeutic) include impacted esophageal FB, sharp or pointed objects, or a battery above the stomach. Consider metal detectors for verification of metal objects.

b) Check x-ray. On A-P film, coins in the esophagus appear round in outline, as the esophagus is floppy and is compressed between the spine and trachea; coins in the trachea appear end-on, as they must pass that way through the vocal cords (film all children who present with a history of coin ingestion, as many children with a coin in the esophagus are asymptomatic).

c) If the patient can manage secretions, a meat impaction can be treated expectantly, but should not be allowed to remain impacted > 12h (time and sedation often allow meat to pass; glucagon 1 mg IV may aid passage, but papain is not recommended).

d) Most patients who have a sensation of a bone caught in their throat after eating fish will not have a bone identified (in these patients, the foreign body sensation is presumably secondary to minor trauma). However, a bone lodged in the esophagus may perforate or cause serious infection. Many bones are lodged on the base of the tongue or tonsils; patients can often localize the position of the bone. Consider a lateral neck x-ray or CT for further evaluation. Examine the oropharynx after spraying with an anesthetic; many bones are visible on exam and can be removed with a hemostat. Consider performing a fiberoptic exam. If the evaluation is normal, the patient can generally be discharged with close ENT follow-up; however, aggressively investigate any patients that have symptoms for more than 48h.

4) Nasal Foreign Body

a) FB often presents only with unilateral rhinorrhea; a risk of aspiration exists and FB must be removed immediately if there is any concern that it may prolapse into the oropharynx. Vegetable matter may swell with fluid.

b) Apply topical vasoconstrictors (phenylephrine and tetracaine, or oxymetazoline spray).

c) Options for removal include suction catheter with funnel tip; alligator clip; hemostat; Fogarty (or Foley) catheter passed above FB and balloon inflated and pulled out; right angle blunt hook; or ear curette. Or, have parent occlude opposite nare and puff into mouth.

5) Respiratory Foreign Body

a) Consider bronchoscopy if suspected foreign body aspiration and choking, wheezing or coughing.

b) If in mainstem bronchus, a FB will cause hyperinflation/air trapping which may be seen in a bilateral decubitus CXR where the "down" hemithorax has no loss of volume (normally, the "down" hemithorax should be hypoinflated with a higher hemidiaphragm as compared to the "up" hemithorax). However, the CXR is often normal in children with airway foreign bodies, and plain films should not be used to exclude an airway foreign body.

CHAPTER 10

GASTROINTESTINAL

I. ABDOMINAL PAIN

*If pain clearly precedes nausea and vomiting, the etiology is more likely to be surgical. Vomiting that precedes pain suggests gastroenteritis, intestinal obstruction, or biliary/ureteral colic.

1) Differential Diagnosis by Location

RUQ: Cholecystitis, hepatitis, hepatic abscess, hepatomegaly from CHF, perforated PUD, pancreatitis, retrocecal appendicitis, zoster, MI, RLL pneumonia, PE.

LUQ: gastritis, pancreatitis, splenic rupture or enlargement, MI, LLL pneumonia, PE.

RLQ: appendicitis, regional enteritis, Meckel's diverticulum, cecal diverticulitis, AAA, ectopic pregnancy, ovarian torsion, PID, endometriosis, ureteral calculi, mesenteric adenitis, incarcerated hernia, volvulus.

LLQ: diverticulitis, AAA, ectopic pregnancy, ovarian torsion, PID, endometriosis, ureteral calculi, psoas muscle abscess, incarcerated hernia, regional enteritis.

Diffuse- porphyria, mesenteric thrombosis, DKA, Addison's, spontaneous bacterial peritonitis, gastroenteritis, sickle cell disease.

2) Differential Diagnosis by Quality of Pain

Acute onset often indicates a vascular etiology (ruptured AAA, mesenteric thrombosis), a ruptured viscus, or obstruction (intestinal, biliary, or renal colic).

Gradual pain is often caused by inflammation (cholecystitis, appendicitis, diverticulitis).

Colicky pain indicates obstruction of a viscus as opposed to a perforation, in which the severe pain persists or worsens.

Constant pain suggests a solid organ process such as hepatitis, pancreatitis, or pyelonephritis.

II. ANORECTAL DISEASE

1) Anal Fissure

a) An anal fissure is a linear tear just below the dentate line extending distally along the anal canal. Over 90% of anal fissures occur in the midline posteriorly.

b) Patients present with rectal bleeding and sharp pain after bowel movements, which subsides.

c) Treat with hot sitz baths 3 x/d and after each bowel movement, increased bran intake, stool softeners, local analgesic, and referral.

2) Anorectal Abscess

a) Almost all abscesses begin with involvement of the anal crypt, which then spreads to the perianal, intersphincteric or ischiorectal space. The abscess may cause severe pain.

b) Only very superficial perianal abscesses which are swollen and fluctuant at the anal verge can be incised and drained in the emergency department. Most abscesses require surgical consult for treatment; even superficial perianal abscesses usually require surgical consult (it may be difficult to determine the depth of the abscess). If diagnosis is in doubt, consider aspiration with an 18-gauge needle.

3) Hemorrhoids

External

a) External hemorrhoids are located below the dentate line and are covered with perianal skin and are usually very painful. If acutely thrombosed, they are hard and tender to palpation.

b) Consider treatment with ice, then inject with lidocaine and epinephrine. Then make an elliptical incision (consider aspirating first), remove clot, and place pressure bandage.

c) Otherwise, if thrombosis is present for less than 48h, swelling is not tense, and pain is tolerable, then treat with hot sitz baths for 15 minutes tid and after each bowel movement. Advise the use of bulk laxatives and bran. Consider stool softeners (Colace 100 mg bid), topical anesthetics (Lidocaine 5% ointment), Witch Hazel, topical steroids (Anusol HC), and systemic analgesics.

Internal

a) Internal hemorrhoids are located above the dentate line and are covered with rectal mucosa. They are usually not painful, not readily palpable, and may ulcerate and cause painless bleeding. They may prolapse, become engorged and strangulate.

b) Treat with ice and assumption of the knee-chest position for 30 min every 2-3h for 2d. Do not sit on doughnut or sitz baths, as this increases venous congestion. Use vasoconstricting suppositories and bulking agents.

c) Definitive treatment may require a nonsurgical procedure (banding or coagulation) or surgical procedure. Incarcerated or strangulated hemorrhoids require an emergent surgical consult.

III. APPENDICITIS

•Etiology•
Obstruction of the appendiceal lumen (by fecaliths, calculi, foreign bodies, or lymphoid hyperplasia) leads to bacterial invasion. Ischemia, necrosis, localized peritonitis and perforation may result.

•Clinical Presentation•
1) Presenting symptoms include abdominal pain, anorexia (seen in 70%), nausea and vomiting, fever (20%), and dysuria (10%). Abdominal pain typically precedes vomiting.
2) The classic presentation of anorexia, nausea, and periumbilical pain localizing to the right lower quadrant (RLQ) over 24h is present in 60%.
3) Appendicitis is unlikely if pain is present > 72h. Recent perforation may temporarily lessen pain.
4) Dysuria may be present if the appendix is located near the bladder or ureter.
5) Children and the elderly are more likely to have atypical presentations. Children have a higher incidence of diarrhea in association with appendicitis.
6) As the uterus enlarges during pregnancy, the appendix becomes dis-

placed from its usual location; by the third trimester, pregnant patients with appendicitis typically have pain in the right flank.

•Evaluation•

1) Check CBC and urinalysis. Check pregnancy test in females.

2) RLQ tenderness is present in the vast majority of patients with appendicitis; many have localized rectal tenderness. The tip of the appendix may extend to any part of the abdomen; a retrocecal appendix is often tender in the right flank or right upper quadrant.

3) Rosving's sign is RLQ pain with LLQ palpation. The psoas sign is pain with right lower extremity elevation against resistance. The obturator sign is pain with right hip flexion and internal rotation.

4) Perform a pelvic exam in females; cervical motion tenderness is present in 30% of patients with appendicitis. Perform a genitourinary exam in males.

5) Spiral CT of abdomen/pelvis is at least 94% accurate for the diagnosis of appendicitis; limited helical CT with rectal contrast (without IV contrast) may be the most accurate and efficient diagnostic imaging method. CT may demonstrate a thickened appendix with an abscess, fluid, or surrounding inflammatory changes.

6) Ultrasound has a sensitivity of 80-94% and a specificity of 90% for acute appendicitis; ultrasound may demonstrate a noncompressible appendix with a dilated lumen and periappendiceal fluid. Ultrasound is the preferred diagnostic test in pregnant patients.

7) WBC >10,000 is seen in most patients with appendicitis.

8) Urinalysis may reveal mild pyuria (from bladder or ureter irritation); isolated hematuria is unlikely with appendicitis.

9) Abdominal films are abnormal in many patients with appendicitis and may show a dilated cecum and/or terminal ileum with air-fluid levels (sentinel or appendiceal ileus), blurring of the distal psoas shadow, or a RLQ appendicolith (distinguished from phleboliths or lymph nodes if solitary, oval, 0.5-2 cm, and in RLQ). However, plain films rarely establish the diagnosis and are not generally recommended.

•Treatment•

1) Treatment is surgical.

2) Establish IV; hydrate with IVNS. Administer antibiotics: cefoxitin or

cefotetan; add clindamycin or metronidazole if the appendix is perforated. Provide analgesia.

3) If diagnosis is unclear, either admit and observe, or, if symptoms are very mild, arrange very close follow-up and return immediately if fever, vomiting, or worsening abdominal pain.

IV. CONSTIPATION

•Etiology•
Constipation may be associated with drugs (anticholinergics, antacids, antidepressants, iron, opioids, calcium channel blockers), diabetes, hypothyroidism, hypercalcemia, spinal cord injury, multiple sclerosis, colorectal tumor or stricture, anal fissure, or hemorrhoids.

•Clinical Presentation•
1) Patients present with a decreased frequency of bowel movements and may have mild abdominal fullness or discomfort.
2) There may be a precipitating factor (drugs, decreased fluid intake).

•Evaluation•
1) Consider plain abdominal films to demonstrate an increased amount of stool and evaluate for possible obstruction or volvulus. Outpatient colonic transit studies can evaluate constipation.
2) The abdomen is generally nontender; a mass may be palpated. Perform rectal exam (evaluate for presence of blood or fecal impaction), and inspect for the presence of anal fissures.

•Treatment •(if pathologic etiologies have been excluded)
Bulk agents : Dietary fiber; methylcellulose; psyllium (Metamucil) 30 g po/d in divided doses.

Lubricants : mineral oil 15-30 ml po qd-bid.

Stool softeners : Docusate (Colace) 100 mg po bid.

Stimulant laxatives: Senekot 1-2 tabs (chronic use may cause motility dysfunction).

Osmotics : Milk of magnesia 15-30 ml po; polyethylene glycol (Golytely, Miralax); sorbitol; lactulose.

Suppository : Bisacodyl (Dulcolax) 10 mg PR.

Enemas : Sodium phosphate (Fleets); tap water.

V. DIARRHEA/FOOD POISONING

A. General Diarrhea/Food Poisoning

•Diarrheal Mechanism•

1) Osmotic- e.g., sorbitol, lactase deficiency.
2) Secretory- e.g., enterotoxins, protozoa, endocrine disorder.
3) Altered motility- e.g., irritable bowel, stress.
4) Altered mucosa- e.g., inflammatory bowel disease, invasive bacteria, enterotoxins, irradiation.

•Etiology• (for infectious diarrhea)

Viral- Viruses account for the majority of acute diarrheal episodes. Rotavirus and Norwalk virus are the most frequent pathogens.

Bacterial

Invasive- bacteria act primarily on the large bowel, causing inflammation and producing blood and mucus in the stools.

Toxigenic- bacteria release a toxin that primarily affects the small intestine, altering electrolyte transport and producing a profuse watery diarrhea.

Parasitic- Pathogens include Giardia, Entamoeba histolytica, Cryptosporidium, and Strongyloides. Parasitic infection is rare outside of specific subpopulations (daycare, campers, and homosexual men).

HIV Patients- may be infected with the usual bacterial pathogens, or CMV, HSV, Cryptosporidium, Isospora, Giardia, and MAI.

•Clinical Presentation• (for bacterial infections)

Infectious/Invasive

1) Incubation period is 1-3d. Typically, there is a gradual onset of symptoms, with a duration of 1-7d.
2) It is associated with fever, abdominal pain, tenesmus, nausea and vomiting, headache, and malaise.
3) If symptoms are caused by an invasive organism, the stool may show blood and WBCs.

Toxigenic

1) Incubation period is 2-12h. Typically, there is a sudden onset of symp-

toms, with a duration of 10-24h.

2) There is generally no fever, and patients may have mild abdominal pain without malaise.

3) Usually, the stool has no blood or WBCs.

•Evaluation•

1) Check stool for blood and WBCs. Typically, invasive bacteria will produce stool WBCs, while toxigenic bacteria will not (although enteroinvasive E. coli and C. difficile, while toxin-producing bacteria, damage the intestinal wall and produce blood and WBCs in the stool). The absence of occult blood may be more accurate than stool WBCs in ruling out an invasive or infectious process.

2) Indications for stool culture include immunocompromised patients, homosexual or bisexual males, public health concerns, presumed invasive etiology, or the presence of WBCs or blood in stool.

3) Consider checking electrolytes.

•Treatment•

1) Consider ciprofloxacin 500 mg bid x 5-7d if fever, abdominal pain, or stool with blood or WBCs.

2) Treat all patients who have Giardia or C. difficile with metronidazole 250 mg tid x 5d.

3) Provide rehydration and antiemetics. Consider Immodium and bismuth (if no blood or WBCs in stool). Avoid Lomotil (it has atropine) and narcotics.

4) Home rehydration: 4 tsp sugar, 3/4 tsp salt, one tsp baking soda, one cup orange juice, dilute to one liter.

B. Specific Bacterial Infections

1) Invasive

Campylobacter- It is usually acquired from chicken, with an incubation period of 2-5d. Consider treatment with antibiotics (quinolones, or erythromycin 30-50 mg/kg/d q8h).

E. coli- Enterotoxigenic e. coli causes the classic traveller's diarrhea without stool WBCs. Enterohemorrhagic e. coli causes diarrhea, vomiting, and abdominal pain with stool WBCs; it may cause hemolytic uremic syndrome or thrombotic thrombocytopenic purpura. Do not give antibiotics for enterohemorrhagic e. coli.

Salmonella- It is usually acquired from dairy, eggs, or pet turtles; it has an incubation period of 8-24h. If patient is toxic and bacteremia is suspected, consider ampicillin 1 gm IV q6h and chloramphenicol 1 gm IV q6h. Otherwise, do not treat with antibiotics, as it prolongs the carrier status.

Shigella- Shigella produces classic dysentery (mucoid, bloody stool), and is acquired from fecal contamination. There is an incubation period of 1-2d. Migration to mesenteric lymph nodes may mimic appendicitis. It often presents with high fever (especially in children, who may present with a febrile seizure). Treat with quinolones, ampicillin 50-100 mg/kg/d in children or 500 mg qid in adults, or Bactrim 8-10 mg/kg/d bid x 5-7d.

Traveller's diarrhea- Most cases are caused by bacteria, usually form enterotoxigenic e. coli. The incubation period is 1-14 days. It causes watery diarrhea and cramping. Treat with ciprofloxacin or Bactrim, loperamide, and bismuth.

Vibrio parahaemolyticus- It is acquired from shellfish, with an incubation period of about 12h. It may be associated with fever. Antibiotics are usually not given.

Vibrio vulnificus- It is acquired from raw oysters and shellfish. It usually occurs in patients with liver disease who present with acute chills, fever (seen in 90%), abdominal pain, and nausea and vomiting. Patients may have cellulitis, bullae or ecchymosis. Treat with tetracycline and ceftazidime.

2) Toxigenic

B. cereus- The short form of B. cereus causes nausea and vomiting with minimal diarrhea <6h after ingestion of fried rice or grains; symptoms last <24h. The long form of B. cereus causes cramping and diarrhea without vomiting 8-16h after exposure.

C. difficile- Broad-spectrum antibiotics (clindamycin, ampicillin, cephalosporins) cause overgrowth of C. difficile, which causes profuse watery diarrhea with WBCs. The stool culture is not helpful, but check for toxin in the stool. Treat with oral vancomycin or metronidazole.

C. perfringens- It is acquired from spores; it may be transmitted through poultry and meats. Patients present with diarrhea and severe abdominal pain, rare fever and emesis. There are no fecal WBCs.

Staphylococcus. aureus- Patients present with explosive nausea and vomiting, abdominal cramping, and slight diarrhea within 2-6h of exposure; symptoms lasts 24h. It can be acquired from any food, especially dairy.

3) Vasomotor Reactions

Scombroid- Scombroid causes flushing, headache, nausea, and diarrhea. It occurs after the ingestion of tuna, mahi-mahi, or dolphin that has not been refrigerated properly. Under certain conditions, histidine in fish is degraded into histamine; patients essentially ingest large amounts of histamine. Symptoms usually occur within 10-30 minutes of ingestion. Treat with H-1 and H-2 blockers.

4) CNS Reactions

Botulism- In botulism, heat labile toxins block neuromuscular endplates. The incubation period is up to 3-4d. 50% of patients with botulism have gastrointestinal symptoms; it may also cause large muscle weakness with cranial nerve disruption. Consider treatment with antitoxin.

Ciguatera – It is a toxin from barracuda, red snapper, or grouper, with an incubation period of 2-24h. Patients present with severe diarrhea, vertigo, ataxia, oral dysesthesias, and reversal of hot/cold sensation. Treatment is supportive; consider mannitol 1 gm/kg. Symptoms may last 1-2 weeks.

Neurotoxic shellfish poisoning- It is acquired from clams and oysters, and occurs in November-March. Patients present with paresthesias, myalgias, and reversal of hot/cold sensation; there are minimal motor or cranial nerve symptoms. Diarrhea and abdominal pain are common. Treatment is supportive.

Paralytic shellfish poisoning- It occurs within several hours of eating molluscs, usually in May-November. Patients present with ataxia, motor paralysis, and cranial nerve palsies. Treatment is supportive.

VI. DIVERTICULAR DISEASE

A. Diverticulitis

•General•

1) Diverticula are herniations of the mucosa and submucosa of the colon.
2) Diverticulitis results from inspissation of fecal material in a diverticulum, with subsequent inflammation and bacterial invasion.
3) The vast majority of diverticula are found in the sigmoid, but can arise in any part of the colon.

•Clinical Presentation•

1) Diverticulitis usually occurs in patients older than 40 years of age.
2) Patients may present with LLQ or suprapubic pain (persistent ache or crampy pain, often worse with defecation), low-grade fever (not universal), malaise, anorexia, mild nausea, or a change in bowel habits.
3) If the inflammation is adjacent to the bladder, the patient may have dysuria.

•Evaluation•

1) Check CBC, electrolytes, BUN/Cr, and urinalysis; consider LFTs and amylase. WBC is usually elevated.
2) Perform abdominal, pelvic and rectal exams. Patients may have localized tenderness, rebound, or guarding (usually in the left lower quadrant). 50% of patients with diverticulitis have hemoccult positive stool.
3) Consider plain films to rule out perforation.
4) Abdominal CT is 93% sensitive and 100% specific (it may demonstrate stranding of pericolonic fat and bowel wall thickening; it may reveal an abscess).

•Treatment•

Inpatient

1) Establish IV. Administer IV fluids. Keep patient NPO.
2) Antibiotic options include Unasyn 3 g IV plus gentamicin; or ampicillin, gentamicin and metronidazole 500 mg every 6h; or clindamycin 300-600 mg every 6h plus gentamicin; or Piperacillin alone.
3) Provide analgesia; meperidine may cause less spasm than morphine.
4) There is no proven benefit of treatment with anticholinergics.

5) Consult surgery if perforation, peritonitis or abscess.

6) Complications include obstruction, abscess, perforation, and fistula.

Outpatient

1) Antibiotic options include Bactrim DS bid; or ciprofloxacin plus metronidazole; or cephalexin 500 mg every 6h.

2) Prescribe a high fiber diet; consider antispasmodics.

•Disposition•

1) Consider outpatient treatment if symptoms are mild, patient is afebrile, and abdominal exam demonstrates minimal tenderness without rebound or guarding.

2) Otherwise, patient should be admitted for IV antibiotics and observation for possible complications.

3) Patients should have an outpatient colonoscopy to rule out colonic malignancy.

B. Diverticulosis

•General•

1) Diverticulosis results from increased intraluminal pressure secondary to chronic constipation and colonic dysmotility.

2) 85% of cases occur in the sigmoid or descending colon.

3) Diverticular hemorrhage is the leading cause of lower GI bleeding.

•Clinical Presentation•

1) Patients are usually older than 40 years of age, and present with recurrent, intermittent LLQ pain and tenderness, constipation or diarrhea, and flatulence.

2) Fever and localized rebound/guarding are absent.

•Treatment•

Treat with local heat, high fiber diet, and consider antispasmodics.

VII. DYSPHAGIA

•Etiology•

Possible etiologies include motility/neuromuscular disorders (e.g. stroke, achalasia, scleroderma, myasthenia gravis, infection) and obstructive disorders (e.g. rings, carcinoma, webs, esophagitis).

•Clinical Presentation•

1) Dysphagia with solids alone usually represents a mechanical obstruction, while dysphagia with solids and liquids is often due to a motility disorder.

2) Esophageal infections usually present with odynophagia.

•Diagnosis•

1) Attempt to distinguish between neuromuscular and obstructive disorders.

2) Consider barium swallow or endoscopy to rule out mechanical obstruction.

•Treatment•

Treatment depends on the etiology.

VIII. GALLBLADDER DISEASE

A. Cholangitis

•General•

Cholangitis is obstruction of the common bile duct (from stasis or stones) with subsequent bacterial infection.

•Clinical Presentation•

1) Charcot's triad (right upper quadrant abdominal pain, fever, and jaundice) is the classic presentation of cholangitis.

2) Patients may present with nausea and vomiting, peritonitis, or shock.

•Evaluation•

1) Check CBC, LFTs, PT/PTT, amylase, electrolytes, BUN/Cr, and blood cultures.

2) Labs may demonstrate an increased WBC, bilirubin, alkaline phosphatase and moderately increased SGPT/SGOT.

3) Abdominal films are usually not helpful, but may show air in the biliary tree.

4) Ultrasound may demonstrate dilation and common bile duct stone.

5) Consider abdominal CT or HIDA scan.

•Treatment•

1) Establish IV. Administer IV fluids.

2) Administer broad-spectrum antibiotics (3rd generation cephalosporin

plus an aminoglycoside; or Unasyn).

3) Urgent surgical and gastroenterology consult.

4) Severely ill patients require immediate biliary decompression with ERCP or surgery.

5) Mild to moderately ill patients may initially be treated medically (antibiotics).

B. Cholecystitis

•Risk Factors•

Risk factors include older age, females, obesity, and increased parity.

•Pathophysiology•

Cholecystitis is inflammation of the gallbladder secondary to cystic duct obstruction. The obstruction is usually from a gallstone, but may be acalculous or from sludge. Inflammation may be sterile or bacterial.

•Clinical Presentation•

1) Patients present with pain, usually in the epigastrium or right upper quadrant; it is initially colicky and then constant and may radiate to the right scapula.

2) There may be associated nausea, vomiting, fever, and RUQ/epigastric tenderness.

3) The patient may have Murphy's sign (patient abruptly stops inspiring during right subcostal palpation).

•Evaluation•

1) Check CBC, LFTs, amylase, urinalysis, electrolytes, BUN/Cr, and blood cultures. Consider abdominal ultrasound.

2) LFTs may be mildly to moderately elevated (significant elevations are unusual unless a common bile duct stone is present). WBC may be elevated.

3) Ultrasound may show gallstones, sludge, a thickened wall, pericholic fluid, or a sonographic Murphy's sign. 90% of acute cholecystitis is associated with gallstones. 5-10% of cases of acute cholecystitis are acalculous, which is more common in the elderly and diabetics, and is associated with trauma, burns, prolonged labor, and major surgery.

4) Consider HIDA scan. One study showed HIDA to be 90-100% sensitive and 85-95% specific (slightly better than ultrasound). In this test, a radionuclide is administered IV and taken up the liver and secreted into the biliary tract. In the normal patient, the gallbladder and cystic duct is visualized within 1h; if the gallbladder is not seen, it suggests obstruction of the cystic duct and cholecystitis.

•Treatment•

1) Establish IV. Administer IV fluids, antiemetics, and antispasmodics (Bentyl).
2) Administer antibiotics (Unasyn; Zosyn; Imipenem; or an aminoglycoside plus 3rd generation cephalosporin).
3) Morphine may increase biliary pressure; consider meperidine for pain.
4) Obtain a surgical consult.
5) Admit.

C. Cholelithiasis

•General•

1) Cholelithiasis is the presence of gallstones in the gallbladder. Symptoms may develop when a gallstone becomes lodged in the cystic or common bile duct.
2) Gallstones may be composed of cholesterol, pigment, or mixed.

•Clinical Presentation•

1) Patients present with RUQ or upper abdominal pain that radiates to the back or shoulder and may be associated with nausea and vomiting; the pain may be steady or colicky. The pain typically begins 30 min-several hours after meals and lasts 1-6h.
2) The physical exam and vital signs are usually normal; the patient may have mild RUQ tenderness. Fever or significant tenderness may indicate the presence of cholecystitis or cholangitis.

•Evaluation•

1) Consider checking CBC, LFTs, amylase, electrolytes, and BUN/Cr. Consider ultrasound.
2) Lab evaluation (LFTs, amylase) is usually normal.
3) Ultrasound is 98% sensitive for gallstones.

•Treatment•

1) Treat biliary colic with ketorolac 15-30 mg IV or with narcotics.
2) If cholecystitis has been excluded, arrange surgical follow-up.

3) If pain persists, consider admission and surgical consultation.

IX. GASTROESOPHAGEAL REFLUX

•Clinical Presentation•

1) Patients present with esophageal pain that is worse with lying or stooping.

2) The pain may radiate to the back, and may be caused by exercise; it is usually worse after meals and transiently improves with antacids.

•Evaluation•

Consider outpatient evaluation with endoscopy. Attempt to exclude other causes of pain.

•Treatment•

1) Instruct patient to elevate head of bed at night. Instruct patient to eat small meals, and to avoid alcohol, tobacco, caffeine, and fatty foods.

2) Medical options include antacids, H-2 blockers, and proton pump inhibitors.

X. GI BLEED

•Etiology•

Upper GI- Upper GI bleed is defined as bleeding proximal to the ligament of Treitz. Etiologies include peptic ulcer disease (duodenal is more common than gastric), mucosal erosive disease, varices, aortoenteric fistula, Mallory-Weiss tear, and esophagitis.

Lower GI- Lower GI bleed is defined as bleeding from a source distal to the ligament of Treitz, and, depending on the location, may present as bright red blood or melena. Etiologies include diverticulosis, A-V malformation, neoplasm, aortoenteric fistula, acute mesenteric ischemia, Meckel's diverticulum, inflammatory bowel disease, hemorrhoids, fissures, infectious diarrhea, trauma, and intussusception.

•Evaluation•

1) Check CBC, type and screen, electrolytes, PT/PTT, and BUN/Cr (BUN may be elevated from absorption of blood from GI tract). Check ECG if any cardiac risk factors. Consider CXR (if clinically indicated) to rule out perforation (although perforation rarely accompanies a major upper GI bleed, as most perforations are anterior and the major duodenal blood supply is posterior).

2) Place NG tube (bile in an otherwise clear NG tube aspirate excludes an active upper GI bleed); a lavage without blood does not rule out a duodenal source of bleeding unless bile is seen in the fluid. There is a 10% misdiagnosis of lower GI bleed in patients with an upper GI source, so perform NG lavage on all patients with upper or lower GI bleed. Hemoccult of NG lavage is not accurate at low pH.

3) Check stool for gross or occult blood; document any abdominal tenderness or distention.

•Diagnosis/Treatment•

1) Establish 2 large bore IVs. Place patient on monitor.
2) Transfuse blood as needed; correct any coagulopathy.
3) Administer an H-2 blocker.
4) Consult GI/surgery.

Diagnosis/Treatment for Upper GI Bleed

1) Consider endoscopy with sclerotherapy (variceal ligation is superior to sclerotherapy).
2) If endoscopy is unavailable or unsuccessful, consider vasoactive agents. In the treatment of esophageal varices, the preferred agent is octreotide 50 mcg IV bolus, followed by 50 mcg/h IV for up to 5d; or consider somatostatin 250 mg IVP every 6h concurrent with 250 mg/h x 48h. These agents temporize and are most useful for varices. If octreotide is unavailable, consider vasopressin 0.2-0.6 units/min IV (usually given with sublingual or patch nitroglycerin, which allows higher doses of vasopressin).
3) If persistent variceal bleeding, consider Sengstaken-Blakemore tubes for tamponade.
4) H-2 blockers have not been shown to be of benefit in the acute setting, but may reduce the risk of rebleeding from gastric ulcers.

Diagnosis/Treatment for Lower GI Bleed

1) Colonoscopy is the procedure of choice for localization of lower GI bleeds (although it is difficult to perform during active bleeding).
2) RBC scanning detects bleeding at 0.1 ml/min, but is not reliable as a localizer of bleeding.

3) Angiogram detects bleeding at 2 ml/min, and may provide a more accurate localization of the bleed.

4) The patient may require an urgent colectomy.

5) 80% of lower GI bleeds stop spontaneously.

•Disposition•

1) Consider admitting all patients with melena.

2) Consider ICU admission if there is active bleeding, SBP <100 mm Hg upon admission to the emergency department, elevated PT, mental status change, or unstable comorbid disease.

3) If the patient presents with a history of bleeding but has a negative NG lavage, trace or normal stool hemoccult, normal Hgb and stable vital signs, then discharge with close follow-up is usually acceptable.

XI. HEPATITIS/JAUNDICE

A. Hepatitis

•Etiology•

Hepatitis refers to inflammation of the liver from infectious (viral, parasitic, bacterial, or fungal) or noninfectious (medications, toxins, or autoimmune disorders) etiologies.

Hepatitis A- It is transmitted via the fecal-oral route, with an incubation period of 15-45 days. There is no chronic carrier state. Acute infection is determined by IgG antibodies, and chronic infection by IgM antibodies.

Hepatitis B- It is acquired through parenteral, sexual, or perinatal exposure, with an incubation period of 4 weeks to 6 months. 10% of adults become chronic carriers. Patients may have arthralgias and urticaria. Patients may develop hepatocellular cancer. Acute infection is manifested by HBsAg and IgM antibody to HBcAg. Patients may have co-infection with hepatitis D.

Hepatitis C- It is acquired through parenteral, sexual, or perinatal exposure, with an incubation period of 15-150 days. 50% of patients become chronic carriers, and 8% develop hepatocellular cancer.

Alcoholic hepatitis- Chronic alcohol abuse may result in inflammatory liver damage.

•Clinical Presentation•

1) Patients may present with malaise, fever, anorexia, nausea and vomiting, diarrhea, right upper quadrant pain, jaundice, pruritis, or mental status change.

2) Patients with alcoholic hepatitis may be asymptomatic, minimally symptomatic with malaise, nausea, and low-grade fever, or may present with hepatic failure (jaundice, coagulopathy, and symptoms of portal hypertension).

3) Manifestations of hepatic failure include dark urine, scleral icterus, ascites, asterixis, and splenomegaly.

•Evaluation•

1) Check CBC, glucose, electrolytes, BUN/Cr, LFTs, PT/PTT, and urine (for bilirubin); consider ammonia level in patients with altered mental status. Check hepatitis panel.

2) In viral hepatitis, there is typically an increase in transaminases with ALT > AST. Bilirubin is usually 5-10 mg/dL (direct and indirect increased in equal proportions). Alkaline phosphatase and LDH may be slightly elevated (a significantly elevated alkaline phosphatase may indicate biliary obstruction). A prolonged PT may indicate impaired liver function. Only conjugated bilirubin is water soluble and appears in the urine.

3) In alcoholic hepatitis, there is usually a moderate increase in the transaminases, with AST > ALT, and an increased bilirubin and WBC. Alcohol abuse usually results in an increased MCV; patients may be anemic, as alcohol is a marrow suppressant.

4) Consider abdominal ultrasound to evaluate for gallbladder disease, biliary obstruction or liver abscess.

•Treatment•

1) Treatment is symptomatic with antiemetics and IV fluids.

2) Patients who are coagulopathic should receive vitamin K.

3) For patients with alcoholic hepatitis, consider D5 NS with 1 g MgSO4, multivitamin, and 100 mg thiamine.

•Disposition•

Admit if severe nausea and vomiting, increased PT, altered mental status, hypoglycemic, elderly, bilirubin >20 mg/dl, or if patient is immunosuppressed.

B. Jaundice

•General•

1) Jaundice is a yellow discoloration of the skin and sclerae; it is caused by an increase in bilirubin production or a defect in bilirubin elimination. Jaundice is usually detectable at bilirubin levels of 2-2.5 mg/dL. Mild jaundice suggests unconjugated hyperbilirubinemia secondary to hemolysis, while more severe jaundice suggests hepatobiliary dysfunction.

2) Elevated unconjugated (indirect) bilirubin results from increased formation or decreased liver uptake of bilirubin; etiologies include hemolytic anemia, hemoglobinopathy, or transfusion reaction.

3) Elevated conjugated (direct) bilirubin results from impaired biliary excretion; etiologies include cholestasis due to infection, toxins, sarcoidosis, cancer, gallstones, bile duct strictures, or pancreatic tumors or cysts.

•Clinical Presentation•

Portal hypertension and ascites suggests a chronic process; abdominal pain and nausea and vomiting suggest acute hepatitis or common duct obstruction. Patients may be asymptomatic.

•Evaluation•

1) Check CBC, LFTs, amylase, PT/PTT, electrolytes, and BUN/Cr. Consider ultrasound, CT, or MRI.

2) Mild hyperbilirubinemia with normal transaminases and alkaline phosphatase suggests hemolysis or Gilbert's syndrome. Significantly elevated transaminases may indicate hepatitis, while disproportionate elevations in alkaline phosphatase suggest a cholestatic process (specifically, a mechanical obstruction such as a common bile duct stone). Only conjugated bilirubin is water soluble and appears in the urine.

•Treatment•

Treatment depends on the etiology.

XII. INFLAMMATORY BOWEL DISEASE

A. Crohn's Disease

•General•

1) Crohn's disease is characterized by focal granulomatous transmural inflammation, potential involvement of any part of the GI tract, skip segments, and rectal sparing (but patients have frequent anorectal complications).

2) There is often small bowel involvement and extraintestinal manifestations. Hepatobiliary disease is common.

•Clinical Presentation•

1) Abdominal pain, anorexia, diarrhea, and weight loss are present in 80% of patients with Crohn's disease.

2) Patients generally have a more chronic course of disease than with ulcerative colitis.

•Diagnosis•

Diagnosis is through colonoscopy.

•Treatment•

1) Consider steroids for acute exacerbations; steroids are not effective in maintaining remission.

2) Newer forms of sulfasalazine may be effective in Crohn's disease of the large bowel.

B. Ulcerative Colitis

•General•

1) Ulcerative colitis is characterized by continuous, diffuse inflammation involving the mucosa and submucosa. It begins in the rectum and extends to the colon. There are no skip segments; there may be crypt abscesses. The small intestine is never involved.

2) It is associated with erythema nodosum and toxic megacolon.

•Clinical Presentation•

1) Patients may present with acute onset of fever, crampy pain (although because inflammation is superficial, it is not usually extremely painful), tenesmus and stool with blood and pus.

2) In severe colitis, patients may develop signs of peritonitis.

3) Physical findings may be subtle or absent in patients taking steroids.

•Evaluation•

1) Check CBC and electrolytes. Consider blood cultures.

2) Check abdominal films.

3) Consider abdominal CT to evaluate for abscess.

•Treatment•

1) If symptoms are severe, admit patient for IV fluids, steroids, bowel rest with nasogastric suction, and antibiotics.

2) Avoid pain medication, as there is risk of toxic megacolon. Antidiarrheals, opioids, and anticholinergics may lead to colonic dilation.

C. Complications

1) Fulminant Colitis

    a) Patients present with severe bloody diarrhea (>8-10 stools/d) and systemic signs (fever, anemia, abdominal tenderness, and tachycardia).

    b) Labs may demonstrate anemia, elevated WBC and ESR, hypokalemia, and metabolic acidosis. Abdominal X-ray may show thumbprinting and thickening of colonic wall with loss of haustration.

    c) Treat with antibiotics, steroids, and surgical consult.

2) Toxic Megacolon

    a) Toxic megacolon typically occurs in severely ill patients with ulcerative colitis.

    b) The abdominal X-ray demonstrates a colon diameter >6-8 cm, with the haustral pattern effaced. Edema may appear as indenting thumbprints with pseudopolypoid projections into the lumen.

    c) Treat with IV fluids, antibiotics, steroids, and surgical consult; consider decompression.

XIII. MESENTERIC ISCHEMIA

•General•

Mesenteric ischemia can result from several different pathological conditions; it can be acute (occlusive or nonocclusive) or chronic. Etiologies include:

1) Acute Arterial Embolus- Emboli cause 75% of acute occlusions; occlusions most commonly involve the superior mesenteric artery.

The median age of patients is 70 years old; risk factors include age, coronary disease, valvular disease, atrial fibrillation, and aortography. The patient usually complains of sudden onset of severe, poorly localized periumbilical pain out of proportion to findings on physical exam and accompanied by nausea and vomiting. 25% of patients have stool with occult blood.

2) **Arterial Thrombosis**- Arterial thrombosis is usually associated with chronic visceral atherosclerosis, peripheral vascular disease, and hypertension. There is a history of abdominal pain after meals in 20-50% of patients. Patients may present with nausea, vomiting, diarrhea, and gradual onset of abdominal pain and distention.

3) **Venous Thrombosis**- Venous thrombosis occurs in younger patients, and is associated with hypercoaguable states. Patients may have an acute or chronic onset.

4) **Non-occlusive Mesenteric Ischemia** - It usually results from low cardiac output states such as hypotension, sepsis, CHF, or shock.

•Clinical Presentation•

1) The patient may present with an abrupt onset of severe, poorly localized pain out of proportion to the findings on physical exam. However, gradual onset of pain is more common; pain may be sudden if an embolus is the cause. The patient may have postprandial pain with weight loss; nausea and vomiting may occur.

2) As transmural necrosis occurs, the parietal peritoneum is irritated, causing peritoneal signs.

3) Translocation of anaerobic intestinal bacteria may lead to secondary sepsis.

•Evaluation•

1) Check CBC, electrolytes, BUN/Cr, LFTs, amylase, phosphate, ABG, lactate, ECG, and abdominal films.

2) Document abdominal exam and any presence of occult blood in the stool.

3) Abdominal X-ray is usually normal, but may have thumbprinting (thickened bowel wall), pneumatosis, portal venous gas, or separation of bowel loops. WBC is usually increased. Metabolic acidosis may be present; an elevated lactate is sensitive but not specific for

advanced ischemia. An elevated phosphate level may suggest mesenteric ischemia (normal levels do not exclude disease).

4) Abdominal CT may suggest mesenteric ischemia. Angiogram is the gold standard for diagnosis.

•Treatment•

1) Establish IV access. Place patient on monitor. Administer oxygen.
2) Fluid resuscitation as necessary.
3) Provide analgesia.
4) Consult vascular surgery.
5) Administer broad spectrum antibiotics.
6) If there are no peritoneal signs, consider obtaining an angiogram.
7) If the patient is unstable with peritoneal signs, an angiogram may be obtained in the operating room. Therapeutic options include intra-arterial papaverine, tPA, embolectomy, and resection.
8) Consider heparin and bowel decompression (nasogastric tube).
9) Admit.

XIV. PANCREATITIS

•Etiology•

1) Alcohol and gallstones are the two most common causes.
2) Other causes include infection, medications, hypertriglyceridemia, and hypercalcemia.

•Clinical Presentation•

1) Patients usually present with constant mid-epigastric or right upper quadrant pain radiating to the back with nausea and vomiting. There is usually an abrupt onset, which reaches maximal intensity in 10-30 min.
2) If hemorrhagic pancreatitis, retroperitoneal blood may produce a Gray Turner sign (blue discoloration of flanks) or Cullen sign (blue discoloration of the periumbilical area).

•Evaluation•

1) Check CBC, electrolytes, BUN/Cr, LFTs, amylase, and lipase. Check ABG for acidosis and hypoxemia. Consider abdominal CT.
2) Amylase is increased in 95% of patients, but lipase is more specific; enzymes are usually three times normal, but the magnitude of eleva-

tion doesn't correlate with the severity of disease. ALT >80 is specific but not sensitive for biliary pancreatitis. Amylase may also be elevated in burns, salivary gland disorders, ectopic pregnancy, small bowel obstruction, and perforated duodenal ulcer.

3) If substantial third space losses are evident (hemoconcentration, oliguria, tachycardia, hypotension), then the pancreatitis is likely severe.

4) A falling Hgb suggests hemorrhagic pancreatitis. If a mass is present, consider pseudocyst.

5) Abdominal CT is the most reliable imaging method for diagnosing pancreatic inflammation and its possible complications (abscess, hemorrhage, pseudocyst).

6) If the patient is severely ill and febrile, consider the possibility of necrotizing pancreatitis.

Prognostic signs (gallstone pancreatitis criteria are in parenthesis)

1) *On admission*: Age >55 (70); WBC >16,000 (18,000); Glucose >200 mg/dL (220); LDH >350 IU/L (400): AST >250 U/L.

2) *At 48h*: Hematocrit drop >10%; BUN rise > 5 mg/dL (>2); calcium < 8 mg/dL; PaO2 < 60 mm Hg; base deficit > 4 mEq/L (>5); fluid sequestration > 6L (>4).

3) If patients have < 3 criteria, the mortality is < 1%; if 3-4 criteria, the mortality is 25%; if 5-6, the mortality is 40%; if > 6, the mortality is 100%.

•Treatment•

1) Bowel rest with a nasogastric tube.
2) Establish IV; administer IV fluids.
3) Provide analgesia (meperidine may cause less spasm than morphine).
4) Administer antiemetics.
5) Surgery may be indicated if gallstones, hemorrhage, abscess, or large pseudocyst.

XV. PEPTIC ULCER DISEASE/GASTRITIS

•General•

1) Peptic ulcer disease (PUD) refers to a duodenal or gastric mucosal defect; the injury results from an imbalance between acid production and the normal protective mucosal barriers. NSAIDS, stress, and etha-

nol may disrupt the protective barrier and predispose the mucosa to injury.

2) H. pylori is the leading cause of PUD.

3) Gastritis and PUD have similar presentations, and the treatment is generally similar.

•**Clinical Presentation**•

1) **Gastric ulcer**- Typically, patients describe a scenario in which pain occurs after eating, followed by vomiting. The pain is usually described as burning, steady and rarely radiates to the back.

2) **Duodenal ulcer**- Typically, patients experience pain, which is relieved after eating. The pain is often described as aching and often radiates to the back.

3) With perforation, most patients have sudden onset of pain. Significant upper GI bleeding does not usually accompany perforation.

•**Evaluation**•

1) Check CBC to evaluate for possible blood loss; consider checking electrolytes and amylase/LFTs.

2) Patients generally have mild epigastric tenderness on exam; document stool hemoccult results.

3) Consider NG tube to evaluate for upper GI bleed.

4) Diagnosis is usually established with endoscopy or an upper GI series; non-invasive tests are available for H. pylori.

•**Treatment**• Options include:

1) Antacids 1-3h after meals and at night; aluminum may cause constipation, Mg may cause diarrhea.

2) H-2 blockers: cimetidine (Tagamet) 400 mg bid or famotidine (Pepcid) 20 mg bid or ranitidine (Zantac) 150 mg bid.

3) Proton pump inhibitors: omeprazole (Prilosec) 20 mg qd or lansoprazole (Prevacid) 30 mg qd or pantoprazole (Protonix) 40 mg.

4) Sucralfate (acts as a barrier).

5) Misoprostol (prostaglandin). In NSAID-related ulcer disease, misoprostol is an effective treatment and protective agent.

6) **H. Pylori**: Cure is achieved in 90-95% with clarithromycin (Biaxin) 500 mg bid, amoxicillin 1 gm bid, and omeprazole 20 mg bid, all x10-14d.

XVI. SMALL BOWEL OBSTRUCTION (SBO)

•Etiology•
Etiologies include adhesions, incarcerated groin hernia, defect in mesentery, and neoplasm.

•Clinical Presentation•
1) Patients may present with abdominal distention, nausea and vomiting, abdominal pain (often episodic), lack of bowel movements (complete obstruction causes obstipation, partial may cause diarrhea), and gas.
2) High obstruction typically presents with pain in the upper abdomen and more frequent episodes of pain.
3) In adynamic ileus, colicky pain is absent, but distention causes discomfort; hiccups are common, and vomiting is rarely profuse.

•Evaluation•
1) Check abdominal films. Check CBC, electrolytes, and BUN/Cr.
2) Consider abdominal CT, which may demonstrate a source of obstruction, and may identify an abscess or inflammatory process. CT may also indicate the presence of strangulation.

Abdominal X-ray
1) In a healthy adult, 1-2 air-fluid levels may be seen, and gas-filled small bowel rarely exceeds 3 cm.
2) In SBO, films may show distention of transverse loops of small bowel (with little or no colon air) with air fluid levels and "strings of beads" (a tiny amount of gas with a large amount of fluid traps the gas bubbles between valvulae and then molecular adhesion causes fluid to surround gas rather than form an air-fluid level, giving the appearance of a string of beads).
3) More than two fluid levels at different heights suggest obstruction (but may also occur with ileus); a few dilated loops located high in the abdomen may indicate distal duodenal or jejunal obstruction.
4) Colonic gas is identified because it is peripheral, with haustrations that are farther apart and that do not involve the entire transverse diameter of bowel (distinctive valvulae are seen better on supine films).
5) If there is a complete obstruction, then there is little or no gas in the

colon (large amounts of colon gas virtually rule out SBO); bowel proximal to an obstruction may be completely filled with fluid and give a pseudotumor appearance.

6) Strangulation is indicated by a thickened bowel wall (true thickness is best evaluated on an upright film).

•Treatment•

1) Nasogastric tube.

2) Establish IV. Administer IV fluids and antiemetics.

3) Obtain surgical consult. Strangulated obstructions are surgical emergencies.

XVII. VOLVULUS

•General•

1) A volvulus results from rotation of bowel about its mesenteric axis, which then compromises arterial blood flow and venous drainage.

2) Volvulus may be associated with congenital defects, mechanical obstruction, inflammation, or neoplasms.

Cecal Volvulus

a) Cecal volvulus usually occurs in patients 25-35 years old who present with an abrupt onset of abdominal pain, abdominal distention, and vomiting.

b) The physical exam usually demonstrates abdominal tenderness and hyperresonance.

c) Check CBC and electrolytes, and type and screen. Check CXR for free air. Abdominal films may demonstrate volvulus in RLQ. Consider abdominal CT.

d) Treat with IV fluids; consider NG tube. Obtain surgical consult; the initial treatment is usually surgical. Give antibiotics (cefoxitin or cefotetan) if perforation or peritonitis is suspected. There is a high mortality.

Sigmoid Volvulus

a) Sigmoid volvulus usually occurs in psychiatric and nursing home patients with a history of chronic constipation. It often presents with abrupt onset of abdominal pain, distention and vomiting.

b) Physical exam usually demonstrates abdominal tenderness and

hyperresonance; rebound tenderness may indicate perforation and/
or peritonitis.

c) Check CBC, electrolytes, BUN/Cr, and abdominal films. Consider
barium enema. Abdominal X-ray shows "bent inner tube" in LLQ;
barium enema shows "bird's beak."

d) Treat with IV fluids; obtain surgical consult. Consider decompression and detorsion with rectal tube, then surgery. Give antibiotics
(cefoxitin or cefotetan) if perforation or peritonitis is suspected.

XVIII. VOMITING

•General•

1) The vomiting center is in the medulla; all emetic stimuli act on this
center. Stimuli include chemical agents (uremia, DKA, toxins), CNS
stimulation, vagal stimulation (myocardial infarction, biliary colic),
and 8th cranial nerve stimulation.

2) Common clinical presentations of vomiting include migraine, gastroenteritis, bowel obstruction, renal or biliary colic, and food poisoning.

3) Vomiting may cause hypokalemia, hypochloridemia, and metabolic
alkalosis.

•Treatment•

1) Consider IV fluids.

2) Determine the underlying cause.

3) Phenothiazines, benzamides, and butyrophenones block dopamine
receptors in the vomiting center; dopamine receptor antagonists may
cause dystonic reactions (promethazine less so). Metoclopramide also
alleviates nausea and vomiting by stimulating gastric emptying. Antihistamines reduce the vestibular stimulation component of nausea
and vomiting. 5 HT$_3$ receptor antagonists cause fewer side effects
than other agents, and may be more appropriate in children. Anti-
emetic options include:

a) Phenothiazines

Prochlorperazine (Compazine)- 25 mg PR q12h; 5-10 mg IV q4h;
2.5-5 mg IM (do not use in children).

Promethazine (Phenergan) – 12.5-25 mg IV; 25 mg PR q6h; 25-50 mg IM q4h.

Trimethobenzamide (Tigan) - 200 mg PR q6h; 200 mg IM q4h.

b) Benzamides

Metoclopramide (Reglan) - 10-20 mg po q4-6h; 10 mg IV (over 15 min)/IM q3-4h.

c) Butyrophenones

Droperidol- 2.5 mg IV/IM.

d) Antihistamines

Hydroxyzine (Vistaril)- 50-100 mg PR q6h; 25-50 mg IM q4h.

e) 5 HT$_3$ receptor antagonists

Ondansetron (Zofran)- 4 mg IV/IM; or 8 mg po bid (4 mg po bid if younger than 12 years).

Dolestron- (Anzemet)- 12.5 mg IV (0.35 mg/kg IV in children).

CHAPTER 11
GENITOURINARY

I. THE ACUTE SCROTUM

•Etiology•
Etiologies of acute scrotal symptoms include torsion, trauma, epididymitis, orchitis, incarcerated hernia, abdominal aortic aneurysm, testicular cancer (which may bleed and cause acute symptoms), renal colic, hydrocele, and Henoch-Schonlein purpura.

A. Epididymitis

•General•
1) E. coli is the predominant causative organism in prepubertal males.
2) In adolescents and patients younger than 35 years old, epididymitis is usually secondary to a sexually transmitted disease (STD).
3) In patients older than 35 years old, epididymitis may be secondary to STD. Obstructive disease may leads to infection with E. coli, Klebsiella, or Pseudomonas. Long-term use of amiodarone is associated with epididymitis.
4) Recent extreme physical exertion (lifting heavy objects) may cause retrograde force of urine through ejaculatory ducts and into the epididymis, causing a chemical epididymitis.

•Clinical Presentation•
The onset of pain is more gradual than with torsion. The patient may have UTI or STD symptoms. Fever is often present; vomiting is rare.

•Evaluation•
1) Check CBC, urinalysis, urine culture, and urethral culture; consider ultrasound. The WBC is usually increased; urinalysis may demonstrate bacteria or WBCs (but may be normal).
2) The exam is characterized by swelling and localized tenderness of the epididymis/posterior testes. Early in the course of the disease, a firm localized mass may be palpated at the inferior portion of the testes. Pain may be relieved with lying down or elevation of the scrotum. Phren sign (decreased pain with elevation of scrotum) does not reli-

ably distinguish epididymitis from torsion.

3) Attempt to rule out testicular torsion. Consider obtaining a testicular ultrasound, as it is often difficult to differentiate epididymitis from torsion; a color Doppler ultrasound usually shows increased flow to the involved testes (unlike testicular torsion). Ultrasound may also reveal an abscess.

•Treatment•

1) Bed rest, scrotal elevation, ice, and analgesics.
2) If presumed to be secondary to STD, administer ceftriaxone 250 mg IM x 1 plus doxycycline 100 mg bid x 10d; or ofloxacin 300 mg bid x 7d.
3) If not presumed to be STD, administer ampicillin 500 mg qid x 14d or Bactrim bid x 14d or ciprofloxacin 500 mg bid for 14d.

B. Testicular Torsion

•General•

1) Torsion typically occurs in early puberty or the first year of life. It is rare after 35 years old. Torsion is associated with a congenital "bell clapper deformity" of the testicle. An undescended testicle is more likely to torse, and may present as a painful inguinal mass without a palpable testicle in the scrotum.
2) Salvage rate: 90% at 5h; 70% at 6-12h; 20% after 12h.

•Clinical Presentation•

1) The typical presentation is sudden, severe, unremitting, unilateral testicular pain. There is often associated nausea and vomiting; the pain is not affected by position. Some patients may have fever; dysuria is unusual.
2) 50% of patients with torsion have a previous history of severe testicular pain with rapid resolution. There may be a history of strenuous physical activity prior to the onset of pain.

•Evaluation•

1) On exam, typically the entire involved testicle is tender, swollen, high riding, and usually has a horizontal axis. There may be loss of the cremaster reflex (normally, stroking of the inner thigh causes reflex elevation of the ipsilateral testes). Pain is not relieved with raising the

scrotum; the epididymis and testes feel like a single mass. Patients may be febrile. However, physical exam without an ultrasound evaluation is unreliable in the diagnosis of testicular torsion.

2) If there is a strong clinical suspicion, arrange an emergent urologic consultation for immediate surgical exploration. If the diagnosis is unclear, consider color flow Doppler, which may demonstrate decreased testicular flow; the sensitivity approaches 90-100%, and the specificity is 100%.

3) If there is a strong clinical suspicion and normal ultrasound, consider exploration.

4) Check urinalysis, which is usually normal but may demonstrate pyuria.

5) Consider obtaining an ultrasound in a traumatic injury to the testes.

•Treatment•

1) Treatment is surgical (urgent).

2) Consider an attempt at manual detorsion. Torsion usually occurs in a medial direction from the top. To de-torse, twist the left testis clockwise, and right testis counterclockwise 180° ("like opening a book").

3) Provide analgesia. Consider applying ice to the affected testicle until surgery can be performed.

C. Torsion of Appendix Testes

1) Torsion of appendix testes usually occurs in patients 7-12 years old.

2) Patients present with sudden onset of pain, which is less severe than with torsion. There are no systemic symptoms. Maximal tenderness is at the site of the appendage; a nodule may be palpable. The blue dot of hemorrhage may be visible through the scrotal skin.

3) Consider ultrasound or exploration to evaluate for possible testicular torsion. Ultrasound usually shows normal or increased blood flow to the involved testicle

4) Treat with elevation, ice, and analgesia; it is not a threat to the viability of the testes.

II. NEPHROLITHIASIS

•General•

1) Kidney stones may result from low urine output, high dietary oxalate (caffeine, citrus), hyperparathyroidism, or gout. Most stones are made

of calcium along with oxalate or phosphate.

2) Struvite stones (which may become staghorn calculi) are formed by urea-splitting bacteria from infection.

3) Some medications may lead to kidney stones by increasing urinary pH or increasing calcium or phosphate excretion (e.g., indinavir, diuretics, and allopurinol).

4) Most stones arise in the kidney and become symptomatic when they become impacted in the ureter.

•Clinical Presentation•

1) Patients usually present with an acute onset of colicky unilateral costovertebral angle (CVA) pain and hematuria. Pain is usually severe, and may radiate to the groin. Nausea and vomiting occur in most patients. Stones in the ureterovesical junction may lead to dysuria and urinary frequency.

2) If fever is present, consider infected hydronephrosis or perinephric abscess.

•Evaluation•

1) Check CBC, BUN/Cr, and urinalysis. Consider imaging for definitive diagnosis.

2) The abdominal exam is usually unremarkable; in patients older than 60 years old, palpate for a possible aortic aneurysm. CVA tenderness is variable, and may suggest proximal stone or infection. Typically, pain from a ureteral stone does not change with palpation.

3) Examine testicles to evaluate for possible testicular etiology for pain.

4) Some suggest imaging all patients in order to document the presence of a large stone, complete obstruction, or solitary kidney. However, if the patient is young, afebrile, has a documented history of nephrolithiasis and the urine is not infected, it is acceptable to relieve pain and arrange follow-up.

5) Obtain abdominal CT if presumed kidney stone and fever (especially if CVA tenderness), to investigate possible perinephric abscess.

•Diagnosis•

1) **Abdominal CT**- Abdominal helical CT is the imaging method of choice, especially in patients over 50-60 years old, as aortic disease may also have CVA pain and hematuria. One study showed that noncontrast

helical CT is 97% sensitive for stones (and also images the aorta); it can also evaluate for possible pancreatitis, appendicitis, or ovarian or bowel conditions. CT precisely identifies stones and the presence of obstruction, but does not evaluate renal function. Certain medications (e.g., protease inhibitors) form stones that are not visualized on CT scan.

2) **BUN/Cr**- Evaluates renal function.

3) **IVP**- An IVP is 96% sensitive for stones; 90% of stones are radiopaque. An IVP provides a clear outline of the entire urinary system and evaluates relative renal function. The most reliable indicator of a stone is a delay in the appearance of the nephrogram or ureter in the 5 min film. The IVP may demonstrate columnization (secondary to poor ureteral peristalsis), a dense nephrogram with delayed excretion, or interruption of the dye column. A delayed nephrogram >2h suggests a clinically important obstruction. Extravasation of dye suggests a decompressed obstruction. An IVP is relatively contraindicated if the creatinine is elevated.

4) **Ultrasound**- Ultrasound is not as sensitive or accurate as helical CT for the diagnosis of kidney stones, but can be used as an alternate method for evaluating the presence of hydronephrosis. Ultrasound cannot always find smaller stones. Ultrasound can also evaluate for possible aortic aneurysm or cholelithiasis.

5) **Urinalysis**- 80-90% of stones present with hematuria; check for infection. Non-opaque stones (e.g. uric acid stones) often are associated with a urinary pH of 5.0 or less; a pH > 7.5 suggests a struvite stone or infection.

•Treatment•

1) Provide pain relief with narcotics or NSAIDS (consider ketorolac (Toradol), as it can be administered parenterally). Although NSAIDS provide good relief for renal colic, some suggest avoiding NSAIDS because of its prostaglandin action or if there is a possibility the patient may need surgery.

2) Hydration is controversial; some suggest that hydration helps "flush out" stones, while others maintain that hydration is not beneficial, and can painfully distend an obstructed ureter.

•Disposition•

1) Obtain an early urology consult and consider admission if infection, large stone (>5 mm), complete obstruction or extravasation, intractable pain, elevated creatinine, or solitary kidney. The belief that an uninfected kidney can tolerate 1 week of complete obstruction may not be valid; some evidence suggests injury occurs after 24h.

2) Large stones should follow-up within 72h; smaller, distal stones can be deferred up to 2 weeks (90% of stones <5mm in diameter pass on their own).

3) If discharged home, advise patient to push fluids and strain urine; prescribe pain medications. Advise patient to return if oliguria, dysuria, worsening pain, persistent vomiting, or fever.

4) At follow-up, patients should have a stone analysis, and a metabolic evaluation for possible hyperparathyroidism, chronic infection, and renal tubular acidosis.

III. URINARY RETENTION

•Etiology•

Penis- phimosis.
Urethra- tumors, strictures.
Prostate- benign prostatic hypertrophy, prostate cancer, prostatitis.
CNS disease- diabetes, multiple sclerosis.
Drugs- antihistamines, anticholinergics, antispasmodics, sympathomimetics.

•Clinical Presentation•

Patients may present with urinary urgency or hesitation, decreased urine flow, or inability to urinate. Patients may present with UTI. Patients may have a distended bladder.

•Evaluation•

1) Check urinalysis, electrolytes, and BUN/Cr (urinary obstruction may result in acute or chronic renal failure). Check post-void residual, which should be less than 125 cc.

2) In women, consider evaluation for an underlying neurologic disorder.

•Treatment•

1) Place urinary catheter. In patients with prostatic hypertrophy, con-

sider using a Coude catheter.

2) If patient has benign prostatic hypertrophy, consider terazosin 2 mg qd.

3) Discontinue medications potentially responsible for urinary retention.

4) If there is no infection and the patient has normal renal function, consider discharge with urine leg bag and close urologic follow-up.

CHAPTER 12
HEMATOLOGY/ONCOLOGY

I. BLOOD PRODUCTS

Cryoprecipitate
1) Each bag of cryoprecipitate contains fibrinogen, von Willebrand factor, factor XIII, and 50-100 units of factor VIII activity.
2) Cryoprecipitate is indicated for the treatment of hypofibrinogenemia or for patients with hemophilia or von Willebrand disease (if factor VIII is not available).
3) Cryoprecipitate should be ABO compatible, but does not need to be crossmatched. The usual dose is 10-20 bags (2-4 bags/10kg).

Fresh Frozen Plasma (FFP)
1) FFP contains all the coagulation factors. There is 1 unit of each factor per ml of FFP; 40 cc/kg raises the activity of all factors to 100%.
2) Indications for FFP include a PT >1.5 x normal, reversal of Coumadin toxicity, active bleeding in the presence of liver disease, and factor deficiency if factor is unavailable.
3) The typical dose is 8-10 ml/kg. Transfused FFP should be ABO compatible (cross-matching is not mandatory).

Packed RBCs
1) Each unit is approximately 250 ml, with Hct 70-80%; each unit should raise the Hgb by 1 g/dl or the Hct by 3%. Packed RBCs have less volume and are less immunogenic than whole blood. Packed RBCs should be typed and cross-matched; if emergency, give O-negative.
2) Packed RBCs can be given as leukocyte poor RBCs (for transplant recipients or patients with previous nonhemolytic transfusion reactions) or washed RBCs (plasma proteins and some leukocytes are removed; it is given to those who are sensitive to plasma antigens).

Platelets
Platelets are generally given as 6 random donor units or one plateletpheresis pack, which should raise the platelet count by 50,000.

II. HEMOPHILIA

•General•

1) Hemophilia is an inherited, X-linked recessive disorder resulting in deficiency of factor VIII or IX; the intrinsic coagulation cascade is disrupted, resulting in easy bruising and bleeding. Patients with factor levels 5-30% of normal have mild disease; levels less than 1% of normal result in severe disease.

2) Hemophilia A is factor VIII deficiency; hemophilia B (Christmas disease) is factor IX deficiency. Hemophilia A and B are clinically indistinguishable.

3) Von Willebrand disease is a deficiency of von Willebrand factor, which facilitates platelet adhesion and is a carrier protein for factor VIII.

•Clinical Presentation•

1) Bleeding in hemophilia is characterized by deep hematomas and hemarthroses that occur spontaneously or with minimal trauma. Bleeding is often delayed; there is usually no bleeding with minor cuts.

2) Back pain may signify a retroperitoneal bleed, and compartment syndromes may result from muscle bleeds.

3) Von Willebrand disease presents with variable bleeding; mucosal bleeding is most common.

•Evaluation•

1) Check CBC, platelets, PT/PTT, and factor levels. If patients have documented hemophilia, determine the type of deficiency, percent factor deficiency, and presence of inhibitors.

2) Patients with hemophilia usually have a prolonged aPTT; bleeding time is normal. Patients with von Willebrand's disease usually have a prolonged bleeding time, the aPTT is variable.

3) Any patient with a new headache or CNS symptoms should be given factor and a head CT should be obtained, as spontaneous bleeding into the CNS can occur.

•Treatment•

1) Moderate hemophilia may respond to DDAVP 0.3 mcg/kg IV.

2) Otherwise, significant bleeding in hemophilia A requires factor VIII (recombinant factor VIII is the preferred source). One unit of factor VIII should raise the level by 2%; the amount given depends on the type of hemorrhage. If mild bleeding, administer 18 units/kg; if moderate bleeding, administer 26 units/kg; if severe bleeding, administer

50 units/kg (i.e., achieve a serum factor VIII level of 100%).

3) Joint or muscle bleeding requires factor VIII level to be raised to at least 40-50% activity; epistaxis requires 80-100%. CNS, GI and genitourinary bleeds require initial levels to be 100%. Mucosal bleeding requires levels of 70-100%; consider antifibrinolytic agents (Amicar 75-100 mg/kg in children, 6 gm in adults) as an adjunct for mucosal bleeding. Lacerations that require sutures mandate factor replacement (50 units/kg).

4) If emergency and factor is not available, administer cryoprecipitate (each bag contains 50-100 units of factor VIII activity) or FFP (which contains all factors; 40 cc/kg will raise activity of all factors to 100%).

5) Treat hemophilia B with Factor IX concentrate (1 unit of factor IX should raise the level by 1%), or FFP.

6) For mild von Willebrand's disease, use DDAVP. If significant bleeding, give factor VIII concentrates containing large amounts of vWF; or, consider cryoprecipitate or FFP.

7) Do not place central lines without prior factor replacement. Do not give IM injections.

III. ONCOLOGIC EMERGENCIES

A. Neutropenic Fever

•General•

1) A decline of the neutrophil count below 500 (or if <1000 with predicted continued decline) is considered neutropenic and a high risk of infection. The highest risk for neutropenia occurs 7-15 days after cytotoxic chemotherapy.

2) In almost all neutropenic patients, infection is accompanied by fever, which is defined as a single oral temp >38.3°C (101°F) over at least 1 hour (some use 38°C (100.4°F) as the cut-off).

3) The GI tract is the most common source of infection; other sites include lung, vascular access sites, skin, and urine. A documented site of infection is found in 60% of neutropenic patients. The offending organism is usually gram-positive.

4) The probability of infection and bacteremia increase as the neutrophil count declines or if there is protracted neutropenia or rapid decline in

neutrophil counts.

5) There is a 5-10% mortality.

•Evaluation•

1) Perform skin, oropharynx, lung and genitourinary exams. Consider infection of any indwelling devices.

2) Check urinalysis, CBC, electrolytes, calcium, magnesium, and LFTs. Obtain cultures of blood (including fungal cultures), urine, and stool. Consider LP if meningitis is suspected. Send diarrhea for cultures and C. difficile toxin. Check CXR; consider abdominal films.

3) Avoid rectal exams.

•Treatment•

1) If patient is febrile or has a history of fever, isolate patient and establish IV.

2) Quickly start antibiotics. Empiric monotherapy regimens include ceftazidime; cefepime; imipenem/cilastatin; or meropenem. Dual therapy regimens include an aminoglycoside plus either an antipseudomonal PCN (e.g. piperacillin) or ceftazidime or cefepime; add vancomycin if obvious catheter-related infection, severe mucositis, hypotension, or known MRSA. Give empiric antivirals only if obvious viral infection (dermatomal rash or chicken pox).

3) If patient is hypotensive, administer aggressive IV fluids and consider steroids; consider removing vascular access devices. Consider vasopressors.

•Disposition•

Generally, all patients with neutropenic fever are admitted.

B. Spinal Cord Compression

1) Epidural spinal cord compression results from direct compression of the cord by a tumor or by tumor involvement of the vascular supply; it may be the initial presentation of malignancy. Common malignancies producing spinal cord compression include lung cancer, prostate cancer, breast cancer, sarcoma, lymphoma and multiple myeloma.

2) Patients present with paraparesis, paraplegia, sensory deficits, ataxic gait, or urinary incontinence or retention. Pain is often the initial symptom and may be described as a deep ache; it is often continuous, progressive, and may increase with recumbency. The patient may have bony tenderness to palpation. Assess rectal tone.

3) Plain films may demonstrate erosion or vertebral body collapse; 30-50% of the bone must be destroyed before it is seen on x-ray. Consider bone scan or MRI.

4) Treat with high dose dexamethasone (20-100 mg) and pain medication. Consult hematology/oncology; consider emergency decompression (surgical), or radiation.

C. Superior Vena Cava Syndrome

1) Superior vena cava syndrome occurs when there is compression, invasion, or obstruction of the superior vena cava. Superior vena cava syndrome typically occurs with small cell lung cancer and lymphoma.

2) Patients may present with facial plethora, upper extremity edema, fatigue, headache, and shortness of breath. Symptoms are often worse upon awakening.

3) CXR may show an enlarged mediastinum; the mass is usually in the right hemithorax. Chest CT is diagnostic.

4) Assess and stabilize the airway. Establish IV, administer oxygen. Treatment includes furosemide, Solumedrol, and radiation.

*Other complications of malignancy include cardiac tamponade; hypercalcemia; SIADH; hyperviscosity syndrome; and adrenal insufficiency.

IV. SICKLE CELL DISEASE

•General•

1) Sickle cell disease results from abnormal hemoglobin synthesis, which causes RBCs to irreversibly sickle when the heme moiety is deoxygenated. Sickled cells produce thrombosis and small vessel occlusion, leading to various crises.

2) Patients who are homozygous for hemoglobin S have sickle cell disease; patients heterozygous for hemoglobin S have sickle cell trait (these patients are usually asymptomatic). Hemoglobin SC is a less severe variant; sickle-b-thalassemia is another variant of varying severity.

3) Patients typically have a chronic hemolytic anemia with Hgb 6-9 gm/

dL and reticulocyte count 5-15%.

•Clinical Presentation•

1) Vaso-occlusive pain crisis is the most common presentation, and patients have often had prior episodes of similar pain. Vaso-occlusive events affect virtually every organ system. Patients may have abdominal pain secondary to mesenteric or visceral infarcts. Neurologic deficits, seizures, or alterations in consciousness may indicate CVA.

2) Hematologic crises (aplastic anemia, splenic sequestration, or acute hemolysis) may present with fatigue, tachycardia, or shock.

3) Infection may present with fever; cough and dyspnea may indicate the acute chest syndrome.

4) Other findings may include icterus, splenomegaly (seen in younger children, but older children and adults typically have a small spleen, which results from recurrent infarction), and an inability to concentrate urine secondary to papillary necrosis.

•Evaluation•

1) Check CBC, reticulocyte count; consider type and screen. Consider LFTs in patients with abdominal pain. Check pulse oximetry. Obtain ECG if chest pain. Document any history of similar presentations.

2) Evaluate for any precipitating factors. If febrile, assume bacterial source, and consider blood cultures, urine culture, and CXR. One study suggested obtaining a CXR on all febrile patients with sickle cell disease, as many patients with positive CXR findings had normal physical exam findings.

3) Obtain CXR if any respiratory symptoms or low pulse oximetry. Consider head CT if any CNS findings. Consider x-ray or bone scan if localized bone tenderness (hip pain with difficulty ambulating may be caused by aseptic necrosis of the femoral head).

•Crises•

1) Vaso-occlusive Crisis

a) Crises occur because sickled RBCs sludge in the microcirculation and cause ischemic injury; the crisis may be precipitated by dehydration, cold weather, hypoxia, or infection. Document any history of similar pain crises.

b) In patients with musculoskeletal pain, consider possible osteomyelitis or avascular necrosis. Abdominal pain is typically diffuse and recurrent, but consider possible cholestasis, cholelithiasis, pancreatitis, or mesenteric infarction; cholelithiasis is a frequent complication, but cholecystitis is relatively rare. Dactylitis is hand or foot swelling from vaso-occlusion; it usually occurs in children, and treatment is supportive.

c) <u>The acute chest syndrome</u> refers to acute pulmonary disease in patients with sickle cell disease; it may be secondary to infectious or non-infectious causes, including pneumonia, pulmonary infarction, and pulmonary embolism. Patients may present with fever, pleuritic chest pain, dyspnea, hypoxia, cough, and possible pulmonary infiltrates on CXR.

d) CNS symptoms suggest infarction. There is an increased incidence of subarachnoid hemorrhage in patients with sickle cell disease.

2) Hematologic Crisis

a) <u>Acute splenic sequestration crisis</u> is secondary to impairment of blood outflow from the spleen from sickled red blood cells (this seldom occurs after age 6 years, as repeated splenic infarcts reduce the spleen to a small fibrous capsule); patients may present with abdominal discomfort, shock, tachycardia, and a sudden enlargement of the spleen with an acutely decreased hemoglobin. Platelets may also be decreased; the reticulocyte count is usually elevated. Treat with IVNS, oxygen, and packed RBCs.

b) <u>Aplastic crisis</u> may cause an anemia in which the reticulocyte count can be as low as 0.5%; the patient appears ill, pale, and is usually non-icteric (no evidence of hemolysis). Aplastic anemia is often caused by infection with Parvovirus B19. Consider treatment with packed RBCs or exchange transfusions (although spontaneous resolution often occurs within 5-10 days).

c) <u>Hemolytic crisis</u> presents with jaundice, decreased Hgb, and increased indirect bilirubin, LDH and reticulocyte count. It may be secondary to infection. Treat with transfusion.

3) Infectious Crisis

Sickle cell disease patients are functionally asplenic, and should be considered immunocompromised; patients are especially susceptible to encapsulated organisms such as S. pneumoniae and H. influenza. Patients may have pneumonia, pyelonephritis, or osteomyelitis (often due to Salmonella), among other infections.

•Treatment•

1) Consider establishing IV access; in order to avoid sodium overload, 0.5 normal saline is used for hydration (renal infarcts decrease the renal concentrating ability). Alternatively, consider oral hydration.

2) Provide analgesia (morphine is the preferred agent; meperidine has more side effects).

3) Administer oxygen only if the patient is hypoxic (oxygen use in nonhypoxic patients may result in suppressed red cell production).

4) If febrile, consider antibiotics.

5) If acute chest syndrome, administer oxygen, albuterol nebulizer, and broad-spectrum antibiotics. If pO2 is greater than 60 mmHg, consider simple transfusion; if pO2 is less than 60 mmHg, give an exchange transfusion.

6) If aplastic crisis or splenic sequestration, give a simple transfusion.

7) If acute ischemic stroke, administer an exchange transfusion to decrease the percent of sickle hemoglobin to less than 25%.

8) Patients with priapism should have their sickle cell hemoglobin reduced to less than 30% with either simple transfusion or exchange transfusion. Also, consult urology for possible corpora aspiration.

•Disposition•

Consider admission if febrile, persistent pain, if in crisis, or if patient appears toxic.

V. TTP (Thrombotic Thrombocytopenic Purpura)

•General•

1) TTP occurs after an inciting event that results in small vessel endothelial damage and platelet/fibrin deposition. It is more common in women.

2) TTP is related to hemolytic uremic syndrome, and is associated with pregnancy, infections, autoimmune diseases, and medications (some chemotherapy agents, ticlopidine, and oral contraceptives).

•Diagnosis•

The diagnosis is generally clinical. Criteria for diagnosis include (the full pentad is seen in only 40%):

1) Microangiopathic hemolytic anemia (with schistocytes and reticulocytosis). Diagnosis is doubtful if there are no schistocytes on smear. Hgb is <6 gm/dL in 30% of patients.
2) Platelets 5000-100,000. (Platelets are < 20,000 in 50% of patients).
3) Renal abnormality (insufficiency, hematuria, proteinuria, or azotemia).
4) Fever.
5) CNS abnormality (the most common complaint).

Other Lab Findings- Other findings may include increased direct bilirubin and LDH and a negative Coombs test. BUN/Cr is usually elevated. PT/PTT is usually normal. The reticulocyte count may be elevated. A DIC panel is usually normal. Urinalysis may show proteinuria and hematuria. Consider head CT. Check pregnancy test.

•Treatment•

1) Establish IV. Place patient on monitor. Administer oxygen.
2) Administer a plasma exchange transfusion with FFP. Use FFP (30 cc/kg) or packed RBCs in hemorrhage.
3) Avoid platelet transfusion (it may worsen the disease).
4) Consider Solumedrol 1 mg/kg and aspirin.

CHAPTER 13
INFECTIOUS DISEASE

I. CELLULITIS

*For impetigo- see Pediatric Infectious Disease

•General•

1) Cellulitis is an infection of the dermis and subcutaneous fat from bacteria that have penetrated breaks in the skin; it is usually caused by infection with group A Streptococcus or Staphylococcus aureus.

2) Erysipelas is a skin infection caused most often by group A Streptococcus through a portal of entry. Peripheral vascular disease is a risk factor.

•Clinical Presentation•

1) The infected skin is pink or red, warm, tender, edematous, and has ill-defined borders that merge smoothly with adjacent skin. High fever suggests bacteremia.

2) If the patient is systemically ill, has numbness in the affected area, color change from red to blue-grey, rapidly advancing border, or tendon or nerve impairment, consider possible necrotizing fasciitis.

3) In erysipelas, the involved skin is elevated, fiery red, indurated and hot, with plaques that are sharply demarcated. The onset of symptoms is usually abrupt, and accompanied by fever and malaise. Erysipelas usually occurs in the lower extremities.

•Evaluation•

1) Consider checking x-ray for gas, as it may indicate that tissues are devitalized and able to support anaerobic bacteria; films may also demonstrate osteomyelitis or foreign body. Ultrasound, CT, or MRI may also be beneficial in evaluating soft tissue. In general, labs and skin cultures are not helpful.

2) Document any presence of lymphangitic spread. Palpate for any tenderness, crepitus, or foreign body. Document neurologic function, distal pulses, and skin temperature.

•Treatment•

1) If the cellulitis is extensive or is complicated by chronic illness, con-

sider IV nafcillin, oxacillin, or cefazolin. If less severe, consider dicloxacillin, cephalexin, or clindamycin. If penicillin allergic, consider macrolides or advanced generation fluoroquinolones. If patient is diabetic, consider Unasyn to cover Staphylococcus, enteric gram negatives, and anaerobes.

2) If infected extremity, immobilize and elevate extremity.

3) If a necrotizing soft tissue infection is suspected, arrange emergent surgical consult for possible debridement; provide aggressive hemodynamic support; and administer broad spectrum antibiotics (e.g., clindamycin plus ceftriaxone).

4) Erysipelas: If mild, treat with oral penicillin. Otherwise, admit for IV penicillin or nafcillin.

5) Consider IV antibiotics for head/neck cellulitis.

•Disposition•

Admit if involvement of >50% of limb or torso, or if 10% of body surface is involved. Also, consider admission if coexisting IDDM, CHF, fever, chronic renal failure, rapidly advancing cellulitis, immunosuppression, impaired nerve function, or failed outpatient treatment

II. DIARRHEA

*See Chapter 10

III. ENDOCARDITIS

•General•

Acute disease more commonly infects previously normal valves (the etiology is often S. aureus); subacute disease infects abnormal valves (the etiology is often S. viridans).

•Clinical Presentation•

1) Acute infection presents as sepsis with or without cardiac failure.

2) Patients may have CNS symptoms secondary to aseptic meningoencephalitis or embolization of vegetations.

3) Subacute disease presents with intermittent fever, malaise, and weight loss.

4) Bacterial meningitis is seen in up to 30% of patients with right-sided disease.

•Evaluation•

1) Check CBC, platelets, ESR, electrolytes, BUN/Cr, and at least 2 sets of blood cultures. Check ECG, CXR, and echocardiogram (transesophageal echocardiogram is preferred).

2) Diagnostic criteria include positive blood cultures and vegetations on echocardiogram.

3) Physical findings suggestive of endocarditis include a new or changed murmur, Osler nodes (tender nodules on tips of toes and fingers), Janeway lesions (nontender plaques on soles and palms), petechiae, and splinter hemorrhages in nails.

•Treatment•

1) Establish IV; administer oxygen; place patient on monitor.

2) Administer antibiotics: if acute disease, administer gentamicin plus vancomycin; if subacute disease, administer ceftriaxone. If prosthetic valve, administer vancomycin plus gentamicin.

3) Treat any complications (e.g., CHF).

4) Admit patient.

IV. EPIDIDYMITIS

*See Chapter 11

V. HERPES ZOSTER

•General•

Herpes zoster occurs when dormant varicella in dorsal nerve roots becomes reactivated. Patients with zoster may develop post-herpetic neuralgia in the distribution of the rash, which can be chronic and severe.

•Diagnosis•

1) The typical rash consists of red vesicular lesions usually limited to one or two dermatomes; it may slightly cross over the midline. The rash may become disseminated.

2) The rash is often painful, and the pain may precede the dermatitis by 7-10 days.

3) If there is involvement of the first division of the 5th cranial nerve, perform a slit lamp exam to evaluate for possible corneal involvement (fluorescein staining will demonstrate a focal dendritic pattern).

•Treatment•

1) Treat all patients older than 13 years with acyclovir (800 mg five times/day for 7 days) or famcyclovir or valacyclovir; it must be started within 48-72h to shorten the duration of the acute infection and associated symptoms. Also, treat all patients (including children) if there is involvement of the first division of the 5th cranial nerve. Anti-virals do not appear to alleviate post-herpetic neuralgia. (Children generally don't get post-herpetic neuralgia). Oral steroids do not prevent post-herpetic neuralgia.

2) If the first division of the 5th cranial nerve is involved, obtain an ophthalmology consult and consider IV acyclovir. If there is corneal involvement, treat with Viroptic eye drops 1 drop every 2h (max 9 drops/d).

3) If severe infection or if the patient is immunocompromised, consider IV acyclovir and admission.

4) Topical steroids or acyclovir ointment are probably of no benefit; Calamine lotion may provide symptomatic relief. Avoid neomycin, as it may cause a severe dermatitis.

VI. HIV- Related Illnesses

A. CNS Disease

•Etiology/Clinical Presentation/Treatment•

*Consider obtaining head CT (consider adding sinus cuts) if patient presents with a new or worsening headache, mental status changes, or fever. Consider performing LP (in addition to regular CSF studies, send fluid for VDRL, India Ink, cryptococcal antigen, and fungal and AFB cultures).

1) **CMV-** CMV may involve the cerebral hemispheres or spinal cord and cause multifocal inflammatory polyneuropathy, inflammatory myositis and retinitis. Check head CT and LP. Treatment is usually ganciclovir or foscarnet.

2) **CNS lymphoma-** Patients with lymphoma typically present with symptoms lasting days to weeks; headache and confusion are common, and patients occasionally have fever. Head CT shows enhancing linear lesions.

3) **Cryptococcus**- Patients may present with mild headache or fulminant meningitis; headache and fever are present in two-thirds of patients. Head CT may demonstrate ring-enhancing lesions with surrounding edema. Obtain CSF and serum cryptococcal antigens (other CSF indices may be normal). Consider obtaining CSF India ink test. Treat with anti-fungals.

4) **Herpes Encephalitis**- Patients may present with confusion, aphasia, apraxia, and fever (behavioral symptoms predominate if infection is in the usual frontotemporal location). Check head CT and LP. Treat with acyclovir.

5) **Progressive multifocal leukoencephalopathy**- It is caused by the JC virus, and is a disease of the white matter of the brain. Patients present with progressive slowing of mentation to abulia. Attempt to exclude other etiologies with CT and LP.

6) **Toxoplasmosis**- Patients usually have a CD4 count <100 cells/uL. A severe frontal headache and fever are present in 50% of patients; a majority have a focal CNS finding on physical exam. Head CT shows multiple hypodense ring-enhancing lesions with surrounding edema. Do not do LP; get serum antibodies. Treat with pyrimethamine and sulfadiazine.

7) **Tuberculosis**- Tuberculosis may cause subacute or chronic meningitis and obstructive hydrocephalus. Head CT may show brain abscesses with surrounding edema.

B. Ophthalmologic Disease

•Etiology/Clinical Presentation/Treatment•

1) **CMV**- Patients may present with floaters, visual field cuts and blurred vision. Fundi may have hemorrhages, cotton wool spots or diffuse whitening. It is usually seen with CD4 count <100 cells/uL. CMV may lead to rapid visual loss. Treat with antivirals and prompt ophthalmologic consult.

2) **Varicella**- Fluorescein may show dendritic branching. Treat with antivirals.

C. Pulmonary Disease

•Etiology/Clinical Presentation/Treatment•

1) **PCP**- Patients present with an insidious onset of dyspnea, dry, persistent cough, intermittent fever, and tachypnea. CXR findings are variable, but may show diffuse bilateral interstitial pneumonia, especially perihilar and basilar. Check ABG, as patient may be hypoxemic and there is often a marked A-a gradient. CD4 count is usually <250 cells/uL. There is often an elevated LDH.

Treatment- Oral options include Bactrim DS 2 qid; or dapsone 100 mg/d plus TMP 20 mg/kg/d divided every 6h; consider clindamycin plus primaquine. Parenteral options include TMP-SMX 15-20 mg/kg/d (based on trimethoprim) or pentamidine 4 mg/kg IV qd. Consider additional coverage for typical pathogens. Admit if patient is acutely ill or pO2 <70. If pO2 <70 or A-a gradient >35, give 40 mg Solumedrol bid (an inflammatory response is needed to maintain PCP). 50% of patients have a reactive airway disease component, so administer bronchodilators. Consider furosemide, as it often improves oxygenation with severe PCP.

2) **TB**- If low CD4 count, TB is more likely to present atypically with primary TB (rather than reactivation TB), with the CXR demonstrating lower and middle lobe infiltrates (cavitation is unusual).

3) **Other causes of pneumonia**- cryptococcus, coccidiomycosis, histoplasmosis, Kaposi's sarcoma, and everyday pathogens seen in patients who are not immunocompromised.

D. Drug reactions

AZT- It may cause anemia or neutropenia.

Dapsone- It may cause methemoglobinemia or hemolytic anemia.

Didanosine, Zalcitabine- It may cause pancreatitis or peripheral neuropathy.

Pentamidine- It may cause pneumothorax, hypotension, and profound arrhythmias.

Protease inhibitor indinavir- It may cause nephrolithiasis.

VII. INFLUENZA

•**General**•

1) Influenza viruses are classified into type A, type B, and type C. Influenza A viruses are responsible for most hospitalizations; however,

influenza A and B are clinically indistinguishable. Influenza C does not cause typical influenza symptoms. Influenza viruses cause annual epidemics that affect all age groups, and have the potential to cause pandemics.

2) Influenza is transmitted by respiratory secretions; there is an incubation period of 1-3 days after exposure.

•Clinical Presentation•

1) Patients often have an abrupt onset of high-grade fever, severe malaise, myalgias, headache and URI symptoms (rhinorrhea, congestion, sore throat, and cough). GI symptoms, if present, are usually minor.

2) Primary influenza pneumonia may present with respiratory failure; it usually occurs on day 3-5 of illness.

3) Infection with influenza predisposes individuals to secondary bacterial infections. Bacterial pneumonia typically occurs 5-10 days after the influenza infection, and is often secondary to S. aureus, S. pneumoniae, or H. influenzae.

•Evaluation•

1) Check pulse oximetry. Consider CXR (which is usually normal).

2) Diagnosis is usually clinical.

3) Diagnosis can be confirmed with a nasal swab culture or rapid antigen detection tests.

•Treatment•

1) Antiviral medications include amantadine (100 mg bid for 7d; 100 mg qd in the elderly; 5 mg/kg/d up to 150 mg in children) and rimantadine (100 mg bid for 7d), which are active only against influenza A. These drugs may also be used for prophylaxis of influenza.

2) Newer antivirals include the neuramindase inhibitors, which are active against both influenza A and B. Zanamivir (Relenza) is administered as 2 inhalations bid for 5d in patients older than 12 years; oseltamivir (Tamiflu) is administered 75 mg bid for 5d in patients older than 18 years. These drugs are only useful if begun within 48 hours of the onset of symptoms. Studies indicate that these medications may reduce the duration of symptoms.

3) Vaccination is recommended for individuals over age 50, nursing home

residents, pregnant women, individuals with cardiopulmonary or renal comorbidities, immunocompromised patients, and health care providers.

VIII. MENINGITIS

•Etiology• (bacterial)

Neonate- Group B streptococcus, E. coli, Listeria.

5-12 weeks of age- Group B streptococcus, E coli, Listeria, S. pneumoniae, H flu.

13 weeks - 6 years old- N. meningitis, S. pneumoniae, TB, H flu.

6 years old - 40 years old- N. meningitis, S. pneumoniae, H. flu, TB.

>40 years old- S. pneumoniae, N. meningitis, H. flu.

Elderly- Listeria.

Head trauma/post neurosurgical procedure- Pseudomonas, enterobacteriacae, S. aureus.

CSF shunts- S. epidermidis.

*Due to the effective vaccine, the incidence of H. flu has decreased dramatically.

•Clinical Presentation•

1) Patients may present with fever, headache, vomiting, malaise, photophobia, mental status change, or nuchal rigidity. Seizures may occur; cranial nerve palsies may be present. While symptoms may develop rapidly, many patients develop symptoms over 1-7 days.

2) Patients may have petechia or the purpuric rash of meningococcemia.

•Differential Diagnosis•

1) If fever and focal CNS signs predominate, consider brain abscess or toxoplasmosis.

2) Also, consider **viral encephalitis**, which may present with mental status changes, seizures or movement disorders. Viral encephalitis typically presents with fever and signs of meningeal involvement such as headache and photophobia, but usually without sensorimotor deficits.

3) Also, consider subarachnoid hemorrhage.

•Evaluation•

1) Check CBC, PT/PTT, electrolytes, glucose, blood cultures, and CSF.

Consider CSF latex agglutination if the patient is currently being treated with antibiotics.

2) Consider obtaining head CT prior to performing LP to exclude other pathology; a CT is mandatory if there are focal CNS signs, papilledema, or focal seizures.

3) Document the neurologic exam and examine the skin for rash. Kernig's sign is bilateral pain and increased resistance to extending knees with hip flexed; Brudzinski's sign is flexion of hips and knees after examiner flexes patient's neck.

CSF

1) Normal CSF has 0-5 WBCs, 0-15% PMNs, glucose 45-65 mg/dL, protein 20-45 mg/dL.

2) Bacterial meningitis shows >1000 WBCs, 90% PMNs. CSF glucose <40 mg/dL or CSF glucose/blood glucose ratio <0.3-0.5 suggests bacterial infection, as does protein >150-170 mg/dL. However, some patients with bacterial meningitis have a predominance of lymphocytes on the initial CSF and only mild changes in glucose/protein. In some cases, the CSF may initially be normal.

3) Viral meningitis shows 100-1000 WBCs, <50% PMNs, glucose 45-65 mg/dL (normal), protein 50-100 mg/dL (slightly elevated); PMNs may predominate in the first 48h and lymphocytes predominate thereafter. There are no bacteria.

4) In AIDS patients, consider obtaining CSF cryptococcal antigen, which is more sensitive than India ink stain for cryptococcal meningitis.

5) In a traumatic LP, there are approximately 1000 RBCs for every 1-2 WBCs. Also, a traumatic LP usually clears. Or:
Number of WBCs introduced/cc = [(Peripheral WBC) x (CSF RBCs)]/(Peripheral RBCs).

6) A Gram stain has a 60-90% sensitivity.

•Treatment• (for bacterial meningitis in adults)

1) If bacterial meningitis is seriously considered, administer antibiotics immediately, and obtain LP as soon as possible (a delay in performing an LP beyond a few hours reduces the likelihood of positive cultures by 20-30%; however, cell counts, morphologies, and CSF protein and glucose generally do not change for up to 24 h after IV anti-

biotics).

2) Antibiotic options include ceftriaxone 2 g IV or cefotaxime 2 g IV; consider adding vancomycin (for resistant pneumococcus). If penicillin allergic, consider chloramphenicol plus vancomycin, ± aztreonam. Consider adding ampicillin 2 g IV for the treatment of Listeria in the elderly, pregnant women, or immunocompromised patients.

3) Steroids decrease the inflammatory response in meningitis. Consider dexamethasone 10 mg IV, which may decrease hearing loss in patients with H. flu or S. pneumoniae meningitis; however, steroids may decrease CSF penetration of antibiotics. Dexamethasone should be administered before the first dose of antibiotics; do not give dexamethasone in patients younger than 6 weeks.

4) Patients are generally admitted. If viral meningitis is obvious (classic CSF findings and viral rash in late summer), consider discharge; otherwise, consider admission for IV antibiotics and possible repeat LP in 12-24h.

IX. OTITIS EXTERNA

•Risk Factors•
Risk factors include swimming, cotton-tipped applicators, and eczema.

•Clinical Presentation•
1) The patient presents with an inflamed external canal, and may have significant exudates.
2) Typically, the patient has pain with external ear movement.

•Treatment•
1) Cortisporin drops (neomycin and steroid) 4 drops every 6h x 10d; if sulfa-allergic administer genoptic drops and neodecadron drops. Continue antibiotics for 2-3 days after cessation of symptoms. 10% of people are sensitive to neomycin; ophthalmic antibiotics are pH-adjusted and thus cause less burning in patients with tubes or perforated tympanic membranes.

2) If the external canal is occluded, place a wick or twist of cotton into the external canal, and instruct patient to instil antibiotic drops onto the wick. If a wick is not placed, clean and irrigate ears with acetic acid drops (Domeboro Otic solution) tid before administering antibi-

otics.

3) Avoid water in ear.

4) Unless there is cellulitis or a concurrent otitis media, systemic antibiotics are not indicated.

5) Diabetics and other immunocompromised patients are at risk for malignant otitis externa (usually caused by pseudomonas). Patients present with severe ear pain and purulent drainage. CT may demonstrate osteomyelitis of the base of the skull or mastoid. Patients with malignant otitis externa are generally admitted; administer ceftazidime or piperacillin, and obtain an urgent ENT consult.

6) If symptoms are unresponsive to antibiotics, consider otomycosis. Treat with solution of clotrimazole and acetic acid.

X. PHARYNGITIS

•General•

1) Pharyngitis is an infection of the posterior pharynx, which may include the tonsils.

2) The majority of cases have a viral etiology. It is important to exclude other more dangerous etiologies of sore throat (e.g., epiglottitis, peritonsillar abscess, and retropharyngeal abscess), and to diagnose group A beta-hemolytic streptococcus (GABHS) infection.

3) Potential complications of GABHS include rheumatic fever and glomerulonephritis.

4) GABHS occurs in <10% of adult cases of pharyngitis and <30% of pediatric cases of pharyngitis; it is rare in children <3 years old.

•Clinical Presentation•

1) It may be difficult to distinguish bacterial from viral etiology on clinical presentation in patients with sore throat. Erythema and lymphadenopathy are sensitive, but nonspecific, indicators of GABHS. Temperature >101°F and exudate are more specific, but less sensitive, indicators of GABHS. Cough is very infrequent with GABHS.

2) Patients with GABHS may have a scarlet fever rash.

3) Chlamydia and mycoplasma most commonly present as headache, pharyngitis, and lower respiratory symptoms. Consider gonorrhea, diphtheria, and syphilis.

•Evaluation•

1) Consider obtaining a rapid strep test (80% sensitive) and throat culture (95% sensitive).

2) Attempt to rule out other pathology, including epiglottitis and peritonsillar abscess; consider the heterophile test for mononucleosis.

•Treatment•

1) If epiglottitis, peritonsillar abscess, retropharyngeal abscess, and gonorrhea have been excluded, consider treatment for GABHS. Options include treating empirically for GABHS, obtaining cultures and treating if positive, or treating empirically and obtaining cultures if there is a concern of spread to siblings, etc.

2) Antibiotic options include Bicillin CR 2.4 million U IM x 1; 1.2 million U IM in children (it has procaine which gives an initial bolus and benzathine which sustains levels). Or, benzathine 1.2 million U IM x 1 (if >60 lbs) or 600,000 U IM (<60lbs); or Pen VK 500 mg TID x 10d (250 mg tid if younger than 12 years); or erythromycin 333 mg tid (in children erythromycin estolate 20-40 mg/kg/d divided tid); or clarithromycin 500 mg bid. Antibiotics are effective in preventing rheumatic fever if given within 9 days of symptoms; antibiotics are not effective in preventing glomerulonephritis, which occurs within 10 days.

3) Steroids (10 mg dexamethasone IM or PO) may help relieve pain and decrease swelling in uncomplicated pharyngitis.

XI. PNEUMONIA

A. Pneumonia

•Etiology • (bacterial)

Community acquired

Typical pathogens: S. pneumoniae (most common), M. catarrhalis, H. influenzae (especially in the elderly, diabetics and COPD patients), S. aureus, and gram negative rods. In older patients, consider S. aureus, Klebsiella, anaerobes, and Pseudomonas.

Atypical pathogens: Legionella, Mycoplasma, and Chlamydia (especially in young patients).

Nosocomial

Gram-negative rods (Klebsiella, Pseudomonas, E. coli), S. aureus, anaerobes, H. flu, S. pneumoniae, and Chlamydia.

•Risk Factors•

Risk factors include alcoholism, asthma, immunosuppression, heart disease, institutionalization, and advanced age.

Risk Factors for Specific Bacterial Agents

<u>H. influenzae/M. catarrhalis</u>: risk factors include smoking or chronic pulmonary disease.

<u>Penicillin-resistant s. pneumoniae</u>: risk factors include advanced age, nursing home patients, alcoholism, immunosuppression, or recent use of beta lactam antibiotics.

<u>Gram-negative Enterobacteriacae</u>: risk factors include advanced age, nursing home patients, alcoholism, or immunosuppression.

<u>Pseudomonas</u>: risk factors include chronic pulmonary disease with chronic broad-spectrum antibiotic use.

•Clinical Presentation•

1) Typically, patients with pneumonia present with fever, cough and dyspnea; purulent sputum does not distinguish between bacterial and viral infections. Crackles are present in 80% of patients with pneumonia. Viral pneumonia may produce coryza, hoarseness, and myalgias.

2) Mycoplasma and Chlamydia usually present with a dry cough. Mycoplasma presents as a flu-like illness with headache, malaise, fever, dry cough, pharyngeal erythema and scattered rales; it may be associated with diarrhea. Mycoplasma generally presents as a bronchitis, whereas Chlamydia is more likely to be pneumonia. Chlamydia usually presents with constitutional and URI symptoms, followed 3-7 days later by symptoms generally limited to the lower respiratory tract; rales and rhonchi are almost always present.

3) A single rigor and rust-colored sputum suggest S. pneumoniae.

4) The elderly often lack cough or fever, and may present with nonspecific complaints such as confusion, weakness, or functional decline.

5) It is generally impossible to differentiate typical from atypical pneumonia from symptoms alone.

•Evaluation•

1) In healthy adults (excluding the elderly) who present with an acute cough illness, pneumonia is unlikely if the patient has normal vital signs (including pulse oximetry), and normal lung sounds; purulent sputum does not indicate a bacterial etiology. These patients generally do not require further evaluation, and should be diagnosed as an acute viral bronchitis, and treated with albuterol inhalers (antibiotics are not recommended).

2) If bacterial pneumonia is suspected, check CXR. Consider checking CBC (although CBC may be normal) and electrolytes; consider blood and sputum cultures. Check pulse oximetry; consider ABG. Consider urinary antigen testing for Legionella.

CXR

It is difficult to attribute radiographic features to specific infectious agents. However, general patterns exist:

1) Viral influenza is characterized by perihilar, interstitial, symmetric, and bilateral infiltrates without pleural effusions.

2) A small effusion suggests H. flu; a massive effusion suggests group A Streptococcus. S. aureus or S. pneumoniae may produce effusions.

3) Mycoplasma has a varied pattern that may include unilateral or multifocal infiltrates or interstitial pattern; there is usually little or no effusion.

4) Lobar infiltrates suggest S. pneumoniae or Klebsiella; patchy multifocal infiltrates suggest S. aureus, mycoplasma, H. flu, or a viral infection.

5) Lung abscesses are generally caused by S. aureus or Klebsiella.

•Treatment•

1) Consider albuterol inhaler and oxygen therapy.

2) If clinically indicated, consider intubation or BiPAP.

3) Patients diagnosed with acute bronchitis (not pneumonia) should be treated with bronchodilators; antibiotic therapy is not recommended. However, a prolonged cough in patients with bronchitis may indicate pertussis, and antimicrobial therapy should be considered for patients at risk for exposure to pertussis (e.g., during outbreaks); therapy is recommended to decrease the spread of pertussis, as antibiotics do

not improve symptoms if started 7-10 days after the onset of the illness.

4) Antibiotic Options for Community-Acquired Pneumonia

a) Initial antibiotic therapy for community-acquired pneumonia should include coverage for the most common typical pathogens (S. pneumoniae, H. influenzae, and M. catarrhalis), as well as atypical pathogens (M. pneumoniae, C. pneumoniae, and Legionella).

b) <u>For empiric outpatient treatment</u>: if otherwise healthy, consider monotherapy with azithromycin, clarithromycin, moxifloxacin, levofloxacin, gatifloxacin or doxycycline.

c) <u>For empiric inpatient treatment</u>: consider combination therapy with either a 2nd or 3rd generation cephalosporin (ceftriaxone is preferred) or a b-lactam/b-lactamase inhibitor, plus azithromycin IV; or monotherapy with IV levofloxacin or gatifloxacin.

d) <u>If patient requires ICU</u>, consider ceftriaxone IV plus levofloxacin IV plus/minus an aminoglycoside; or ceftriaxone IV plus azithromycin IV plus/minus an anti-pseudomonal agent.

e) <u>If nursing home patient or chronic alcoholic</u>, consider monotherapy with levofloxacin IV or combination therapy with ceftriaxone IV plus azithromycin IV.

f) <u>If severe infection in a patient with structural lung disease</u>, pseudomonas should be covered. Consider levofloxacin IV plus cefepime IV plus an aminoglycoside; or, consider azithromycin IV plus ciprofloxacin IV plus an aminoglycoside IV

g) <u>If suspected aspiration</u>, consider ceftriaxone IV plus azithromycin IV plus clindamycin IV; or levofloxacin IV plus either clindamycin IV, ticarcillin/clavulanate IV, or ampicillin-sulbactam IV.

h) <u>If the patient is immunocompromised</u>, consider levofloxacin IV plus vancomycin IV; or consider ceftriaxone IV plus vancomycin IV plus azithromycin IV.

i) Macrolides provide excellent atypical coverage, but S. pneumoniae is increasingly resistant; erythromycin has poor H. flu coverage. Doxycycline has excellent atypical coverage, but S. pneumoniae and H. flu have increasing resistance. Beta lactams have good S. pneumoniae, staph, H. flu and anaerobic coverage but do not cover atypicals. Cephalosporins do not cover atypicals. Bactrim has good gram-negative rod coverage, but poor atypical coverage and S. pneumoniae and H. flu are increasingly resistant.

j) S. pneumoniae has increasing resistance to penicillin, beta-lactamase inhibitors (Unasyn) and macrolides.

•Disposition•

Consider admission if pO2 <60, abnormal vital signs, elderly, acute comorbidity, new mental status change, absolute neutrophil count <1000, BUN >30, or sodium <130 mEq/L.

B. Aspiration Pneumonia

1) Aspiration usually results from impaired airway protection (altered level of consciousness or abnormal swallowing). Aspiration of gastric contents may result in a chemical pneumonitis, causing obstruction, ventilation-perfusion mismatch, and significant hypoxia (often within minutes). Secondary bacterial infection often follows.

2) Community acquired aspiration may involve both aerobes and anaerobes; nosocomial infection may involve anaerobes, Pseudomonas, and methicillin resistant Staphylococcus.

3) On CXR, the posterior segment of the right upper lobe and the superior segment of the right lower lobe are most commonly involved; the right middle lobe and lingula are not commonly involved, as these branch anteriorly from the bronchial tree, and patients usually aspirate when they are supine.

4) Prophylactic antibiotics may cause superinfection, but start antibiotics (consider clindamycin, Unasyn, or 3rd generation cephalosporin; consider adding amikacin to cover Pseudomonas) if new fever, new or expanding infiltrate >36h after aspiration, leukocytosis, purulent sputum, if patient deteriorates, or if small bowel obstruction and suspected aspiration of fecal material. Steroids are not helpful.

C. Specific Pathogens

1) H. flu- H. flu is more common in COPD patients and alcoholics. Patients often present with sudden onset fever, cough with sputum production, and dyspnea. CXR may show multi-lobar infiltrates with effusions. Treat with fluoroquinolones.

2) Klebsiella- Klebsiella usually occurs in nursing home patients and alcoholics; it may occur in COPD patients. It often presents as sudden onset of cough productive of "currant jelly" sputum, rigors, and malaise. CXR may show a lobar infiltrate. Treat with a third generation cephalosporin or extended spectrum quinolone.

3) **M. catarrhalis**- It is more common in COPD patients. It often presents with a one-week prodrome of cough with sputum production, and fever. CXR may show diffuse infiltrates or lobar consolidation. Treat with macrolides, quinolones, second and third generation cephalosporins, extended spectrum penicillins, or Bactrim.

4) **Pseudomonas**- Pseudomonas often produces a severe, rapidly progressing disease, usually in elderly, immunocompromised or institutionalized patients. CXR may show bilateral lower lobe streaky infiltrates and effusions. Treat with ceftazidime and an aminoglycoside.

5) **S. aureus**- S. aureus occurs most frequently in IV drug abusers, COPD patients, and post-influenza. Patients often present with gradual onset of dyspnea, fever, and purulent sputum. CXR may show multilobar infiltrates and effusions. Treat with penicillinase resistant antibiotics and, if severe, vancomycin.

6) **S. pneumoniae**- It is the most common etiology of community acquired pneumonia. Patients may present with sudden onset of fever, cough, a single rigor, and rust-colored sputum. It is associated with lobar or segmental pneumonia; CXR may also demonstrate a pleural effusion and 'round' infiltrates. Treat with macrolides or extended spectrum quinolones; consider vancomycin if severe.

7) **Tuberculosis (TB)**- TB can result in latent or active infection. Latent infection is more common, and may become reactivated secondary to immunological stress. Asymptomatic patients with latent infection are not contagious. Active disease may present with fever, cough, hemoptysis, weight loss, and night sweats. Diagnosis is generally with sputum and CXR. Primary pulmonary TB often presents with lower lobe infiltrates and moderate pleural effusions. Reactivation TB often presents with bilateral apical infiltrates and cavitations without lower lobe infiltrates or effusions. Initial 4 drug therapy is usually recommended (isoniazid, rifampin, ethambutol, and pyrazinamide).

8) **Atypical Pathogens**

Atypical pneumonias are often relatively benign infections. They usually present with an insidious onset of low-grade fever, nonproductive cough, constitutional symptoms, and a protracted clinical course. If the patient demonstrates extrapulmonary symptoms, consider atypical pathogens, as no typical bacterial pneumonias are associated with extrapulmonary symptoms. Pharyngitis favors Mycoplasma or Chlamydia and makes Legionnaire's disease unlikely; earache is associated with Mycoplasma. Diarrhea is associated Mycoplasma and Legionnaire's disease. Also, a pulse-temperature deficit (relative bradycardia) often occurs with Legionnaire's disease.

a) <u>Chlamydia Pneumoniae</u>- It most often presents with mild symptoms of sore throat followed by a cough with fever. CXR may show subsegmental infiltrates. Treat with macrolides or extended spectrum quinolones.

b) <u>Legionnaire's Disease</u>- It is most likely to present as a severe community acquired pneumonia, usually during the summer in the elderly. It is associated with cardiopulmonary disease, post-surgical transplant patients, altered mental status, elevated transaminases, hyponatremia, and hypophosphatemia. It may present as a mild cough with low-grade fever, or as fulminant respiratory distress with multisystem organ failure; there is often a relative bradycardia. Patients often present with malaise, headache, abdominal pain, vomiting, and diarrhea. CXR may show a patchy localized infiltrate; one-third of patients have effusions. Consider urine antigen testing for diagnosis. Treat with erythromycin 1 gm every 6h (however, erythromycin may cause ototoxicity, so consider azithromycin 500 mg IV/po or levofloxacin 500 mg IV/po).

c) <u>Mycoplasma Pneumoniae</u>- It is more common in children and young adults, and occurs throughout the year. It is usually associated with an insidious onset of cough, malaise, pharyngitis, and headache. The patient generally appears nontoxic; the otoscopic exam may reveal bullous myringitis. CXR may show unilateral infiltrates or patchy multifocal infiltrates; there may be hilar adenopathy or effusions. Most cases resolve after several weeks. Treat with macrolides or extended spectrum quinolones.

XII. RHEUMATIC FEVER

•General•

1) Rheumatic fever results from group A streptococcal infection, and causes cardiac damage (especially valvular).
2) Rheumatic fever also involves the skin, joints, and CNS.
3) Rheumatic fever occurs about 2 1/2 weeks after a streptococcal infection, and virtually always in patients younger than 30 years old; the peak incidence is 5-15 years old. The incidence of rheumatic fever has declined significantly.

•Evaluation•

1) Check CBC, ECG, CXR, and ESR; consider echocardiogram.
2) Evaluate for new murmur or CHF.

•Diagnosis•

Jones criteria

Major Criteria- carditis, polyarthritis, chorea, erythema marginatum, and subcutaneous nodules.

Minor Criteria- fever, arthralgias, elevated ESR, prolonged PR interval.

*The diagnosis requires 2 major criteria or 1 major plus 2 minor criteria. The patient may also have supportive evidence (recent scarlet fever, throat culture positive for group A Strep, increased ASO).

•Treatment•

Treatment includes penicillin, aspirin, and, if carditis, prednisone.

XIII. SEXUALLY TRANSMITTED DISEASES

A. Pelvic Inflammatory Disease (PID)

•General•

1) PID refers to a spectrum of infections that ascend from the female genital tract, and includes endometritis, salpingitis, tubo-ovarian abscess, and peritonitis.
2) PID is most commonly associated with Chlamydia and N. gonorrhea. Other bacteria include Bacteroides, E. coli, H. influenzae, Mycoplasma, and Gardnerella.

•Diagnosis•

The minimum criteria for diagnosis include lower abdominal tenderness, adnexal tenderness, **and** cervical motion tenderness; additional minor criteria include temperature >38.3°C, vaginal discharge, elevated erythrocyte sedimentation rate, and elevated C-reactive protein.

•Clinical Presentation•

1) Unless an abscess is present, most patients report diffuse pelvic pain and bilateral abdominal and adnexal tenderness. Patients may have a vaginal discharge and fever.

2) N. gonorrhea/Chlamydia occur more frequently during the first week after the onset of menses; PID is much less likely if the patient is postmenopausal or on oral contraceptive pills. Pregnancy is protective against acquiring new pelvic infections.

3) Chlamydia is asymptomatic in 80% of women. The incubation period is 1-3 weeks; cervicitis is the most common presentation, which may progress to PID.

4) Endocervicitis is the most common presentation of gonorrhea; 20% of patients have retrograde spread, which may result in PID (salpingitis, endometritis, tubo-ovarian abscess, or a perihepatitis known as Fitz-Hugh-Curtis syndrome).

5) Disseminated N. gonorrhea may present with petechial or pustular lesions (usually on the distal extremities), asymmetric arthralgias, fever, endocarditis, tenosynovitis, and septic arthritis.

•Evaluation•

1) Check cervical cultures, urinalysis, CBC, wet prep, and pregnancy test. 95% of patients with PID have a cervical os that is leaking pus. Consider ultrasound for evaluation of possible tubo-ovarian abscess.

2) Consider evaluation for other STDs, including HIV and syphilis.

•Treatment•

1) PID

    a) <u>Hospitalized</u>: Cefoxitin 2 g IV q6h or cefotetan 2 g IV q12h; either one plus doxycycline 100 mg IV q12h. Alternate: clindamycin 900 mg IV q8h plus gentamicin 2 mg/kg IV.

    b) <u>Outpatient</u>: Ceftriaxone 250 mg IM once plus doxycycline 100 mg bid x 14d; or ofloxacin 400 mg bid x 14d plus either metronidazole 500 mg bid x 14d or clindamycin 450 mg qid x 14d; or azithromycin 500 mg IV followed by 250 mg po qd x 7d.

2) Urethritis, cervicitis, proctitis (treat for both Chlamydia and N.

gonorrhea):

a) <u>Chlamydia</u>: Azithromycin 1 gm po once; or doxycycline 100 mg bid x 7d; or ofloxacin 300 mg bid x 7d; if pregnant, erythromycin 500 mg qid x 7d or amoxicillin 500 mg tid x 10d or azithromycin.

b) <u>N. Gonorrhea</u>: Ceftriaxone 125 mg IM once; or ciprofloxacin 500 mg po once or ofloxacin 400 mg po once. If bacteremia, arthritis, or disseminated GC: ceftriaxone 1 g IV qd x 2-3d, followed by ciprofloxacin.

•Disposition•

1) Have a low threshold for treatment.

2) Admit if possible appendicitis or ectopic pregnancy, suspected abscess, pregnant, adolescent, HIV positive, or failed outpatient treatment (some advocate inpatient treatment for all, to avoid later complications).

3) Uncomplicated cases do not need follow-up cultures.

4) Instruct patient to avoid intercourse until symptoms have resolved and antibiotic therapy has been completed. Instruct patient to advise all partners to be tested.

B. Other STDs

1) **Bacterial Vaginosis-** It is associated with Gardnerella vaginalis and anaerobic bacteria. Patients present with a malodorous discharge with fishy odor. The pH of the discharge is >4.5, and has a positive amine odor test and the presence of clue cells. Treat with metronidazole gel 0.75% 5 g intravaginally bid x 5d or Clindamycin 2% cream 5 g intravaginally qhs x 7d; or metronidazole 2 gm once, or 500 mg bid x 7d.

2) **Chancroid-** It is an ulcerative disease caused by H. ducreyi. Patients present with a very painful ulcer with lymphadenopathy; in men, it usually occurs on the penis. Treat with ceftriaxone 250 mg IM once or azithromycin 1 gm x 1 or ciprofloxacin 500 mg bid x 3d.

3) **Human Papilloma Virus-** It may cause condyloma acuminata; refer patient to a dermatologist.

4) **Herpes Simplex-** HSV-1 is the cause of genital herpes in 15% of cases, HSV-2 causes the rest. It is transmitted from secretions or infectious lesions, and has an incubation period of 2-16 days; asymp-

tomatic shedding occurs in 1-8% of patients. Local paresthesias and irritation occur 12-48h prior to the appearance of tender, grouped, small vesicles with a red base. In women, lesions are located on vulva/vagina and are weeping, shallow, ulcerated, and usually without vesicles. In men, vesicles are typically located at the base of the scrotum. Treat first episode with acyclovir 400 mg (800 mg if proctitis) tid x 10d or valacyclovir 1 gm bid x 10d; treat recurrent disease with acyclovir 400 mg tid x 5d or 800 mg bid x 5d, or valacyclovir 500 mg bid x 5d. Prevent recurrence with acyclovir 400 mg bid or valacyclovir 500 mg qd.

5) **Lymphogranuloma Venereum**- It results from Chlamydia, and is rare. Initial lesions are similar to HSV, then a painful lymphadenopathy develops with fever and malaise. Over 1-3 weeks, the nodes enlarge into bubos. Treat with doxycycline 100 mg bid x 21d.

6) **Syphilis**- The average incubation period is 14-28 days. In the primary stage, the patient has a painless ulcer or chancre that is circular with sharp edges and is associated with local lymphadenopathy. Secondary symptoms occur 6 weeks after the primary chancre heals and include flu-like symptoms with a maculopapular rash involving the soles and palms. Then, the latent phase occurs, followed by a tertiary stage, which is manifested by CNS and cardiac symptoms. Lab findings may include a positive RPR and VDRL. Treat early syphilis (primary, secondary or early latent) with penicillin G 2.4 million U IM once; treat late stage with penicillin G 2.4 million U IM q week x 3.

7) **Trichomonas**- It often presents with vulvar irritation and a malodorous yellow-green discharge. Diagnose with wet mount. Treat with metronidazole 2 gm po once (do not give metronidazole during the first trimester of pregnancy- use clotrimazole vaginal suppositories).

8) **Vaginal Candidiasis**- Patients present with vulvar pruritis, erythema, and occasional thick cottage cheese discharge. Diagnose with KOH prep. Treat with topical clotrimazole or miconazole; or fluconazole 150 mg po once.

C. Prophylaxis After Sexual Assault

1) Patients should be screened for STDs, and either treated prophylactically or if the results are positive.

2) Prophylaxis should cover chlamydia (azithromycin or doxycylcine), gonorrhea (ceftriaxone of ciprofloxacin), and bacterial vaginosis/trichomoniasis (metronidazole).

3) Consider the morning after pill (two OCP pills at presentation and two pills 12h later).

4) Consider hepatitis vaccination and immune globulin and HIV prophylaxis (zidovudine 300 mg bid or 200 mg tid plus lamivudine 150 mg bid for 28 days). Arrange for HIV antibody testing on day 1, and at 6, 12, and 24 weeks.

XIV. SINUSITIS

•General•

1) Acute sinusitis may be viral or bacterial in origin, and occurs with obstruction of the normal draining mechanisms from edema or inflammation. An upper respiratory infection or allergic rhinitis may predispose patients to sinus obstruction and subsequent bacterial infection.

2) Common bacterial pathogens associated with acute bacterial sinusitis include S. pneumoniae and H. influenzae. Chronic bacterial sinusitis is associated with S. aureus and anaerobes.

•Clinical Presentation•

1) Patients may present with low grade temperature, purulent nasal discharge, and frontal/maxillary sinus tenderness, pain, or fullness. Leaning forward often worsens the pain.

2) Patients may have a concurrent periorbital cellulitis.

•Diagnosis•

1) Most cases of acute sinusitis are viral; it can be difficult to differentiate bacterial from viral sinusitis. The diagnosis of bacterial sinusitis is usually reserved for patients who have symptoms for longer than 7d, have maxillary pain or tenderness in the face or teeth (especially if unilateral) and have purulent nasal discharge. In general, sinus films/CT are not recommended for uncomplicated sinusitis.

2) Plain films have a poor sensitivity for maxillary sinusitis; sensitivity increases if mucosal thickening is added as a criterion, but the specificity is then diminished.

3) On CT, mucosal thickening as the sole abnormality is less suggestive of sinusitis, as it is an incidental finding in 10-40% of asymptomatic patients. Complete sinus opacification or air-fluid levels are convincing evidence of bacterial sinusitis.

•Treatment•

1) Reserve antibiotics for patients who have symptoms for longer than 7d, have maxillary pain or tenderness in the face or teeth, and have purulent nasal discharge. Antibiotic options include amoxicillin, levofloxacin, doxycycline, clarithromycin, azithromycin, cefaclor, Augmentin, or Bactrim for 10-14 days.

2) Oral decongestants (pseudoephedrine) may be given if no history of labile hypertension or prostatic hypertrophy; topical decongestants (oxymetazoline or phenylephrine) may be given for the first 3-5 days.

3) Antihistamines are contraindicated (they may thicken secretions), although consider antihistamines if allergic symptoms are prominent.

4) Consider nasal saline irrigations and guaifenesin.

5) If chronic sinusitis, consider intranasal steroids.

XV. TETANUS

•General•

1) Tetanus is caused by Clostridium tetani, an anaerobic organism whose spores are ubiquitous. A break in the skin allows spores to enter the body and eventually produce a neurotoxin; the incubation period is days to months, usually <2 weeks.

2) Generalized tetanus occurs when the toxin disseminates hematogenously and is taken up at nerve ends and travels via retrograde transmission to the CNS and blocks inhibitory neurons, resulting in tetany; localized disease may occur at the site of inoculation.

•Clinical Presentation•

1) Tetanus presents with an acute onset of muscular contractions, spasms, and hypertonia. The toxin causes trismus, muscle rigidity, opisthotonos, risus sardonicus, and intermittent convulsions.

2) Patients may develop respiratory complications.

•Evaluation•

1) Tetanus is a clinical diagnosis.

2) Check ECG, electrolytes, and glucose. Consider an evaluation for infection.

•Treatment•

1) Establish IV access. Place patient on monitor. Administer oxygen.
2) Treatment includes wound debridement, tetanus immune globulin, and either metronidazole or penicillin. Admit to a monitored setting.
3) <u>Routine wound management</u>: for clean, minor wounds administer tetanus toxoid if the patient has had an uncertain number of previous doses of toxoid (or less than 2 previous doses); administer toxoid and tetanus immune globulin for all other wounds. If the patient has had 3 previous doses of toxoid, administer the toxoid if the last immunization was more than 10 years ago for clean, minor wounds or more than 5 years ago for all other wounds.

XVI. TICK-BORNE ILLNESSES

A. Lyme Disease

•General•

1) Lyme disease is a spirochetal infection (Borrelia burgdorferi) transmitted by the bite of an infected Ixodes tick.
2) Infection occurs during tick season (May-September); most cases occur in the northeast United States and Wisconsin.

•Clinical Presentation•

1) **Early Lyme Disease**- It most often presents as erythema migrans. Erythema migrans occurs in 80% of patients with Lyme disease, usually 7-10 days after the tick bite. It develops at the site of the bite and expands over days to weeks; the average size is 16 cm. It is usually flat, and central clearing occurs in a minority; it is usually not found on the distal extremities. The rash may be accompanied by headaches, fevers, and myalgias. Respiratory and GI complaints are generally not associated with Lyme disease.
2) **Early disseminated Lyme Disease**- It usually presents as multiple erythema migrans lesions, but may include cardiac, neurologic or joint involvement. Early disseminated disease may present within 1 or 2 weeks of exposure, and may include lymphocytic meningitis, cranial neuropathy (usually of the facial nerve), encephalitis, radiculoneuritis,

or a migratory polyarthritis; Lyme carditis may present with weakness and palpitations and may cause atrioventricular block or myopericarditis.

3) **Late Lyme Disease**- It usually manifests as neurologic disease (peripheral neuropathies or chronic encephalopathy) or arthritis (usually monoarticular involving the knee).

•Diagnosis/Evaluation•

1) The diagnosis is mostly clinical (taking into account geography, season, and patient history); serology results are not useful if only a rash is present.

2) Obtain serology only if disseminated disease is present.

3) If suspected neurologic involvement, obtain CSF; if suspected cardiac involvement, obtain ECG.

•Treatment•

1) Remove the tick: using a forceps, grasp tick close to the skin and apply upward pressure; consider injecting intradermal lidocaine and epinephrine beneath the tick.

2) If erythema migrans or mild early disseminated disease, treat with amoxicillin 500 mg tid for 3 weeks, or doxycycline 100 mg bid for 3 weeks (do not use doxycycline in pregnant women or children younger than 8).

3) If severe disease (severe neurologic disease or significant A-V block), treat with IV ceftriaxone 2 g daily for 2-4 weeks.

4) If significant A-V block, admit to telemetry; consider pacemaker.

5) Prophylaxis of routine tick bites is generally not indicated, although consider prophylaxis in pregnant patients and those with engorged Ixodes ticks. A longer duration of attachment increases the likelihood of infection. If the patient lives in an endemic area and the tick was attached for a prolonged time, some recommend a single dose of doxycycline 200 mg (not recommended for pregnant patients or children younger than 8).

B. Rocky Mountain Spotted Fever

•General•

1) An infected dog or wood tick (Dermacentor) transmits the parasite

Rickettsia rickettsii, usually between April and September. It is widely distributed in the United States, but most cases occur in the south-eastern and south central states.

2) The rickettsiae are released from the tick in as little as 6h after attachment. The incubation period is 3-12 days.

•Clinical Presentation•

1) Typically, fever is present, often with headache and malaise. Gastrointestinal symptoms and pneumonitis are common. A red petechial or maculopapular rash occurs within 10 days of symptom onset and often starts on the wrists, ankles, palms or soles. Patients may have bilateral periorbital edema and edema of the dorsal hands and feet.

2) The organism causes a severe vasculitis and may result in arrhythmias, noncardiogenic pulmonary edema, GI bleeding, encephalitis, and other neurologic complications.

•Diagnosis/Evaluation•

1) The diagnosis is clinical (it can be confirmed with serology during convalescence).

2) Consider CXR, ECG, CBC, LFTs, CPK, ESR, electrolytes, and BUN/Cr.

•Treatment•

1) Establish IV. Monitor patient. Administer oxygen.

2) Begin early, presumptive treatment with doxycycline (100 mg po/IV bid) or tetracycline.

3) Admit.

XVII. URINARY TRACT INFECTION (UTI)

A. UTI

•Etiology•

Pathogens include E. coli (80% of cases), S. saprophyticus (11%), Klebsiella, Proteus, Pseudomonas, and Enterococcus.

•Clinical Presentation•

1) Patients typically have symptoms of dysuria with urinary urgency and frequency; lower abdominal discomfort may be present. Hematuria may be present.

2) Fever, chills, vomiting, and flank pain may indicate upper urinary tract involvement.

3) Vaginal discharge suggests vaginitis, cervicitis, or pelvic inflammatory disease; a pelvic exam should be performed.

4) <u>Complicated UTI</u>- A complicated UTI is defined as upper urinary tract symptoms, recent UTI, symptoms for longer than 7 days, coexisting pregnancy, diabetic patients, recent instrumentation (catheter), anatomic or functional urinary tract abnormality, immunocompromised patients, recent antimicrobial use, resistant pathogens, or age >65 years.

•Evaluation•

1) Perform an abdominal exam. Consider a pelvic exam in women, especially if sexually active.

2) Check rapid urine screen for leukocyte esterase and nitrite. Consider urine microscopy and culture. Consider CBC and BUN/Cr if pyelonephritis is suspected.

3) Check a pregnancy test in women of childbearing age.

<u>Urinalysis</u>

1) The urine is infected if it shows 5-10 WBCs plus ≥ 1 bacteria, or the presence of leukocyte esterase and nitrites. Esterase and nitrites are indirect evidence of pyuria and bacteriuria (esterases result from the breakdown of WBCs, and nitrates are converted to nitrites by gram-negative organisms). Nitrites become positive if bacteria act on nitrate for >6h (thus, the first morning void is the most sensitive). Hematuria is present in 40% of cases.

2) Urinary frequency dilutes the number of WBCs.

3) Nitrates are present in most infections of patients with indwelling urinary catheters, but are not present with colonization; multiple organisms without pyuria suggests colonization.

•Differential Diagnosis•

Pyelonephritis, vaginitis (symptoms of external dysuria), urethritis (more common with multiple sex partners).

•Treatment•

1) **Uncomplicated UTI**. Antibiotic options (depending on local resistance) include:

   a) Nitrofurantoin 100 mg q6h for 7 days (covers E. coli and S. saprophyticus; it has no effect on vaginal or bowel flora.)
   b) Trimethoprim 100 mg q12h for 3 days (adds some Proteus and Klebsiella coverage but affects normal flora).
   c) Trimethoprim-sulfamethoxazole (Bactrim DS) 160mg/800mg bid x 3d (adds all Proteus and Klebsiella coverage).
   d) Cephalexin 250 mg qid mg bid.
   e) Amoxicillin 500 mg bid.
   f) Fosfomycin 3 gm once
   g) Fluoroquinolones (e.g., norfloxacin 400 mg q12h, ciprofloxacin 500 mg bid, or levofloxacin 250 mg qd) for 3 days; consider fluoroquinolones if there is a high resistance to TMP/SMX.
2) **Complicated UTI**. Antibiotic options include:
   a) Fluoroquinolones (e.g., norfloxacin 400 mg q12h, ciprofloxacin 500 mg bid, or levofloxacin 250 mg qd) for 7-14 days
   b) Ampicillin plus gentamicin
   c) Ceftazidime or cefepime
3) **If pregnant**, consider cephalexin, amoxicillin, or nitrofurantoin; consider TMP/SMX during the first or second trimesters. Asymptomatic bacteriuria may progress to pyelonephritis and should be treated.
4) For dysuria, consider pyridium 200 mg tid x 2d.
5) For spasm pain, consider Urispas 100 mg, 1-2 tid/qid.
6) Asymptomatic bacteriuria is frequent in the elderly; multiple studies have shown that if the patient appears well and is asymptomatic (even if the patient has a urinary catheter), antibiotics are of no benefit.
7) Catheterized patients should have a fresh catheterized specimen obtained. If the patient is asymptomatic, bacteriuria is generally not treated. Febrile patients with suprapubic discomfort, or elderly patients with vomiting or mental status changes, should be treated.

B. Pyelonephritis

•General•
Pyelonephritis is an infection of the renal parenchyma and pelvis.

•Clinical Presentation•
Patients present with fever, flank pain, exquisite costovertebral angle tenderness, vomiting, and malaise; some patients may have no symp-

toms of cystitis.

•Evaluation•

1) Check CBC, BUN/Cr, and urinalysis (which may show white blood cell casts). Obtain urine culture; routine blood cultures are unnecessary.

2) Consider ultrasound to evaluate for obstruction or abdominal CT to evaluate for abscess.

•Treatment•

1) If mild (patient is not toxic, can tolerate liquids, has mild tenderness, and is not pregnant), consider outpatient treatment for 10-14 days with a fluoroquinolone, or TMP/SMX (if known susceptibility).

2) Otherwise, admit patient and administer gentamicin 1.5 mg/kg plus 1 gm ampicillin IV, or ceftriaxone 1 gm IV plus gentamicin, or a fluoroquinolone.

3) If pregnant, consider ampicillin plus gentamicin, TMP/SMX (except during the 3rd trimester), aztreonam, or cefazolin.

4) If elderly, consider ampicillin plus aztreonam.

CHAPTER 14
LEGAL ISSUES
COBRA/EMTALA

General
COBRA is an acronym for the Consolidated Omnibus Reconciliation Act of 1986, a bill passed by the US Congress. A section of this bill is the EMTALA (Emergency Medical Treatment and Active Labor Act) statute. The intent of this statute was to remedy a common practice in which uninsured or underinsured patients were refused medical treatment or transferred inappropriately (usually to a public hospital). COBRA was enacted to expressly guarantee the right of equal access for all patients.

COBRA only applies to hospitals that participate in Medicare, and applies to all patients within these hospitals. All physicians (not just emergency medicine physicians) that treat patients in a Medicare-participating hospital are subject to the legal duties of COBRA. Institutions that do not meet the legal definition of a hospital are exempt from COBRA (although some hospital-owned facilities may be subject to COBRA).

EMTALA Regulations
1) The hospital must provide an appropriate medical screening exam to any individuals who present to the hospital requesting an evaluation of a medical condition. The purpose of the exam is to identify any emergency medical conditions that exist; therefore, the exam must include any appropriate ancillary services or speciality consultations that are routinely available in the emergency department. An emergency medical condition is vaguely defined as a condition that presents as acute symptoms of sufficient severity (including severe pain), such that the absence of immediate medical attention could reasonably be expected to result in risk to the patient's health. A triage evaluation is not a medical screening exam. The statute does not specifically state who should provide the screening exam. If no emergency

181

medical condition exists, the hospital has no further COBRA obligations.

2) If the screening exam identifies an emergency medical condition, then the hospital has an obligation to stabilize the patient. Stabilization is vaguely defined as treatment of the medical condition such that no deterioration of the condition is likely to result from discharge or transfer of the patient; stabilization is therefore subjective and open to different interpretations. Patients in labor are considered unstable until the baby and placenta have been delivered. Once the patient has been stabilized, the hospital has no further COBRA obligations.

3) A patient may be transferred if the following criteria are met:
   a) The patient has been stabilized.
   b) The patient requires a higher level of care, and the risks outweigh the benefits.
   c) The patient requests to be transferred.

4) If a patient has not been stabilized, the patient may not be transferred unless the following criteria are satisfied: the transfer is appropriate; the patient requests the transfer and is aware of the risks; a physician has signed a certification that the medical benefits from treatment at another facility outweigh the risks from transfer; the receiving facility has available space and qualified personnel and has agreed to accept the patient; and the transferring hospital provides all appropriate medical records.

5) Hospitals and physicians who violate EMTALA regulations risk fines and penalties. Also, the accepting hospital is required to report any violations that the transferring hospital may have committed.

CHAPTER 15

METABOLIC/ELECTROLYTE DISORDERS

I. ACID-BASE DISORDERS

1) Formulas for Compensatory Responses

Metabolic acidosis: $pCO2 = (1.5 \times HCO3) + 8 \pm 2$.

Metabolic alkalosis: $pCO2 = (0.9 \times HCO3) + 9 \pm 2$.

Acute Respiratory acidosis: amount of HCO3 increase = $(0.1 \times$ amount of pCO2 increase); HCO3 is increased 1 mEq for every 10 mm Hg increase in pCO2.

Chronic Respiratory acidosis: amount of HCO3 increase = $(0.4 \times$ amount of pCO2 increase); HCO3 is increased 3.5 mEq for every 10 mm HG increase in pCO2.

Acute Respiratory alkalosis: amount of HCO3 decrease = $(0.2 \times$ amount of pCO2 decrease); HCO3 falls 2 mEq for each 10 mm Hg fall in pCO2.

Chronic Respiratory alkalosis: amount of HCO3 decrease = $(0.4 \times$ amount of pCO2 decrease); HCO3 falls 5 mEq for each 10 mm Hg fall in pCO2.

2) Metabolic Acidosis- etiology

Anion gap = Na - (HCO3 + Cl).

Increased anion gap metabolic acidosis: Methanol, uremia, DKA, paraldehyde, infection, INH, lactic acidosis, ethylene glycol, alcohol ketoacidosis, salicylates.

Normal anion gap metabolic acidosis: Uterosigmoidostomy, saline, endocrine (hypo-aldosteronism), diarrhea, carbonic anhydrase inhibitor (acetazolamide), hyper alimentation, renal tubular acidosis).

3) Metabolic Alkalosis- etiology

It is usually from excessive diuresis (loss of K, H, and Cl) or excessive loss of gastric secretions (loss of HCl). Mineralocorticoids may cause alkalosis.

4) Osmolality (calculated) = $2(Na) + glucose/18 + BUN/2.8$.

Osmol gap = measured osmolality-calculated osmolality (normal is 5-15).

Etiology of osmolar gap: ethanol, isopropanol, methanol, ethylene glycol, mannitol, lactate.

II. CALCIUM

A. Hypercalcemia

•Etiology•
Etiologies include primary hyperparathyroidism, malignancy, adrenal insufficiency, pheochromocytoma, thiazides, Vitamin D intoxication, and tuberculosis.

•Clinical Presentation•
1) Patients may present with fatigue, polyuria, nausea and vomiting, constipation, and arrhythmias.
2) Patients may also present with anorexia, abdominal pain, pancreatitis, nephrolithiasis, lethargy, coma, or hyporeflexia.

•Evaluation•
1) Check glucose, electrolytes, calcium, magnesium, phosphate, BUN/Cr, and ECG; consider amylase.
2) Ionized calcium is the physiologically relevant level, so either check ionized calcium or adjust the total calcium for changes in the protein (40% of calcium is bound to protein and a 1 gm/dL drop in albumin reflects a 0.8 drop in the serum calcium level). The formula for the corrected calcium is: corrected calcium mg/dL = measured total calcium mg/dL + 0.8 (4.4- measured albumin g/dL).
3) The ECG may demonstrate a short QT interval, prolonged PR and QRS intervals, or complete heart block.

•Treatment•
1) If calcium is less than 13 mg/dL, treatment is oral/IV rehydration. Normal saline infusion improves extracellular volume and glomerular filtration, and increases urinary calcium excretion.
2) If calcium is 13-15 mg/dL, administer IV normal saline and furosemide (furosemide produces a saline diuresis and concomitant calcium excretion; *administer only after adequate hydration*). Avoid thiazide diuretics, as they decrease renal calcium excretion. Replace potassium with KCl as needed.
3) If calcium is greater than 15 mg/dL, in addition to IVNS and furo-

semide as above, consider calcitonin 4 U/kg SC/IM (it inhibits bone resorption and increases excretion of calcium; it is the anticalcemic agent with the most rapid onset of action). Consider biphosphonates, which inhibit bone resorption: etidronate (Didronel) 7.5 mg/kg IV over 4h, or pamidronate. Mithramycin is generally not used in the ED secondary to hepatic and renal toxicity.

4) Steroids are effective if the hypercalcemia is caused by myeloma, lymphoma, or sarcoidosis, as they decrease intestinal absorption.

5) Dialysis is required for patients with renal failure and severe hypercalcemia.

B. Hypocalcemia

•Etiology•
Etiologies include shock, sepsis, renal failure, pancreatitis, surgical hypoparathyroidism, medications, and rhabdomyolysis.

•Clinical Presentation•
Patients may present with paresthesias (usually around the mouth or fingertips), weakness, tetany, Chvostek's sign (twitch at corner of mouth after tapping facial nerve in front of ear), Trousseau's sign (carpal spasm with blood pressure cuff >SBP for 3 min), bronchospasm, arrhythmias, or confusion.

•Evaluation•
1) Check glucose, electrolytes, calcium, magnesium, phosphate, BUN/Cr, and ECG.

2) Hypocalcemia is defined as serum calcium less than 8.5 mg/dL or an ionized calcium less than 2.0 mEq/L or 1.0 mmol/L; adjust serum calcium for albumin levels.

3) ECG may show prolonged QT interval.

•Treatment•
1) If severe and acute, establish IV, place patient on monitor, and administer 10 ml of 10% calcium chloride IV over 10 min.

2) Otherwise, administer oral calcium therapy.

III. POTASSIUM

A. Hyperkalemia

•Etiology•

Etiologies include acidemia, tissue necrosis (rhabdomyolysis), hemolysis, renal failure, potassium sparing diuretics, GI bleed, and Addison's disease.

•Clinical Presentation•

1) Patients may present with weakness, fatigue, paresthesias, or arrhythmias. Hyperkalemic paralysis is a rare complication.
2) Symptoms are often nonspecific; hyperkalemia may be an incidental lab finding.

•Evaluation•

Check electrolytes, BUN/Cr, glucose, calcium, and ECG. Consider ABG if acidosis is suspected.

ECG- The ECG may demonstrate sequential changes:
1) Peaked T waves (earliest sign, suggests a K > 6.0 mEq/L) and shortened QT intervals.
2) Decreasing P wave amplitude (suggests a K >7.0 mEq/L) until the P wave disappears (K >8.5 mEq/L).
3) A-V conduction blocks (increased PR interval), brady/tachyarrhythmias.
4) Progressively widening QRS.

•Treatment•

1) Establish IV; place patient on monitor. Start immediate treatment if there are any ECG changes; levels > 6.5 mEq/L (even without ECG changes) should also be treated. Treatment attempts to stabilize the myocardium, shift potassium intracellularly, and facilitate potassium excretion.
2) Calcium gluconate 10 cc IV of a 10% solution, may repeat x 2 prn every 5-10 min. Or, calcium chloride 5 cc IV of a 10% solution (one ampule of calcium chloride has 3 times the calcium of one ampule of calcium gluconate). Calcium is usually given if K > 7.0 mEq/L. Administer slowly and with extreme caution if patient is on digoxin, since it potentiates the toxic effects of digoxin. Calcium protects the myocardium by antagonizing the effects of hyperkalemia on cardiac conduction. Onset is in 3 min; it is effective for 1 hour.
3) Sodium bicarbonate 44 mEq IV over 2-5 min causes alkalosis, which

forces potassium into cells; may repeat once in 10 min. Onset is in 10 min; it lasts 1-2 hours. Bicarbonate is usually given if K >6.5 mEq/L. Bicarbonate has been shown to be ineffective in reducing potassium in dialysis patients.

4) Glucose 50-100 mg IV with regular insulin 10-20 U IV, then 20% glucose solution with 40-80 U insulin; onset is in 30 min. It is usually given if K >6.5 mEq/L. Insulin shifts potassium into cells, and glucose prevents hypoglycemia.

5) Albuterol nebulizer treatment; onset is in 30 min. It works by shifting potassium into cells.

6) Kayexalate 25 mg po/PR exchanges sodium for potassium. Use caution, as the sodium content in Kayexalate may precipitate CHF in cardiac patients.

7) Furosemide 40 mg IV.

8) Dialysis.

B. Hypokalemia

•Etiology•

Etiologies include alkalemia, renal loss (from hyperaldosteronism, hypercalcemia, or renal tubular acidosis), and GI loss.

•Clinical Presentation•

Patients may present with arrhythmias, muscle weakness (including paralysis), or ileus.

•Evaluation•

1) Check electrolytes, Mg, Ca, phosphorus, BUN/Cr, and ECG; consider ABG.

2) The ECG may demonstrate low voltage, flat T waves, depressed ST segments, a prominent U wave, or a prolonged QT interval.

•Treatment•

1) Before replacing potassium, ensure adequate urine output.

2) If mild-moderate hypokalemia (K >2.5 mEq/L), treat with oral potassium (40-80 mEq/day in divided doses) or KCl IV 10 mEq/hour.

3) If K < 2.5 mEq/L, admit patient to monitored setting and administer IV potassium. If symptoms are severe (manifesting with paralysis or arrhythmias), administer up to 20-40 mEq/hour IV.

4) Hypokalemia often occurs in association with hypomagnesemia, which may need correction.

IV. SODIUM

A. Hypernatremia

•Etiology•

Hypovolemic Hypernatremia- It may result from extrarenal water losses from skin, GI, or respiratory tracts; or renal water losses from diuretics or intrinsic renal disease.

Euvolemic Hypernatremia- It may result from impaired thirst, extrarenal insensible water loss (hyperventilation), or renal water loss from diabetes insipidus.

Hypervolemic Hypernatremia- It may result from iatrogenic causes or mineralocorticoid excess.

•Clinical Presentation•

Patients may present with confusion, lethargy, thirst, ataxia, seizures, or coma.

•Evaluation•

1) Check glucose, electrolytes, BUN/Cr, and plasma and urine osmolalities.

2) Evaluate the patient's volume status.

•Treatment•

1) If patient is severely volume depleted or hypotensive, establish IV, place patient on monitor, and administer IVNS.

2) Calculate and replace the water deficit. Lower sodium no faster than 1-2mEq/L/h. A rapid decrease in sodium may cause cerebral edema and seizures.

3) If the patient has central diabetes insipidus, consider desmopressin (DDAVP) intranasally 10-40 mcg/24h divided tid.

B. Hyponatremia

•Etiology•

Decreased Extracellular Fluid (ECF)- It may result from extrarenal losses (with urinary sodium <20 mEq/L) from sweating, vomiting, diarrhea, third spacing with burns, peritonitis, Addison's disease, or renal tubular acidosis. Or, it may result from renal losses (with urinary sodium >20 mEq/L) from loop diuretics or osmotic diuretics.

Normal ECF- It may result from SIADH, myxedema, or Addison's disease.

Increased ECF- If urinary sodium is >20 mEq/L, renal failure is the likely etiology. If urinary sodium is <20 mEq/L, etiologies include cirrhosis, CHF, and renal failure.

•Clinical Presentation•

Patients may present with confusion, lethargy, seizures, or coma.

•Evaluation•

1) Check glucose, electrolytes, BUN/Cr, and plasma and urine osmolalities.
2) Check urine electrolytes.
3) Evaluate the patient's volume status.
4) Elevated glucose or triglyceride may cause psuedohyponatremia; there is a 1.6 mEq/L decrease in sodium for every 100 mg/dL increase in glucose over 100 mg/dL.

•Treatment•

1) Treatment depends on the etiology.
2) If the patient has severe hyponatremia with seizures or coma, consider 3% NaCl, 300-500 ml over 6-8h; consider concurrent furosemide, which causes excretion of a hypotonic urine. The goal is to increase the sodium to 120-125 mEq/L.

CHAPTER 16
NEUROLOGY

I. ALTERED MENTAL STATUS IN THE ELDERLY

•Etiology•
Dementia
1) Dementia is a chronic loss of intellectual function with alterations in both short-term and long-term memory; it is a global, progressive impairment of cognitive function without alteration of consciousness.
2) Dementia develops over months or years; there is widespread neuronal degeneration.
3) Dementia is usually from Alzheimer's or multi-infarct dementia; consider subdural hematoma, tumor or depression.

Delirium
1) Delirium is an acute organic brain dysfunction characterized by global cognitive impairment and a decrease in the level of consciousness; long-term memory may be spared.
2) Delirium is usually secondary to metabolic, infectious or structural disease. Consider drug toxicity (virtually any drug), especially anticholinergics (increasing age is accompanied by chronic cholinergic deficiency in the CNS, thus anticholinergics can precipitate delirium; peripheral signs may be limited); examples of anticholinergic medications include diphenhydramine, meperidine, cimetidine, tricyclic antidepressants, and anti-Parkinsonians. Consider aspirin or steroid intoxication. Consider infection, HHNK, stroke, MI, trauma, and seizure.

•Evaluation•
1) Check ECG, pulse oximetry, CBC, electrolytes, glucose, BUN/Cr, urinalysis, CXR, head CT, and alcohol level; consider ABG, urine toxicology, LP, and TSH.
2) Specific abnormalities in the vital signs may point to the diagnosis.

•Treatment•
1) Identify and treat the underlying pathology.
2) Treat agitation with haloperidol (Haldol) 0.5-2.0 mg IM/IV/po or

droperidol (Inapsine) 5 mg IM/IV. Haldol lowers the seizure threshold, may worsen anticholinergic toxicity and may cause dystonic reactions. Droperidol 2.5 mg IM/IV is associated with QT interval prolongation and Torsades de Pointes, and should only be administered if an ECG demonstrates no QT interval prolongation and other options have proved ineffective.

3) Consider lorazepam (Ativan).

4) If acute brain syndrome or toxic/metabolic disorders have been excluded, consider appropriate psychiatric consultation and disposition.

II. BELL'S PALSY

•Etiology•
It is probably caused by herpes simplex. Consider Lyme disease.

•Diagnosis•
1) Bell's palsy is a peripheral nerve lesion that presents with an acute onset of facial nerve paralysis/paresis. There is usually ipsilateral frontalis muscle involvement and weakness of the ipsilateral half of the face, although any of the five branches of the facial nerve may be involved. A proximal lesion may affect salivation, taste, and lacrimation. Bell's palsy should have no other associated neurologic deficits.

2) Distinguish between central (stroke, tumor) and peripheral etiologies for facial palsy. A central lesion presents with the relative sparing of the frontalis muscle, as this muscle has bilateral innervation; thus the weakness of a central lesion is partial and involves the frontalis and orbicularis muscles less than the muscles in the lower part of the face. Also, consider central CNS etiology if diplopia, dysphagia, hoarseness or facial pain; weakness progressing to paralysis over weeks/months with twitching suggests neoplasm.

3) Evaluate the parotid gland, as inflammation/neoplasm may cause facial nerve paralysis. Check ears for external otitis, mastoiditis, and herpetic vesicles. Perform a complete neurologic exam.

4) **Ramsey-Hunt-** It is a facial nerve palsy associated with a zoster infection of the outer ear and the nerves of the internal auditory canal. The patient may have antecedent pain. The prognosis is worse than Bell's palsy. Treatment is similar to Bell's palsy.

•Treatment•

1) Prednisone taper over 2 weeks.
2) Consider acyclovir 400 mg po 5x/d for 10d.
3) Lubricant eye drops, eye patch.

III. GUILLAIN-BARRE SYNDROME

•General•

1) Guillain-Barre is an acute ascending, progressive, inflammatory poly-neuropathy with muscular weakness and mild distal sensory loss; it often follows an acute febrile episode.
2) 85%-95% of patients have a full recovery (often weeks to months after symptoms stop progressing).

•Clinical Presentation•

1) Patients present with a relatively symmetric weakness, usually accompanied by paresthesias; it usually begins in the legs and progresses to the arms. Deep tendon reflexes are lost; weakness is always more prominent than sensory symptoms. Maximal weakness typically occurs 2 weeks after the initial onset of symptoms.
2) Patients may have autonomic dysfunction; cranial nerves may be involved. Mental status remains normal.

•Differential Diagnosis•

The differential includes organophosphates, botulism, tick paralysis, lead poisoning, diphtheria, myasthenia gravis, tetanus.

•Diagnosis•

1) The diagnosis is generally clinical. CSF with elevated protein (>400 mg/L) and very few cells suggests Guillain-Barre. Nerve conduction studies may demonstrate reduced conduction velocities. Imaging of the brain is not usually required.
2) Consider obtaining forced vital capacity (FVC) to help guide disposition and predict which patients may be at risk for respiratory compromise (consider ICU admission if FVC < 20 ml/kg, and consider intubation if FVC < 15 ml/kg).

•Treatment•

1) If severe (any respiratory compromise, rapidly progressing symptoms, or severe autonomic dysfunction), establish IV, place patient

on monitor, administer oxygen, and admit to ICU (5% of patients require intubation).

2) Plasmapheresis and IVIG are the only effective treatments.

3) Steroids are not effective.

IV. HEADACHE

•Etiology/Clinical Presentation•

1) Cluster Headache

   a) Cluster headaches are characterized by daily constricting unilateral pain, nonthrobbing, and usually in the distribution of the trigeminal nerve; there is never an aura. Headaches usually occur at night, often recurring at the same time each night. Maximal pain occurs in the orbital or temporal region. There is usually associated ipsilateral lacrimation, rhinorrhea or conjunctival injection and the patient is usually agitated. Symptoms typically last 30 min-2h.

   b) 90% of cluster headaches occur in males.

2) Headache Secondary to Increased Intracranial Pressure

   a) The headache is secondary to mass/edema.

   b) Patients present with a new headache worsening over 4-6 weeks; it is worse with awakening, bending forward, and Valsalva.

3) Migraine

   a) <u>Migraines without aura (common migraine)</u>- These account for 75% of all migraines. Diagnosis requires at least 2 of the following characteristics of pain: a.) unilateral; b.) pulsating; c.) moderate or severe; or d.) aggravated by physical activity. In addition, pain must be accompanied by at least one of the following: a.) nausea or vomiting; or b.) photophobia or phonophobia.

   b) <u>Migraines with aura (classic migraine)</u>- These account for 20% of all migraines. Auras are usually visual, but the patient may experience facial or extremity paresthesias or motor phenomena. Typically, an aura occurs 1 hour before the headache and is completely reversible.

   c) Patients may have scotomas often 'marching' across the visual field; zigzags are commonly described at the leading edge of the scotoma. The duration is typically 15-20 minutes and is usually followed by a headache. However, some are acephalgic migraines, which may be difficult to distinguish from retinal tears.

   d) It is unlikely to be a migraine if it is a new or different headache and the patient is older than 35 years. Most patients have their first headache before 30 years of age, usually in adolescence.

   f) Migraines are associated with stress, menses, foods with tyramine, nitrates/MSG, estrogen, and caffeine withdrawal.

4) Subarachnoid Hemorrhage

   a) Patients present with a sudden onset of severe headache. Most patients have some depression of consciousness; the majority of patients have neck stiffness.

   b) See also <u>Neurology; Subarachnoid Hemorrhage</u>.

5) Temporal Arteritis

   a) The average age of patients is 70 years. It is associated with polymyalgia rheumatica.

   b) The pain is usually unilateral and piercing; systemic symptoms are often present. The patient may have jaw or neck pain. Blindness can develop secondary to ischemic papillitis.

   c) The exam usually reveals tender temporal arteries; ESR is usually >50. Definitive diagnosis is through a biopsy of the artery.

6) Tension-type Headache

   a) Tension-type headaches cause a constant, constricting, band-like pain, usually located in the back of neck/occiput/frontal regions. The pain is bilateral, and usually nonpulsatile; there is usually no associated nausea, vomiting or photophobia.

   b) Symptoms worsen as the day progresses, and may persist for weeks/months.

•Evaluation•

1) Document mental status and CNS (including cerebellar) exam; examine the fundi and the temporal arteries.

2) Through history, physical exam, and diagnostic studies, attempt to exclude significant pathology; consider head CT, LP, ESR, carbon monoxide level, and eye pressure evaluation.

3) Signs that may indicate serious pathology include a headache associated with focal neurologic or meningeal signs; new or different headache; fever; worst headache of life; mental status change; sudden onset of severe headache; or if the patient is immunocompromised or on anticoagulants. Always consider carbon monoxide poisoning (especially if several members of the same household have similar symptoms).

•Treatment•

1) Cluster Headache- Oxygen 8L/min or 100% face mask is effective (the mechanism of action is unknown); also, consider sumatriptan, DHE with metoclopramide, prochlorperazine, or narcotics.

2) Migraine- Options include:

a) Dopamine antagonists

Phenothiazines-Prochlorperazine (Compazine)- 10 mg IV; complete relief is achieved in 74% of patients. IV administration is more effective then IM (74% cure vs. 50%).

*Metoclopramide (Reglan)-*10 mg IV; it is as effective as compazine. IV administration works best.

b) Serotonin agonists

Sumatriptan (Imitrex); dosage options include 6 mg SC (may be repeated in 1h; the maximum dose is two 6 mg injections in 24h), or 100 mg po, or 5-20 mg intranasally (may be repeated in 2h). Sumatriptan relieves pain in 77% of patients within 1h; 40% have a recurrence in 24h. If the initial dose doesn't work, a repeat dose probably won't. Avoid the use of sumatriptan with ergotamines, or if the patient has coronary artery disease. Sumatriptan provides better initial relief than DHE, but has a higher recurrence rate. Newer triptans are also available.

DHE (dihydroergotamine)- 0.75-1.0 mg IV/SC. Administer 15 minutes after metoclopramide or prochlorperazine; a second dose may be administered. DHE is contraindicated if the patient has coronary artery disease.

Ergotamine- Dosage options include 2-4 mg po; 2 mg pr; 2-4 mg SL; it is used as an abortive agent.

c) NSAIDs

Consider oral or parenteral (ketorolac) NSAIDs.

d) Narcotics

Narcotics may be administered as a last resort.

e) Oral Medications

Oral medications include Cafergot (ergotamine/caffeine) 100 mg two to six tabs, max 10/wk; Midrin 100-325 mg; or Fiorinal.

f) Prophylaxis

Prophylactic medications include tricyclic antidepressants, beta-blockers, or methysergide.

3) Temporal Arteritis- Treat with prednisone 60-80 mg/d (steroids given 1-2 weeks before surgery have no effect on the results of the biopsy).

4) Tension-type Headache- Treat with NSAIDs and muscle relaxants.

V. MULTIPLE SCLEROSIS

•General•

Multiple sclerosis is an inflammatory demyelinating disease of the CNS; it is immune-mediated. Plaques of demyelination throughout the CNS slow conduction.

•Clinical Presentation•

1) Multiple sclerosis is characterized by at least two CNS findings separated in space and time. The average age of onset is 30 years.

2) The most common symptoms are focal paresthesias, weakness or clumsiness, visual disturbances, fleeting ocular palsy, and difficulty with bladder control. Patients may also have optic neuritis (blurry vision/visual loss in one eye, pain with movement), or heaviness, stiffness or pain in the extremities.

3) Brainstem involvement is manifested by nystagmus, impaired ocular motility, loss of balance, dysarthria, tic douloureux, or numbness.

4) Patients may present with an exacerbation of chronic symptoms, and a possible infectious etiology should be investigated.

•Differential Diagnosis•

The differential includes small infarcts, CNS tumor, amyotrophic lateral sclerosis, syphilis, pernicious anemia, systemic lupus.

•Evaluation•

1) Perform a complete neurologic exam. Among other findings, patients may demonstrate an afferent pupillary defect, internuclear ophthalmoplegia, spasticity, and Babinski's sign.

2) In patients with known multiple sclerosis who present with worsening symptoms, consider lab evaluation and head CT. Consider an evaluation for infection (especially UTI), as infection may exacerbate any neurologic symptoms.

3) Definitive diagnosis of multiple sclerosis includes brain and spine MRI, CSF evaluation, and somotosensory evoked potentials.

•Treatment•

1) Consider steroids for multiple sclerosis exacerbations.
2) Interferon may be of benefit.
3) Treat any infection.
4) Treat fever, as high temperatures worsen signs and symptoms.

VI. MYASTHENIA GRAVIS

•General•

Myasthenia gravis results from an antibody-mediated depletion of acetylcholine receptors.

•Clinical Presentation•

1) Patients present with symmetrical, descending fatigable muscle weakness; it usually affects the extraocular muscles first, then other bulbar muscles and limbs. Ptosis (which may be asymmetrical) and diplopia are the most common presentations of myasthenia. There is no sensory impairment or loss of reflexes.

2) Patients with a history of myasthenia gravis may present with worsening symptoms (myasthenic crisis), which may be secondary to infection (typically pneumonia); or, patients may present with a cholinergic crisis (salivation, lacrimation, urination) from excess medication.

•Evaluation•

1) The tensilon test (edrophonium) is used to diagnose myasthenia gravis. Edrophonium inhibits acetylcholinesterase, improving strength; it has an onset of 30 seconds and duration of 5-10 minutes. Patients should be monitored during the test. An initial dose of 0.1-0.2 mg is administered, as some patients demonstrate sensitivity. For diagnosis, a dose of 2 mg IV is administered; unequivocal improvement of weakness is a positive test. If there is no change, additional doses of 3mg and then 5 mg are administered. (Patients may experience salivation, nausea, or fasciculations; if hypotension or bradycardia, administer atropine.)

2) The patient's response to edrophonium may help distinguish a cholinergic crisis from a myasthenic crisis (the patient in cholinergic crisis will worsen after administration of edrophonium).

3) If the patient has ocular myasthenia or mild weakness, consider administering edrophonium in the ED to make the diagnosis.

4) Patients in myasthenic crisis should undergo an evaluation for infection. Check CBC, electrolytes, glucose, ECG, CXR, and urinalysis. Consider obtaining forced vital capacity (FVC) to help guide disposition and predict which patients may be at risk for respiratory compromise.

5) Most patients demonstrate anti-acetylcholine receptor antibodies; repetitive nerve stimulation testing may also aid in the diagnosis.

•Treatment•

1) If the patient has worsening weakness or is in myasthenic or cholinergic crisis, establish IV and place patient on cardiac monitor. These patients should be admitted to a monitored setting, as patients may quickly develop respiratory weakness or bulbar dysfunction with an inability to handle secretions. Ensure an adequate airway; if rapid sequence intubation is necessary, a rapid onset non-depolarizing paralytic agent (e.g., rocuronium) is preferred.

2) If there is a question of cholinergic toxicity, discontinue acetylcholinesterase inhibitors.

3) Myasthenia exacerbations most commonly result from inadequate treatment with cholinesterase inhibitors. Edrophonium has a 10 min half-life, and repeated doses may be necessary until oral medications take effect. Provide supportive measures. Consider plasmapheresis and IV immune globulin. Treat any infection.

4) Long-term medications include oral pyridostigmine and immunosuppressive agents (prednisone, azothioprine). Plasmapheresis may be helpful; thymectomy may also be beneficial.

VII. SEIZURES

A. Seizures

•Classification•
1) Generalized Seizures

Generalized seizures are characterized by synchronous involvement of both hemispheres; consciousness is almost always impaired. Types of generalized seizures include:

a) Absence/petit mal seizures- brief episodes of loss of consciousness that may appear as staring or lip smacking. There is no aura or postictal period. It generally occurs in patients less than 20 years old.

b) Atonic seizures- drop attacks with sudden loss of muscle tone and brief or no loss of consciousness.

c) Clonic seizures- continuous jerking motions with altered consciousness.

d) Myoclonic seizures- brief muscular contractions with jerking of extremities; there is no altered mental status.

e) Tonic seizures- stiffening of muscles with altered consciousness.

f) Tonic-clonic/grand mal seizures- sudden loss of consciousness, followed by rhythmic jerking; the seizure is followed by a postictal period.

2) Partial (Focal) Seizures

Partial seizures arise from a focus of brain activity; they may remain focal or spread and progress to a generalized seizure. The presence of an aura implies a focal seizure (which may generalize); postictal (Todd's) paralysis also suggests a focal onset. Types of partial seizures include:

a) Simple seizures- it may have motor, sensory, or autonomic components; there is no impairment of consciousness.

b) Complex partial seizures- consciousness or mentation is affected, sometimes producing hallucinations, automatisms, or affective disorders.

•Etiology•

1) Neonates, children- etiologies include birth trauma (subarachnoid or intraventricular hemorrhage), hypoxia, meningitis, CNS malformations, phenylketonuria, metabolic derangements, febrile seizures, and toxins.

2) Adolescents, young adults- etiologies include stroke (vascular tumor causing embolism or infarction), substance abuse, noncompliance, withdrawal, or trauma.

3) Older adults- etiologies include cerebrovascular disease, medications, infection, metabolic derangements, trauma, or withdrawal from alcohol/drugs.

•Diagnosis•

1) Seizures have an abrupt onset and termination, are usually not provoked by environmental stimuli, have purposeless movements, usually last 1-2 minutes, and are stereotyped.

2) Patients have lack of recall.

3) Except for petit mal or simple partial seizures, seizures are followed by post-ictal confusion.

•Evaluation•

1) Perform complete neurologic and cardiac exams. Evaluate for signs of trauma (especially cervical spine injury). Check for signs of meningitis (fever, nuchal rigidity or petechiae); check for a bulging fontanel in infants.

2) In patients with a previous seizure history who present with a typical seizure (and the patient has had a full recovery), check medication levels; other tests are unnecessary.

3) Obtain a head CT if atypical seizure, status epilepticus, abnormal CNS exam, persistent altered mental status, protracted headache, history of malignancy, recent head injury, on anticoagulants, or HIV positive. Consider electrolytes, calcium, toxicology screen, and glucose.

4) Perform an LP if meningitis is suspected.

5) If first-time seizure- If not related to trauma, hypoglycemia, or alcohol or drug use, consider CBC, electrolytes, calcium, urinalysis, toxicology screen, head CT (with and without contrast), and LP.

•Treatment•

1) Administer benzodiazepines if the patient is still seizing (see status epilepticus below).

2) If first-time seizure- If the evaluation is negative and the patient has fully recovered, then hospitalization is usually unnecessary. Patients with remote symptomatic seizures (seizures thought to be caused by previous neurological illness or injury) have a 50-65% risk of recurrence and should probably be started on anticonvulsants; it is unclear if medications are beneficial for idiopathic first-time seizures.

3) Chronic medications include:

a) Phenytoin (Dilantin) 1.0-1.5 g IV loading dose (15-18 mg/kg) with cardiac monitoring or 1000 mg po in two divided doses over 12h, then 200 mg bid (oral loading of Dilantin may not be effective in patients at high risk for another seizure, as 30% of patients given a 1 gm load have subtherapeutic levels 8h after administration); fosphenytoin is similar to phenytoin, but may be given more rapidly or IM.

b) Carbamazepine (Tegretol) 200 mg, then 600-1200 mg/d divided tid.

c) Phenobarbital 10 mg/kg IV over 20 min (monitor respirations); po loading 180 mg bid x 3d then 90-180 mg qd.

d) Valproate (Depakote) 750-2000 mg/d divided bid.

e) Ethosuximide (Zarontin) 15 mg/kg/d load, then 500 mg po qd.

f) Gabapentin (Neurontin) 300 mg po qhs, increased to 300-600 mg tid.

g) Topiramate (Topamax) 50 mg po qhs, increased to 200 mg bid.

h) Clonazepam (Klonopin) 0.5-2mg po tid.

•Disposition•

If the patient is discharged, avoid swimming, driving, and hazardous tools.

B. Status Epilepticus

•General•

1) Status epilepticus is defined as either continuous seizure activity (one definition is 30 minutes; some define status epilepticus as continuous seizure activity for >5min), or ≥2 seizures without full recovery between seizures.

2) In patients who have not regained consciousness 20-30 minutes after a seizure, consider subtle status epilepticus, in which the patient has minimal or very subtle motor manifestations of the seizure.

3) Status epilepticus causes an increase in catecholamines, which may result in hypertension, tachycardia, hyperglycemia, and lactic acidosis.

•Evaluation•

1) Check glucose, CBC with differential, electrolytes, BUN/Cr, calcium, magnesium, medication levels, toxicology screen, and alcohol level.

2) Consider head CT and LP.

•Treatment•

1) Establish IV. Administer oxygen. Place patient on monitor. Assess and stabilize the airway.

2) Consider administering glucose D50 50 ml and thiamine 100 mg IV.

3) Administer benzodiazepines. The first line agent is lorazepam (Ativan) 0.05- 0.15 mg/kg IV (max 2 mg/min). Otherwise, consider diazepam (Valium) 0.15 mg/kg IV over 2 min, max 30 mg. (Diazepam has a slightly faster onset but much shorter effective half-life than lorazepam.) Respiratory depression and decreased blood pressure are related to the speed of administration. If unable to obtain IV access, consider intranasal or intramuscular midazolam (Versed) 10mg, or diazepam 0.5 mg/kg pr or lorazepam 0.1 mg/kg pr.

4) Concurrently with benzodiazepines, administer phenytoin (Dilantin) 18 mg/kg IV at 50 mg/min (may administer up to a total of 30 mg/kg if the patient is still seizing). Fosphenytoin can be given in equivalent doses, up to 150 mg/min IV; if necessary, fosphenytoin may be given IM.

5) If status continues after phenytoin is administered, consider phenobarbital 10 mg/kg IV, max 30 mg/kg (the initial rate is 100 mg/min, and subsequent rates are 50 mg/min; bolus with 10 mg/kg with additional doses of 5-10 mg/kg); consider intubation. Further options include lidocaine 1-2 mg/kg at 50 mg/min then maintenance at 50 ug/kg/min, total 3 mg/kg; midazolam drip 0.1-0.3 mg/kg bolus, then 0.1-0.4 mg/kg/h; or pentobarbital 5-15 mg/kg IV (may repeat x 2) load slowly then 0.5-5 mg/kg/h. If long-acting paralytics are used, continuous EEG monitoring should be employed to evaluate for persistent seizures.

6) If meningitis is suspected, consider empiric antibiotics.

7) Specific treatment for possible overdoses:

Cocaine- Lorazepam.

Isoniazid- Lorazepam and 5 mg pyridoxine (do not administer Dilantin).

Theophylline- Lorazepam, thiopental, and consider hemoperfusion.

Tricyclics- Lorazepam and bicarbonate.

8) Admit to ICU.

C. Pseudoseizures

Psuedoseizures account for up to 20% of all intractable seizures, and have the following characteristics: a prodrome of increased stress/anxiety; it rarely occurs in social isolation; patients manifest unresponsive behavior in the absence of motor manifestations, and slow, writhing or in-phase limb movements; there is a longer duration; it frequently occurs in adolescent or young women; ictal behavior varies during the seizure and the patient is frequently responsive to the environment; and there is a low incidence of injury. It can occur in patients with epilepsy.

VIII. STROKE/TIA (Transient Ischemic Attack)

A. Stroke

•General•

1) Stroke may be defined as a sudden loss of blood flow to an area of the brain, resulting in a corresponding neurological deficit. Rapid diagnosis of ischemic stroke is essential for patients who are candidates for fibrinolytic therapy.

2) Presenting symptoms depend on the area of the brain involved; symptoms may include hemiparesis, visual loss or change, ataxia, dysarthria, aphasia, sensory deficits, or mental status change.

3) Strokes can be ischemic (80% of all strokes; ischemic strokes may be thrombotic, embolic, or secondary to hypoperfusion) or hemorrhagic (associated with chronic hypertension, amyloidosis and younger age).

4) No clinical presentation reliably distinguishes hemorrhagic stroke from ischemic stroke. Headache occurs in a majority of hemorrhagic strokes, but occurs in only 10-20% of ischemic strokes. Hemorrhagic strokes are more likely to be associated with seizures, vomiting, altered mental status, and hypertension. Stuttering deficits suggest a thrombotic stroke.

•Physical Exam•

1) Perform neurologic (including cerebellar and cranial nerve) and cardiovascular (including carotid) exams. The physical exam should attempt to rapidly confirm and define the presence of a stroke syndrome, and exclude other etiologies of the presenting neurologic deficit. The National Institute of Health Stroke Scale can be used to quan-

tify the neurologic deficit.

2) Upper extremity weakness is best tested by pronator drift. A broad-based gait or positive Romberg (done with eyes open) indicates cerebellar dysfunction. Reflex findings are always significant if asymmetrical.

3) Dominant hemisphere functions include speech and math; nondominant functions include special orientation and body image.

4) Midbrain and pontine dysfunction are associated with extraocular muscle palsies, as the nuclei for cranial nerves III, IV, and VI occupy a large area of the pons and midbrain.

5) Loss of sensation on one entire side of the body suggests a lesion above the brainstem; facial findings on one side and extremity findings on the opposite side indicate a lesion in the brainstem.

6) A stocking glove distribution of sensory loss indicates a peripheral lesion; cape-like distribution of motor or sensory loss is associated with a lesion in the spinal cord (e.g. syringomyelia or a traumatic central cord syndrome).

7) There are several major neuroanatomic stroke syndromes, which result from disruption of their corresponding vascular supply. These include:

8) **Ischemic Stroke Syndromes**

   a) <u>Anterior Cerebral Artery Occlusion</u>- It affects frontal lobe function, resulting in mental status and behavioral change, gait disturbance, and contralateral lower extremity weakness.

   b) <u>Middle Cerebral Artery Occlusion</u>- It presents with contralateral weakness (usually the weakness is more pronounced in the upper extremity than the lower extremity) and numbness, ipsilateral hemianopia, possible dysarthria, and gaze preference toward the side of the lesion. If the lesion is in the dominant hemisphere (the left hemisphere is dominant in all right handed people and in 80% of left handed people), the patient may have a receptive or expressive aphasia. If the lesion is in the non-dominant hemisphere, the patient may have neglect of the involved side.

   c) <u>Posterior Cerebral Artery Occlusion</u>- It may produce cortical blindness, homonymous hemianopia, or mental status changes.

   d) <u>Vertebrobasilar Artery Occlusion</u>- It may cause dizziness, vertigo, diplopia, dysphagia, ataxia, cranial nerve palsies, and bilateral limb weakness. A hallmark is crossed neurological deficits: ipsilateral cranial nerve palsies and cerebellar signs, and contralateral hemiplegia and sensory deficits (the posterior circulation supplies the brainstem, cerebellum, and the visual cortex).

e) <u>Basilar Artery Occlusion</u>- It causes quadriplegia, coma, and the "locked-in" syndrome.

f) <u>Lacunar Infarcts</u>- It usually results in pure motor or sensory deficits; it usually involves the terminal vasculature of the subcortical cerebrum or brainstem. It often occurs in patients with small vessel disease secondary to diabetes or hypertension. Lacunar strokes generally do not cause impairments of speech or level of consciousness.

9) Hemorrhagic Stroke Syndromes

a) <u>Intracerebral Hemorrhage</u>- It causes contralateral weakness, numbness, hemianopia, and, if the dominant hemisphere is involved, aphasia (if the non-dominant hemisphere is involved, the patient may have neglect of the involved side).

b) <u>Cerebellar Hemorrhage</u>- It causes sudden onset of dizziness, vomiting, and severe truncal ataxia. Brainstem herniation may cause a rapid decrease in the level of consciousness, followed by apnea and death.

c) <u>Other</u>- The patient may also present with symptoms ranging from mild headache to coma.

•Evaluation•

1) Obtain head CT as soon as possible. An ischemic CVA may appear on CT by 6-12h, but more often at 24-48h.

2) Check ECG, glucose, electrolytes, BUN/Cr, PT/PTT, CBC, and CXR.

•Treatment•

1) Establish IV. Place patient on cardiac monitor. Administer oxygen. Assess and stabilize the airway.

2) If there are signs of herniation, intubate the patient and temporarily hyperventilate. If intubation is necessary, use etomidate, midazolam, or a decreased dose of thiopental (avoid hypotension); use lidocaine to decrease the gag response. If paralysis is necessary, first adminis-

ter a defasciculating dose of the paralytic.

3) Arrange admission; consider telemetry.

4) Further treatment options depend on the results of the head CT.

5) Treatment for Ischemic Stroke

  a) <u>Although controversial, assess patient for possible fibrinolytic therapy- see below.</u>

  b) Heparin is an unproven intervention. However, consider administering heparin for small or progressive strokes, especially in the vertebrobasilar distribution. Do not administer bolus heparin (there is an increased risk of hemorrhage). Do not administer heparin if the patient is hypertensive or if the physical exam indicates a large hemispheric stroke. Recent cardioembolic strokes are at risk for hemorrhagic transformation, so consider holding heparin for 48h in these patients (however, consider anticoagulation if there is only a minor deficit).

  c) Obtain an early neurosurgical consult if there is an infarct >50% of the middle cerebral artery territory or cerebellum, as these are likely to cause significant edema and herniation (a decompressive craniectomy may help).

  d) Steroids are not effective for edema caused by ischemia. If there is significant edema on CT (especially if it is accompanied by a decreasing level of consciousness), consider temporary hyperventilation, furosemide and mannitol to decrease intracranial pressure.

  e) Seizure prophylaxis is generally not indicated.

  f) Avoid hyperglycemia (it fuels anaerobic metabolism, increasing lactic acid production).

  g) Aspirin 325 mg is an effective preventive measure for stroke. Ticlopidine 250 mg bid may be given if aspirin allergic; it has a 2.4% risk of neutropenia.

  h) Administer antipyretics as needed.

6) Treatment for Hemorrhagic Stroke

  a) If edema is evident on CT (especially if accompanied by a decreasing level of consciousness), consider temporary hyperventilation, furosemide, and mannitol (1-2 g/kg). The patient may require surgical decompression.

  b) Steroids are not indicated in hemorrhagic strokes.

c) Reverse any anticoagulants or bleeding disorder.

d) Many recommend seizure prophylaxis with phenytoin.

7) Hypertension Treatment for Hemorrhagic Stroke

    a) If SBP > 230 or DBP > 120 mm Hg: Administer nitroprusside 0.5-10 mcg/kg/min or nitroglycerin drip 10-20 mcg/min.

    b) If SBP 181-230 or DBP 106-120 mm Hg: Consider labetalol 10 mg IV; may repeat or double every 10-20 min (max 300 mg).

    c) If hypertensive relative to prestroke condition: Consider lowering pressure to premorbid levels.

8) Hypertension Treatment if Ischemic Stroke, No Fibrinolysis

    a) If DBP > 140 mm Hg: Administer nitroprusside 0.5 mcg/kg/min.

    b) If SBP > 220 or DBP 121-140, or MAP > 130 mm Hg: Consider labetalol 10-20 mg IV over 1-2 min; may repeat or double every 20 min (max 150 mg).

    c) If SBP < 220 or DBP <120 or MAP < 130 mm Hg: Defer therapy unless aortic dissection, AMI, severe CHF, or hypertensive encephalopathy.

9) Fibrinolytic Therapy

    a) <u>Inclusion Criteria</u>: Clearly defined onset <3h; measurable CNS deficit; no intracranial hemorrhage on head CT; age over 18 years.

    b) <u>Exclusion Criteria</u>: On oral anticoagulant, PT>15, INR>1.7; heparin within 48h with increased PTT; history of intracranial hemorrhage or aneurysm; neoplasm; major surgery within 14d; seizure at onset of stroke; glucose <50 mg/dL or >400 mg/dL; uncontrolled HTN >185/110 mm Hg. Also, patients with early infarct signs on CT (peri-infarct edema, mass effect, sulcal effacement, or hemorrhage), should not receive tPA.

    c) <u>Relative contraindications</u>: GI or GU bleed within 21 days; stroke or serious blunt head trauma within 3 months; noncompressible arterial stick or LP within 7 days; rapidly improving or minor symptoms; platelet count <100; patient pregnant or lactating.

    d) <u>tPA protocol</u>: 0.9 mg/kg (max 90 mg), 10% as bolus, 90% over 60 minutes; do not administer anticoagulation or antiplatelet agents.

    e) <u>HTN Treatment if receiving tPA</u>

      Pre-treatment: if blood pressure >185/110 mm Hg, treat with nitroprusside or 10-20 mg labetalol x 1-2 within 1h; if this does not maintain blood pressure <185/110 mm Hg, do not administer tPA. *During treatment*: if DBP >140 mm Hg, start nitroprusside; if SBP >230 mm Hg or DBP 121-140 mm Hg, administer labetalol 20 mg IV, may repeat or double every 10 min (max 150 mg). If SBP 180-230 mm Hg or DBP 105-120 mm Hg, administer labetalol 10 mg, may repeat or double every 10-20 min (max 150 mg). Consider labetalol drip of 2-8 mg/min

f) <u>Complications</u>- For bleeding/coagulopathy, treat with protamine if heparin was given; if tPA was given, use amicar 5 g, cryoprecipitate 10-15 bags, and 1-2 U platelets (if CNS bleed). If patient is on Coumadin, administer vitamin K and FFP. If CNS bleed, consult neurosurgery.

B. Transient Ischemic Attack (TIA)

•General•

1) TIA is defined as a temporary loss of focal cerebral function secondary to vascular occlusion.

2) By definition, TIA symptoms last <24h; in one study, the median duration was 8 minutes for vertebrobasilar symptoms and 14 minutes for carotid distribution symptoms. TIA symptoms lasting over 1h will completely resolve in under 24h in only 14% of patients; 25% resolve within 5 min, and 50% resolve within 30 min.

3) The most common etiology is atherosclerosis. Less common etiologies include hypercoagulable states, arterial dissection, arteritis, aneurysm, and AVM; up to 30% of TIAs are cardioembolic.

4) Patients with TIAs have up to a 16-fold increased risk of stroke in the following year.

•Clinical Presentation•

1) Presenting symptoms depend on the area of the brain involved. Distinguish between anterior circulation symptoms (motor or sensory deficits of extremity or face, aphasia, homonymous hemianopia, amaurosis fugax) and posterior circulation symptoms (possible motor or sensory dysfunction, but usually in association with diplopia, dysarthria, ataxia, or vertigo).

2) Generally, symptoms are focal, acute in onset, and all symptoms begin at the same time.

3) Isolated nausea, vertigo, or dizziness is seldom caused by vertebrobasilar insufficiency; other symptoms are usually present.

4) Isolated syncope, confusion, amnesia or seizure is unlikely due to TIA.

•Evaluation•

1) Check CBC, glucose, electrolytes, PT/PTT, ESR, RPR, ECG, and head CT. Consider MRI/MRA.

2) If the diagnosis is not clear, consider echocardiogram, LP, and carotid ultrasound.

3) Document the presence of any neurologic deficit, cardiac arrhythmia or carotid bruit

•Treatment•

1) Consider antiplatelet therapy with aspirin 325 mg po qd. Ticlopidine (Ticlid) 250 mg po qd is comparable to aspirin, but the effect may take several days. Clopidogrel 75 mg/d is another option.

2) There is no evidence that heparin will prevent stroke if there is no clear etiology of the TIA. However, consider heparin (80 U/kg bolus, then 18 U/hr; reduce the loading dose in the elderly) or Coumadin if the patient has recurrent symptoms on aspirin, crescendo TIAs, or if there is a cardiac source (e.g., if the patient is in atrial fibrillation).

3) Do not anticoagulate septic cardiac emboli.

•Disposition•

1) Consider admitting all patients, especially high-risk patients (crescendo TIAs, cardiac source, multiple TIAs in past 2 weeks, severe deficit associated with TIA or persistent TIAs despite anticoagulation). If the patient is high-risk, consider anticoagulation and admission to a telemetry unit.

2) If the patient is low-risk, consider discharge with close follow-up and expedited outpatient evaluation; discharge on aspirin or ticlopidine 250 mg bid.

IX. SUBARACHNOID HEMORRHAGE

•General•

1) Etiologies include a berry aneurysm (which may be congenital or degenerative), AVM, mycotic aneurysm, and trauma.

2) The incidence increases in 20-30 year olds and peaks at 60 years; 80% of subarachnoid hemorrhages occur between ages 40-65 years.

3) Risk factors include smoking, cocaine use, pregnancy, and African-American race.

•Clinical Presentation•

1) Patients may present with a sudden, exploding, bursting headache, nausea, vomiting, altered mental status, and nuchal rigidity. 50% of patients have an altered mental status or syncope.

2) Warning symptoms (sentinel headaches) occur in 30-50% of patients, usually 1-3 weeks earlier.

3) Nuchal rigidity is the most common physical finding, but takes 3-12h to develop.

4) Focal CNS findings are unusual; seizures occur in 3-25% of patients.

5) Increased systolic blood pressure occurs in 35-50% of patients. The patient may be febrile secondary to thermoregulatory dysfunction caused by bleeding.

Hunt and Hess Classification of Subarachnoid Hemorrhage

Grade 1: Asymptomatic or minimal headache and slight nuchal rigidity.

Grade II: Moderate to severe headache, nuchal rigidity, no neurologic deficit other than cranial nerve palsy.

Grade III: Drowsiness, confusion, or mild focal deficit.

Grade IV: Stupor, moderate to severe hemiparesis, possible early decerebrate posturing.

Grade V: Deep coma, decerebrate rigidity, moribund appearance.

•Evaluation•

1) Obtain head CT, ECG, CBC, platelets, glucose, electrolytes, BUN/CR, and PT/PTT (hyponatremia and volume contraction are common). Consider CXR, type and crossmatch, and ABG.

2) Head CT- It is approximately 90% sensitive, although 3rd and 4th generation CT scanners may have up to a 93-99% sensitivity in the first 12 hours after symptom onset. Sensitivity declines with time. 15% of alert patients with subarachnoid hemorrhage have a normal CT scan. Anemic patients may have false negative CT scans.

3) Lumbar Puncture (LP)- If the head CT is negative, perform an LP. If positive, the LP usually shows >100,000 RBCs and xanthochromia. (Xanthochromia appears 6-12h after the onset of bleeding, persists up to 3 weeks, and is present in all cases; lab analysis is required. Xanthochromia is the yellow discoloration of the supernatant caused by lysis of red blood cells; RBCs from a traumatic tap do not have time to degenerate, and therefore do not produce xanthochromia). There is no absolute number of RBCs that defines subarachnoid hemorrhage; check for a decline in the number of RBCs from tube 1 to tube 4 of the LP (although there is no absolute percentage decline that rules out subarachnoid hemorrhage). LP is most sensitive 12h after the onset of bleeding, and may be negative in the first 2h. *Always do CT first*

4) <u>ECG</u> may show peaked or deep inverted T waves, with prolonged QRS and QT intervals (from increased catecholamines). Arrhythmias occur in 40% of patients. 20% have evidence of ischemia.

5) Consider cerebral angiogram.

•Treatment•

1) The goals are the prevention of rebleeding, vasospasm (which occurs in 50% of patients, usually beginning in 3-5 days), and hydrocephalus.

2) Establish IV access (avoid dehydration). Place patient on monitor. Administer oxygen. Assess and stabilize the airway.

3) Elevate the head to decrease intracranial pressure.

4) If there are signs of herniation, intubate the patient and temporarily hyperventilate. If intubation is necessary, use etomidate, midazolam, or a decreased dose of thiopental (avoid hypotension); use lidocaine to decrease the gag response. If paralysis is necessary, first administer a defasciculating dose of the paralytic.

5) If herniation is suspected, consider mannitol 1-2 g/kg and furosemide.

6) Administer antiemetics (prochlorperazine), narcotics, and sedatives as needed.

7) Consider dexamethasone 10 mg IV, then 4 mg q6h (although it has not been shown to improve outcome).

8) Administer phenytoin if the patient has a seizure (prophylactic anticonvulsant use is controversial).

9) If the diastolic blood pressure is greater than 120-130 mm Hg, ad-

minister labetalol.

10) Administer nimodipine 60 mg every 4h if the patient is not comatose (start in ED or within 12h); it improves outcome after vasospasm but does not decrease its incidence.

11) Consult neurosurgery and admit to a monitored setting.

X. SYNCOPE

•Definition•

Syncope is defined as a sudden, transient loss of consciousness with loss of postural tone.

•Etiology/Clinical Presentation•

1) Cardiac Etiology

Arrhythmia/Reduced cardiac output

a) Syncope may be secondary to arrhythmia, or obstruction to flow (e.g., myopathy, aortic stenosis, pulmonary embolus, myocardial infarction, tamponade, pulmonary hypertension, pulmonic stenosis, or aortic dissection).

b) Patients present with an abrupt onset usually without preceding symptoms (although patients may have brief weakness, chest pain, or palpitations). There is a prompt resolution. It may occur while the patient is recumbent (as opposed to vasovagal syncope).

c) Exertional syncope suggests aortic stenosis (or prosthetic aortic valve dysfunction which requires urgent investigation); it may indicate a critical narrowing of the outflow tract (or cardiomyopathy). In these patients, exercise results in a pathologic increase in left ventricular pressure that then causes a reflex decrease in systemic vascular resistance, causing hypotension and syncope.

d) Stokes-Adams attacks occur when patients develop heart block and asystole occurs before a ventricular escape rhythm begins; presyncope or syncope occurs during the asystole period. The ECG may show a left bundle branch block or a right bundle branch block with left atrial hypertrophy.

2) Non-Cardiac Etiology

A. Neurocardiogenic/vasovagal

a) Peripheral venous pooling (e.g. with prolonged upright posture, especially if dehydrated) may decrease preload and precipitate a maladaptive reflex which results in paradoxical vasodilation and bradycardia; this occurs because vigorous contraction of a volume depleted heart activates left ventricular stretch receptors and the Bezold-Jarisch reflex, in which the medulla interprets the activation of the stretch receptors as hypertension and thus decreases sympathetic tone and activates the parasympathetics.

   b) This may lead to hypotension, cerebral hypoperfusion, and syncope; the patient may experience lightheadedness, nausea, and diaphoresis. Usually the patient has progressive warning symptoms (which allow the patient to protect himself during a fall) and a prompt recovery after assuming a supine position. Neurocardiogenic syncope may also be precipitated by fear, pain, or anxiety. Exclude other etiologies, especially if the patient is older than 40 years and presents with a first episode of syncope.

   c) A similar process occurs with cough and micturition syncope (or Valsalva), in which cough or micturition cause mechanical reduction of venous return and a decrease in sympathetic tone and/or a surge in parasympathetic tone.

   d) Other causes include carotid hypersensitivity and reflex syncope (pain of visceral origin stimulates the vagus nerve, causing bradycardia).

B. Orthostatic hypotension

   a) It usually occurs in elderly patients, diabetics, alcoholics, and Parkinson's patients who have defective vasomotor reflexes and suddenly rise from a recumbent position. Patients become lightheaded and hypotensive with blurred vision; symptoms resolve with the assumption of a recumbent position.

   b) It is often precipitated by drugs (e.g. nitrates, diuretics, antiarrhythmics, or antihypertensives) and autonomic disorders.

C. Hypovolemia/blood loss

   Intravascular depletion may lead to hypotension and syncope. Examples include ruptured abdominal aneurysm and ruptured ectopic pregnancy.

D. Neurologic

   a) Syncope may result from decreased global perfusion, focal involvement of the brainstem, or seizure.

b) Vertebrobasilar TIAs may rarely cause syncope, but usually with other symptoms (e.g. dysarthria, vertigo, and diplopia); carotid TIAs usually do not cause syncope, as the reticular activating system is not involved.

c) A seizure presents with an abrupt onset and is followed by a postictal period. Typically, there are no premonitory vasovagal symptoms. An abrupt onset may also be cardiogenic; tongue biting, incontinence, and clonic jerks may occur with any syncope.

d) Also, consider subarachnoid hemorrhage.

E. Miscellaneous

Other etiologies include hypoglycemia (which almost always occurs with hypoglycemic agents), hyperventilation (usually presyncope and reproducible), toxic etiologies, and psychogenic.

•Evaluation•

1) Check glucose, stool hemoccult, pregnancy test and ECG. Electrolytes and CBC are of little benefit (bleeding significant enough to cause syncope should be detectable on clinical grounds).

2) Palpate the abdomen for aneurysm. Auscultate for the murmur of aortic stenosis or cardiomyopathy. Look for signs of pulmonary hypertension. Document a complete cardiac and neurologic exam.

3) Look for evidence of trauma or hypovolemia (trauma may indicate a less benign etiology, as benign syncope usually has premonitory symptoms, allowing the patient to protect himself).

4) Document the patient's activity and position prior to syncope. Document any symptoms preceding the syncopal event. Post-syncopal convulsions or confusion may indicate a seizure.

5) If symptoms develop slowly, consider vasovagal syncope, hyperventilation or hypoglycemia; if symptoms occur over a period of seconds, consider arrhythmia (e.g. sudden A-V block), postural hypotension, or carotid sinus syncope. If a patient has syncope or faintness with bradycardia, it is important to distinguish between a reflex vasovagal episode and cardiogenic or Stokes-Adams bradycardia.

6) Consider a Holter monitor, event monitor, echocardiogram, telemetry, and tilt table test. Consider head CT if focal CNS signs.

7) Red flags include chest pain or palpitations; no warning symptoms;

occurs when supine; family history of sudden cardiac death; elderly; abnormal CNS exam; long QT interval; WPW; or if it is associated with exercise.

•Disposition•

1) Admit and monitor patients who have a history of CHF or ventricular arrhythmias, associated chest pain, a physical exam consistent with CHF or valvular disease, or an ECG that shows ischemia, arrhythmia, bundle branch block, or a prolonged QT interval. Dilated cardiomyopathy associated with syncope has a very high risk for sudden death.

2) Consider admission for patients older than 60 years, any patient with a history of CAD or congenital heart disease, a family history of sudden death, or younger patients with exertional syncope.

3) In younger patients without cardiac disease and a normal ECG, there is no increased risk of sudden death.

4) Near syncope should be treated the same as syncope.

XI. VERTIGO

•Etiology/Clinical Presentation•

*Distinguish between peripheral and central etiologies of vertigo.

1) **Peripheral Vertigo/Labyrinthine Dysfunction**- Patients present with a sensation of intense spinning or swaying, nausea and vomiting, possible diarrhea, and diaphoresis; the vertigo is usually brief and episodic. Movement or a change of position aggravates it; there is usually an acute onset. Patients may describe a feeling of impulsion- a sensation of being pulled to one side of the ground. There is possible tinnitus and hearing loss. The nystagmus is fatigable, unidirectional, and is inhibited by ocular fixation. Other CNS deficits are absent. Etiologies include:

   a) <u>Benign Positional Vertigo</u>- Benign positional vertigo is thought to result from floating debris in the posterior semicircular canal of the ear; it is the most common cause of vertigo and has a good prognosis. The Hallpike (Nylen-Barany) test is diagnostic and helps distinguish peripheral from central vertigo: with the patient in a sitting position, support the head and rapidly assume a supine position, first with the head straight, then with 45 degrees to the left and right; the neck should be extended slightly over the edge of the bed when the patient is placed supine. With peripheral vertigo, the vertigo and nystagmus are reproduced with a latency of 2-20 seconds, the duration is less than 1 minute, and the nystagmus is unidirectional; the nystagmus and vertigo fatigue with repeated testing. With central vertigo, there is no latency of nystagmus, the nystagmus lasts longer than 1 minute, and is multidirectional and nonfatiguing.

  b) <u>Acute Labyrinthitis</u>- It produces peripheral vertigo with hearing loss. It may be secondary to infection, trauma, ischemia, or drugs.
  c) <u>Meniere's Disease</u>- It causes recurrent severe vertigo with tinnitus and progressive sensorineural hearing loss.

2) Central Vertigo- Symptoms are ill defined, less intense than peripheral vertigo, and not positionally related; symptoms are usually chronic and continuous. Nausea and vomiting are less common than with peripheral vertigo. The patient may have brainstem and cerebellar symptoms (e.g. diplopia, dysphagia, ataxia, hemiparesis). The nystagmus is often nonfatiguable and multidirectional. Hearing is usually unimpaired. Etiologies include a cerebellar infarct, hemorrhage, tumor (including acoustic neuroma), vertebrobasilar arterial insufficiency, CNS infection, or multiple sclerosis.

•Evaluation•

1) Perform a complete neurologic exam, including cranial nerves and cerebellar exam; evaluate for truncal and limb ataxia. Perform a cardiac exam. Check the tympanic membranes.
2) Lab evaluation is usually unnecessary. Obtain MRI/MRA or head CT with thin cuts of the posterior fossa if a cerebellar bleed, cerebellar infarct or cerebropontine angle tumor is suspected.
3) Consider carbon monoxide poisoning if dizziness, headache and nausea.

•Treatment•

1) Meclizine 25 mg po/IV every 6h or diazepam 2-10 mg po every 6-8h.
2) If the patient has benign positional vertigo, a canalith-repositioning procedure (the Epley maneuver) may be attempted:

a) Have patient seated with head turned 45° toward the affected ear and lower the patient into a supine position (maintaining the head at 45°), and hang head off the end of the bed.

b) Maintain the patient in this position for 4 minutes or until symptoms resolve.

c) Next, turn the patient's head 90° toward the opposite ear and maintain until symptoms resolve; then ask the patient to roll onto the shoulder on the side of the unaffected ear. Next, turn the patient's head, so he is looking at the floor; maintain until symptoms resolve.

d) Maintaining the position of the head, return patient to seated position, turn patient's head to midline and tilt head 30° toward chest, and maintain for 4 minutes.

e) Have patient remain upright for 1-2 days.

CHAPTER 17
OB/GYN

I. DELIVERY

A. Normal Delivery Procedure

1) Place patient in the dorsal lithotomy position, slightly on the left side to avoid caval compression; perform a midline episiotomy if needed (avoid extension into the rectum).

2) As the head emerges, place your left hand over the head to control delivery; with your right hand under a sterile towel, apply pressure through the perineum and gently lift the infant's chin. As the head is delivered, allow it to restitute to one side; palpate the neck region and slip the nuchal cord over the head (if the cord is tight, place two clamps close together and cut in between).

3) Wipe the mouth and nose, and aspirate with bulb.

4) Place both your hands on either side of the head and apply gentle downward traction to ease the anterior shoulder under the pubis (if there is resistance, apply suprapubic pressure- not fundal), then upward traction to deliver the posterior shoulder.

5) Hold the infant with one hand behind the neck and use your anterior hand to grasp the legs by placing your index finger between the legs and the middle finger and your thumb around each leg.

6) Maintain the infant below the level of the placenta prior to clamping the cord with 2 clamps. Cut the cord in between the clamps with a sterile scissors.

7) Massage the uterus. Administer 10 U oxytocin. Consider methergine if excessive bleeding.

B. Shoulder Dystocia- Delivery Procedure

*Typically, the head is pulled tightly to the perineum (the turtle sign). To extricate the infant, attempt, in order:

1) McRoberts maneuver (maternal legs sharply flexed). Evacuating the bladder by straight catheterization may aid delivery.

2) Generous episiotomy.

3) Suprapubic (not fundal) pressure.

4) Rotate one or both shoulders toward the anterior surface of the fetal chest to displace the anterior shoulder from the pubis.

5) Deliver the posterior arm by making a large proctoepisiotomy, and attempt delivery or rotate the infant.

6) Fracture the clavicle or humerus.

C. Breech Delivery Procedure

1) If footling (a foot is the presenting part), pull feet through the vulva, make a wide episiotomy, and use gentle traction to deliver the hips. If frank breech (buttocks are the presenting part), allow spontaneous delivery to the umbilicus, and make a wide episiotomy. At this point, the infant's back is anterior. Gently handle the pelvis and back (not the abdomen), and deliver the scapulae, and then rotate the infant's back laterally.

2) Rotate one shoulder anteriorly and deliver the first shoulder by lowering the body.

3) Rotate the infant in the opposite direction and deliver the next shoulder beneath the symphysis pubis. If the arm does not pass, reach in and follow the shaft of the humerus to the elbow, grasp the forearm and sweep across chest and through introitus.

4) If the shoulders cannot be delivered by the previous method, deliver the posterior shoulder first by using upward traction on the lower extremities. Then, deliver the anterior shoulder with downward traction.

5) To deliver the head, place the infant's back under the symphysis pubis and apply suprapubic pressure to maintain flexion of the head; with the infant on your hand and forearm, place your fingers over the maxilla. Place 2 fingers from your other hand onto the neck. Grasp the shoulders and apply downward traction and flex the head to complete delivery.

D. Post-Partum Hemorrhage

*It is defined as >500 cc blood loss in the first 24h after delivery. The most common etiologies are uterine atony, an abnormally adherent placenta, cervical/uterine lacerations, and bleeding disorders. Treatment includes:

1) Establish 2 large bore IVs. Place patient on monitor. Administer oxygen.
2) Check CBC, platelets, PT/PTT, type and crossmatch.
3) Administer IVNS; transfuse blood as needed.
4) Inspect the cervix and vagina for the presence of lacerations. Bimanual palpation of the uterus may reveal bogginess or uterine atony. Examine the placenta for any missing sections, which may indicate retained placenta.
5) Perform uterine massage.
6) If the placenta does not spontaneously separate, it may be secondary to placenta accreta; the patient should be transferred to labor and delivery for definitive management (improper attempts at removal may result in uterine inversion or massive bleeding).
7) Administer oxytocin (Pitocin) 10 U IM or 10-40 U in 1L NS at 100-200 cc/h after delivery of the placenta (it may cause hypotension). Or, consider Methergine 0.2 mg IM after delivery of the placenta.
8) Arrange an emergent OB/GYN consult.

II. DYSFUNCTIONAL UTERINE BLEEDING (non-pregnant)

•General•

1) Dysfunctional uterine bleeding (DUB) refers to abnormal bleeding not related to organic causes (e.g., pregnancy, neoplasm, or bleeding dyscrasias). DUB is usually hormonal in etiology (either abnormal endogenous hormone production or exogenous birth control pills).
2) Menorrhagia is defined as a menstrual cycle in which bleeding is excessive or prolonged; metrorrhagia is bleeding at irregular intervals.
3) DUB may occur in anovulatory or ovulatory cycles.
4) In anovulatory cycles (90% of DUB is anovulatory), the corpus luteum does not form, and subsequent normal progesterone secretion does not occur. This results in continuous unopposed production of estradiol, which in turn stimulates growth of the endometrium. Without progesterone, normal orderly shedding of the endometrium does not occur, and the endometrium outgrows its blood supply, causing

irregular and prolonged bleeding (the amount of bleeding depends on the level of chronic circulating estrogen; low levels result in spotting, whereas higher levels may cause heavy bleeding). In addition, vasodilatory prostaglandins play a role in DUB, causing further excessive bleeding.

5) Ovulatory bleeding is usually secondary to prostaglandin dysfunction or prolonged progesterone secretion, which results in irregular shedding of the endometrium.

6) DUB may be associated with obesity, eating disorders, hyperprolactinemia, stress, or polycystic ovarian syndrome.

•Evaluation•

1) Check CBC, platelets and pregnancy test. If severe bleeding, consider PT/PTT and type and screen.

2) Perform a pelvic exam.

3) Attempt to exclude treatable disorders, including infection, tumors, fibroids, cysts, endocrine disorders, trauma, and bleeding disorders.

•Treatment•

1) If the patient is younger than 35 years, consider oral contraceptive pills (OCPs) that have high dose estrogen and progesterone (e.g., Ortho-Novum); estrogen will regulate endometrial growth and control bleeding. If heavy bleeding, give two pills bid x 1-2d, then one pill bid x 1-2d, then one pill qd; if mild bleeding, consider prompt OB follow-up or starting the patient on regular OCP cycle and /or NSAIDs (prostaglandins induce follicle rupture and dilate the endometrium; NSAIDS may lower prostaglandins and decrease bleeding).

2) Progestins have an anti-estrogen effect; consider medroxyprogesterone 30-40 mg/d x 1 week, then taper. Reserve progestins for patients with a definite diagnosis of anovulatory DUB.

3) If severe bleeding, establish IV, administer oxygen, and place patient on monitor. Consider Premarin 25 mg IV every 4-6h and blood transfusion. Chronic bleeding and long-term OCPs may result in an atrophic endometrium; IV estrogen may induce endometrial cell proliferation, stop bleeding, decrease capillary permeability, and increase fibrinogen, factors V and IX and platelet aggregation. Arrange emergent OB/GYN consult.

4) If severe bleeding persists, consider inserting a Foley catheter through the cervical os and inflate to tamponade bleeding.

5) Consider dilatation and curettage.

6) Avoid uterine contracting agents such as ergotamine.

III. ECTOPIC PREGNANCY

•Risk Factors•

Risk factors include a previous ectopic pregnancy or tubal surgery, in-vitro fertilization, current IUD, diethylstilbestrol (DES) exposure, history of pelvic inflammatory disease, use of progestin-only birth control pills, and smoking.

•Clinical Presentation•

1) The triad of pain (seen in 96%), amenorrhea (80%) and vaginal bleeding (64%) is present in only 50% of patients. The character of the pain is variable. Ectopic pregnancy may be an incidental finding.

2) Bleeding is usually mild; heavy bleeding with clots is atypical.

3) Fever is rare.

4) If hemoperitoneum is present, the patient may have left shoulder pain or tenesmus; the patient may present in hemorrhagic shock. The patient may present with syncope.

5) 5-10% of ectopic pregnancies are associated with the shedding of a decidual cast.

•Evaluation•

1) Check ultrasound (US), CBC, quantitative HCG, type and crossmatch. Perform abdominal and pelvic exams. Tenderness is usually unilateral, but may be contralateral to the ectopic pregnancy (representing the corpus luteum); tenderness may be absent. The pelvic exam reveals a mass in 50% of patients.

2) HCG

a) The serum test detects levels as low as 5 mIU/ml; the ELISA urine test detects levels of 25-50 mIU/ml. The HCG at the time of missed menses (13-14 days after conception) is 50-300 mIU/ml, which should double every 2 days, reaching 100 mIU/ml by 4 weeks gestational age, and peaking at 100,000 at 11 weeks. The HCG correlates directly with the mass of viable trophoblastic tissue.

    b) A low HCG level does not preclude rupture (one study showed that 29% of ectopic pregnancies with an HCG <1000 mIU/ml were ruptured and that 36% had no adnexal tenderness).

    c) Women with lower HCG values (< 1000 mIU/ml) have a 3-4 times greater risk for an ectopic pregnancy. In one study of proven ectopic pregnancies, the HCG level at the time of diagnosis ranged from 11 to 28,930, with 35% of ectopics <550 mIU/ml.

3) Ultrasound

    a) On transvaginal ultrasound, an intrauterine pregnancy (IUP) is seen 5 weeks after the last menstrual period (with HCG 1000-2000 mIU/ml); on transabdominal ultrasound, the HCG must be ≥6500 mIU/ml.

    b) On transvaginal ultrasound, look for a gestational sac (seen at 5 weeks, HCG 1200-1500 mIU/ml), the double sac sign, the yolk sac (seen at 6 weeks, HCG ≥2500 mIU/ml), and the fetal pole (seen at 6.5 weeks, HCG 5000 mIU/ml) with heart beat (7 weeks, HCG 12,000-14,000 mIU/ml).

    c) Possible indications of an ectopic pregnancy may include a solid or cystic adnexal mass, free fluid in the pelvis, a tubal gestational sac, and an empty uterus. One study showed that up to 40% of ectopic pregnancies can be detected by experienced technicians even with an HCG <1000 mIU/ml

    d) The incidence of heterotopic pregnancies has increased significantly; the general population has an incidence of 1:4000-7000, while patients who have undergone assisted reproduction have an incidence up to 1:100.

4) Progesterone- A viable pregnancy stimulates the production of progesterone by the corpus luteum. A level <5 ng/ml suggests a nonviable pregnancy; 80% of ectopic pregnancies have a progesterone <15 ng/ml. If the progesterone is >25 ng/ml, then only 2.5% of pregnancies are abnormal.

•Treatment/Disposition•

1) If ultrasound identifies an ectopic pregnancy- establish 2 large bore IVs, check CBC, type and screen, place patient on monitor, transfuse blood as needed, and consult OB/GYN for possible immediate laparotomy or admission for medical therapy (methotrexate).

2) **If HCG >1500-2000 and US is indeterminate**, it is an ectopic pregnancy or recently completed abortion. Consider observing the patient (or, if the patient is very stable and low risk, consider discharge with close OB/GYN follow-up), and re-checking HCG levels and ultrasound. If the HCG rises or plateaus, then an ectopic pregnancy is confirmed. Falling titers indicate a completed abortion or a spontaneously resolving ectopic pregnancy (which occurs in 5% of ectopic pregnancies); however, there is a much slower decline in titers in resolving ectopic pregnancies. Or, consider immediate laparotomy, especially if there is a suggestive physical exam or the US shows free fluid or a complex adnexal mass. Or, consider dilation and evacuation (as there is no fear of aborting a viable gestation) to identify chorionic villi, which will confirm a recent abnormal intrauterine pregnancy.

3) **If HCG <1500-2000 and no IUP is seen on US**, the differential diagnosis includes early IUP, abnormal IUP, completed abortion, or ectopic pregnancy. If the patient is high risk or there is a suggestive physical exam, consider observation. In all patients, follow the HCG levels and arrange a repeat US. Consider laparoscopy, especially if US shows free fluid or a complex adnexal mass.

IV. PLACENTAL ABRUPTION; PLACENTA PREVIA

A. Placental Abruption

•General•
1) Placental abruption is defined as separation of the normal placenta from the uterus after the 20th week of gestation and prior to birth.
2) Placental abruption accounts for 30% of 3rd trimester bleeding.

•Risk Factors•
Risk factors include hypertension, trauma, maternal age greater than 35 years, smoking, and cocaine use.

•Clinical Presentation•
1) Patients present with vaginal bleeding in the 3rd trimester (although the bleeding may be concealed behind the adherent membranes) and abdominal or back pain.
2) Patients may present with uterine contractions and fetal distress or

fetal death.

3) DIC may result.

•Evaluation•

1) Check CBC, platelets, electrolytes, PT/PTT, DIC panel, type and screen and RH, and ultrasound.

2) Avoid a digital pelvic exam unless placenta previa has been excluded.

3) Ultrasound may verify the diagnosis and determine fetal viability. While an ultrasound may not diagnose abruption, it can determine the location of the placenta and exclude placenta previa.

4) Arrange fetal heart monitoring, which may show signs of fetal distress.

•Treatment•

1) Establish IV. Place patient on monitor. Administer oxygen. Arrange continuous fetal monitoring.

2) Transfuse packed RBCs and FFP as needed.

3) Arrange an emergent OB/GYN consult.

4) If the mother or fetus becomes unstable, immediate delivery by C-section is indicated. If abruption is minimal, close observation may be an option.

B. Placenta Previa

•Definition•

The placenta is implanted over the internal cervical os.

•Risk Factors•

Risk factors include multiple gestations, advanced maternal age, increased parity, and previous c-section.

•Clinical Presentation•

Patients present with sudden profuse vaginal bleeding in the latter half of pregnancy, without abdominal pain (as the lower uterine segments thins out during the 3rd trimester, the placenta may separate, resulting in bleeding).

•Evaluation•

1) Check CBC, platelets, PT/PTT, type and screen and RH, and ultrasound.

2) Ultrasound is 95% sensitive for diagnosing placenta previa.

3) Avoid a digital pelvic exam (the exam should be performed in an OR equipped for possible C-section). The uterus is usually nontender.

•Treatment•

1) Establish 2 large bore IVs; transfuse as needed.

2) Arrange an emergent OB/GYN consult.

3) Arrange continuous fetal monitoring.

4) If severe bleeding, or if the patient is near-term and in labor, then delivery is indicated (usually c-section).

5) If the patient is pre-term, and bleeding is controlled, consider tocolysis with terbutaline 0.25-0.5 mg SC q 2h.

V. PREECLAMPSIA/ECLAMPSIA

•General•

1) Preeclampsia is defined as hypertension (SBP >140 mm Hg or 30 mm Hg above pre-pregnancy level; DBP >90 mm Hg or 15 mm Hg above pre-pregnancy level) associated with proteinuria (1-2+ on urinalysis or > 300 mg/24h), and often edema (more than just lower extremity dependent edema; usually of the face and hands).

2) Eclampsia is defined as preeclampsia associated with seizures or coma.

3) Preeclampsia usually occurs after the 20th week of pregnancy. It occurs in the third trimester unless there is a molar pregnancy or prior history of hypertension or renal disease. It may develop for up to 2 weeks post partum. 85% of preeclamptics are primagravidas.

4) The criteria for severe preeclampsia include BP ≥160/110 mm Hg, proteinuria >5 g/24h, oliguria, cerebral or visual disturbances, pulmonary edema, epigastric or right upper quadrant pain, or the HELLP syndrome (Hemolysis, Elevated LFTs, Low Platelets).

•Risk Factors•

Risk factors include a prior history of preeclampsia/eclampsia, hypertension, molar pregnancy, primagravidas, extremes of maternal age, and diabetes.

•Clinical Presentation•

1) The patient may be asymptomatic. The presence of headache, altered mental status, visual changes, pulmonary edema, epigastric or right upper quadrant pain, oliguria, or seizure defines severe disease.

2) Up to 10% of severe preeclamptics develop the HELLP syndrome; vigorous palpation of the liver in these patients may rupture a sub-capsular liver hematoma.

•Evaluation•

1) Check electrolytes, BUN/Cr, LFTs, urinalysis, CBC, platelets, PT/PTT, and a peripheral blood smear.

2) A head CT is indicated if headache, focal CNS signs, altered mental status, or seizure.

3) Consider ultrasound to assess the fetus.

•Treatment•

1) Establish IV. Place patient on monitor. Assess and stabilize the airway.

2) If severe preeclampsia or seizures, induce delivery.

3) For hypertension: If >160/110 mm Hg (although severe symptoms may require treatment at a lower BP), start hydralazine 5-10 mg IV every 20 min (max 60 mg) or labetalol 50-100 mg IV or nitroprus-side.

4) If seizure, or for seizure prophylaxis in severe preeclampsia: Mg 4-6 gm IV over 5-20 min, then 1-2 g/h for prophylaxis. Monitor the patellar reflexes (hyporeflexia usually precedes more serious adverse effects of Mg therapy). Magnesium toxicity may manifest as respiratory depression and cardiac arrest; treat magnesium overdose with 1 gm calcium gluconate IV over 2 min.

5) Consider lorazepam if status epilepticus.

6) If mild preeclampsia, generally admit the patient for bed rest and Ob/Gyn evaluation. If patient is term, delivery is indicated.

VI. SPONTANEOUS ABORTION

•Classification•

Complete- All tissue is passed and the os is closed.

Inevitable- The cervix is dilated but no tissue has passed.

Incomplete- The cervix is dilated and some tissue has passed but some remains.

Missed- There is no evidence of fetal life, but no cervical dilation or passed tissue.

Septic- The patient is febrile, with pelvic pain; it usually occurs after instrumentation.

Threatened- Bleeding without cervical dilation.

•Clinical Presentation•

1) Patients present with vaginal bleeding, a history of amenorrhea, and variable uterine cramping (bleeding and cramping are worse with incomplete or inevitable abortion).

2) Pain usually occurs after the onset of bleeding, and is generally midline.

3) Document any history of fever or prior instrumentation.

•Evaluation•

1) Using a sterile technique, determine the patency of the cervical os and the size of the uterus. Document any uterine or adnexal tenderness or mass. Document the presence or absence of fetal heart tones. Document any fever.

2) If tissue is present, float tissue in saline and observe for a branching pattern of the placenta, firm structure, and purple and white flecks. Send tissue to pathology for diagnosis.

3) Consider CBC, type and RH, quantitative HCG, and ultrasound.

4) An ultrasound is indicated in incomplete, inevitable, complete, septic or missed abortions, to evaluate for retained products. Consider ultrasound if there is a question of ectopic pregnancy, if the uterine size is inconsistent with dates, if there is evidence of a molar pregnancy, or for prognostic information of a threatened abortion. If a heartbeat is detectable on ultrasound, then continuation of the pregnancy is very likely.

5) If a prior intrauterine pregnancy is documented and bleeding has stopped, an ultrasound is usually not necessary.

•Treatment•

1) **Complete**- Consider an ultrasound to evaluate for retained products; consider curettage.

2) **Inevitable/incomplete**- Consider dilation and curettage on all patients through 14 weeks; beyond 14 weeks curettage in the OR is usually necessary. If heavy bleeding, consider 30-40 U of pitocin.

3) **Missed**- Obtain ultrasound. Most 1st trimester missed abortions will abort spontaneously; consider expectant management or suction curettage. 2nd trimester missed abortions require dilation and evacuation or induction of labor.

4) **Septic**- Admit patient, obtain ultrasound, and administer antibiotics.

5) **Threatened**- Treat expectantly; if bleeding more briskly than normal menses or more than minimal cramping, observe for 2-3h. Consider checking a baseline HCG (falling levels indicate fetal demise or missed abortion). Bed rest may decrease bleeding and cramping, but there is no evidence that it affects outcome. Advise patient to return if heavier bleeding (>1 pad/h), severe cramping, or tissue passage; follow-up within 1 week.

6) **Rh Sensitization**

   a) Rh incompatibility may occur when an Rh negative mother is exposed to RBCs from an Rh-positive fetus (which may occur during abortion, trauma, or delivery).

   b) If the patient is Rh negative with no previous history of sensitization (pregnancy or transfusion), give Rhogam (anti-D immune globulin Rh IgG) 50 mcg if ≤12 weeks gestational age and 300 mcg if >12 weeks gestational age. If there is a history of previous sensitization, obtain an Rh antibody titer and, if negative, give Rhogam; if positive, Rhogam is not indicated (the mother has already been sensitized, and should be referred to OB/Gyn for fetal evaluation).

   c) Rhogam is probably indicated in a threatened abortion in Rh-negative patients; alternatively, if necessary, the patient can receive it later in pregnancy or when she aborts.

   d) If the patient is aborting and is Rh positive, Rhogam is not indicated.

7) The patient should wait three normal menses before attempting pregnancy (to allow the uterine lining to regenerate). Avoid coitus until all bleeding has stopped, to minimize the risk of infection.

•Prognosis•

1) Vaginal bleeding occurs in the 1st trimester in 20% of pregnancies; of these, half will abort. In those pregnancies that continue, there is no increase in fetal anomalies, but the risk of a suboptimal pregnancy

(low birth weight, prematurity) doubles.
2) If the patient is aborting and there is no history of previous spontaneous abortion, the risk of miscarriage with the next pregnancy is unchanged.

CHAPTER 18

OPHTHALMOLOGY

I. CELLULITIS

A. Periorbital (Preseptal) Cellulitis

•General•
1) Pathogens include H. flu and S. pneumococcus.
2) It usually occurs in children younger than 5 years, with a peak incidence at 6 months -2 years.

•Clinical Presentation•
1) Patients present with fever, erythema and edema of the lids, chemosis, orbital pain, and conjunctivitis.
2) **Extraocular muscle use is unrestricted**.
3) Patients may have recent facial trauma, facial infection or otitis media.

•Evaluation•
Consider LP and CT, to exclude meningitis and more extensive ocular involvement.

•Treatment•
1) If very mild, consider cefaclor 40 mg/kg/d divided q8h po.
2) Otherwise, administer nafcillin 100-200 mg/kg/d IV divided q6h and Unasyn 1.5-3 gm IV for anaerobic coverage; or cefuroxime 100-150 mg/kg/d IV divided q8h.

B. Orbital Cellulitis

•General•
1) Orbital cellulitis is an abscess posterior to the septum; pathogens include S. aureus, S. pneumoniae, and H. flu.
2) The patient is usually older than 6 years. It usually occurs from a sinus infection.

•Clinical Presentation•
1) Patients present with proptosis, orbital discomfort, ophthalmoplegia,

fever, redness and edema of lids, chemosis, and impaired vision.
2) Patients may have axial displacement of the eye. It is usually unilateral.

•Evaluation•
Obtain CT or MRI to rule out a retro-orbital abscess. Consider LP to exclude coexisting meningitis.

•Treatment•
1) Establish IV.
2) If younger than 6 years, administer cefuroxime 100-150 mg/kg/d IV divided q8h.
3) Otherwise, administer nafcillin or vancomycin (40-60 mg/kg/d) divided q6h plus ceftriaxone or cefotaxime (150-200 mg/kg/d divided q6-8h).
4) Consult ophthalmology.

II. CONJUNCTIVITIS

•Etiology•
The most common etiologies of conjunctivitis include viruses, S. aureus, S. pneumoniae, H. influenzae, N. gonorrhea, Chlamydia, Herpes, and allergic conjunctivitis.

•Clinical Presentation•
1) Patients present with a red, inflamed eye, and may have some orbital discomfort and matting of the eyelashes in the morning.
2) Visual acuity is normal.
3) Viral conjunctivitis and Chlamydia are associated with preauricular adenopathy.

•Diagnosis•
1) Conjunctival injection (with or without discharge) is present on exam. The pupil, cornea, and anterior chamber are normal.
2) Viral conjunctivitis presents with watery discharge. Bacterial conjunctivitis presents with purulent discharge. N. gonorrhea presents with a hyperacute copious purulent discharge. Chlamydia presents with diffuse injection, corneal punctate lesions, and mucoid discharge, and may be accompanied by urethritis or cervicitis. Allergic conjunctivitis presents with tearing, nasal congestion, and itchy, burning eyes

with mucoid discharge.

3) Consider a slit lamp exam to exclude foreign body, corneal abrasion, or herpes infection (with fluorescein staining, herpes will demonstrate a focal dendritic pattern). Check visual acuity.

•Treatment•

1) Cold compresses. Provide education on proper hygiene to prevent spread.

2) Most conjunctivitis is viral, but it is difficult to differentiate viral from bacterial conjunctivitis; consider treating all viral or bacterial conjunctivitis with antibiotic drops. Options include sulfacetamide, Polytrim (polymyxin/trimethoprim), Polysporin (polymyxin/bacitracin), tobramycin, or ciprofloxacin 2 drops every 6h. S. aureus is increasingly resistant to sulfa; gentamicin and neomycin can be toxic to the cornea.

3) If gonorrhea (hyperacute exuberant purulent discharge), arrange an immediate referral, irrigate the eyes, administer ceftriaxone 1 gm IV and doxycycline 100 mg po bid x 14d, and apply topical bacitracin.

4) Chlamydia requires systemic treatment with doxycycline 100 mg bid for 7d or azithromycin 1 gm; also treat with topical antibiotics.

5) If allergic, treat with topical antihistamines (Livostin 2 drops qid) and vasoconstrictors (Naphcon-A 1-2 drops bid/qid prn).

6) Consider herpes keratoconjunctivitis, which is treated with topical antivirals such as trifluridine (1 drop 5x/d x 10d) or vidarabine 3%. Consider oral acyclovir or famciclovir. Arrange an urgent referral.

III. CORNEAL ABRASION

•Clinical Presentation•

1) Patients may present with a red, painful eye, often with lacrimation.

2) Patients may have a foreign body sensation, photophobia and blurry vision.

•Diagnosis•

1) Always evaluate for a foreign body and evert the lid; check visual acuity.

2) Diagnose a corneal abrasion by slit lamp exam with fluorescein staining.

3) <u>A corneal ulcer</u> may be secondary to bacteria (usually after corneal trauma) or viruses (which usually occur on intact corneal epithelium). It occurs most often in patients who wear contact lenses (usually with pseudomonas). Ulcers are an ophthalmologic emergency. The ulcer is usually round and white, with sharply demarcated borders. It will usually stain brightly with fluorescein; the dendritic pattern of herpes infection may be present. It may have an associated exudate.

•Treatment•

1) Treat with antibiotic ointment or drops for 3-5 days. Options include sulfacetamide, Polytrim (polymyxin/trimethoprim), Polysporin (polymyxin/bacitracin), tobramycin, or ciprofloxacin 2 drops every 6h.

2) If the patient wears contact lenses, there is an increased incidence of Pseudomonas; use ciprofloxacin, gentamicin or tobramycin drops. Do not patch. Follow-up in 1 day. Discontinue contact lens use until abrasion has healed.

3) Patching probably does not help or hurt, although any patient who wears contact lenses should never be patched.

4) Consider a cycloplegic (Cyclogyl) if severe pain. Topical ketorolac (Acular) may reduce pain.

5) Prescribe oral pain medication.

6) Arrange ophthalmology follow-up.

7) Tetanus vaccine is probably unnecessary.

8) If an ulcer is present, obtain an emergency ophthalmology consult; treatment includes frequent application of broad-spectrum antibiotics (aminoglycosides and fluoroquinolones).

IV. GENERAL EYE SYMPTOMS/MEDICATIONS

A. Differential Diagnosis by Symptoms

1) Decreased vision

a) <u>Monocular Decreased Vision</u>- Etiologies include optic neuropathy (Marcus-Gunn pupil; papillitis; ischemic disease); amaurosis fugax (retinal artery occlusion); acute glaucoma; vitreous hemorrhage; space occupying lesion; central vein occlusion; retinal detachment; and anterior conditions (iritis, keratitis, etc.).

b) <u>Binocular Decreased Vision</u>- Etiologies include trauma (occipital);

cerebral vascular occlusions; temporal arteritis; toxic; hypertension; and pituitary apoplexy.

2) Diplopia (Double Vision)

a) Binocular (central) diplopia resolves with one eye covered; monocular (peripheral) diplopia persists when the uninvolved eye is covered.

b) If binocular, it is secondary to disruption in eye movement. Etiologies include a central event with 3rd, 4th or 6th nerve palsy; multiple sclerosis; trauma; infection; myasthenia gravis; or Guillain-Barre.

c) If monocular, it is usually secondary to a refractive error of the eye. Consider lens dislocation, cataract, trauma, or corneal edema (e.g. from glaucoma). Symptoms may be confused with blurry vision.

3) New flashes or floaters

They suggest a retinal tear or vitreous hemorrhage.

4) Painful Eye

a) Non-injected- Etiologies include optic neuritis, cluster headache, sinusitis, and dental pain.

b) Injected- A corneal etiology (abrasion, keratopathy, ulcer, herpes) should be apparent with fluorescein exam. If the corneal staining is normal, check the intraocular pressure (an elevated pressure indicates glaucoma). If the pressure is normal, inflammatory cells in the anterior chamber suggest iritis or endophthalmitis (especially in the setting of trauma); if there are no inflammatory cells in the anterior chamber, consider scleritis or episcleritis.

c) Photophobia suggests iritis, an acute corneal lesion, or meningeal irritation. If the pain is completely relieved with a topical anesthetic, then the condition is usually confined to the cornea/conjunctivae.

B. Medications

*Caps on eye drops are color-coded: red caps are mydriatics; green caps are miotics; blue and yellow caps are beta-blockers; white caps are anesthetics.

1) Mydriatics/cycloplegics

Cyclopentolate (Cyclogyl) 1%- produces mydriasis and cycloplegia within 30 min and may last 24h.

Phenylephrine (Neo-Synephrine) 2.5% (do not use 10%, as it may cause myocardial infarction)- produces mydriasis without cycloplegia within 15 min and lasts for 3h.

Tropicamide (Mydriacil) 0.5-1% - produces cycloplegia and mydriasis within 15 min and may last 6h.

2) Topical Anesthetics

Proparacaine 0.5% lasts 15 min and has onset of 20 sec.

Tetracaine 0.5% lasts 30 min and has onset of 20 sec.

V. GLAUCOMA- Acute narrow-angle

•General•

Acute narrow-angle glaucoma occurs when the pupil dilates and obliterates a preexisting narrowing of the anterior chamber angle, and outflow of humor is blocked. Intraocular pressure then increases, with possible damage to the optic nerve.

•Clinical Presentation•

1) Patients may present with conjunctival injection, mild-to-severe pain, visual blurring, and headache.

2) Patients may also have nausea and vomiting and a perception of halos.

•Diagnosis•

1) The eye exam demonstrates a shallow anterior chamber with a possible inflammatory reaction and corneal edema; the pupil is poorly reactive and mid-dilated.

2) Intraocular pressure is elevated, usually 40-80 mm Hg (normal is 10-20 mm Hg); the eye feels rock-like.

3) Visual acuity is decreased.

•Treatment•- (for acute angle-closure glaucoma)

1) Treatment is directed at lowering intraocular pressure.

2) Acetazolamide 500 mg IV decreases the secretion of aqueous humor by the ciliary body, thereby decreasing intraocular pressure.

3) Apply topical pilocarpine 2-4% (2% is used in patients with light-colored eyes, and 4% is used in patients with dark-colored eyes) every 15 min until pupillary constriction is achieved. Pupillary constric-

tion facilitates aqueous humor outflow; it may not work well with high intraocular pressure because the eye is ischemic. Administer pilocarpine prophylactically to the unaffected eye.

4) Timolol 0.5% topical solution, 1 drop every 30 min for 2 doses; it decreases aqueous production. Also, apraclonidine 0.5% 2 drops is an alpha-agonist that decreases aqueous production.

5) Consider prednisolone 1% 1 drop every 30-60 min to reduce inflammation.

6) Consider Mannitol 1 g/kg over 45 min to reduce vitreous volume.

7) Arrange an urgent ophthalmology consult.

VI. LID DISORDERS

A. Blepharitis

1) Blepharitis is inflammation of the eyelid margins from seborrhea, S. aureus infection, or gland dysfunction; it may be associated with conjunctivitis.

2) Treat with topical polysporin, and consider 6 weeks of doxycycline (50-200 mg/d) to improve gland function (especially if severe symptoms).

B. Chalazion

1) A chalazion develops secondary to blockage of the eyelid glands and subsequent granulomatous inflammation; it is usually painless. It usually occurs away from the lid margin. Chalazia are often chronic, and lack the acute suppurative inflammation found in a hordeolum.

2) Treatment is same as for hordeolum, although definitive treatment may involve steroid injection or excision.

C. Hordeolum (stye)

1) A hordeolum develops secondary to blockage of the eyelid glands and subsequent localized infection; it may involve the sebaceous glands of the eyelid margin/eyelash follicle (external hordeolum or stye) or the Meibomian glands within the eyelid tarsus (internal hordeolum). The etiology is usually S. aureus.

2) It is painful and erythematous; there is no intraocular pathology.

3) Treat with warm compresses 3-4 x/d and gentamicin ointment; fol-

low-up in 2 days if no resolution. Consider drainage with an 18-gauge needle. If left untreated, it may spontaneously resolve, or it may progress to chronic granulation and form a chalazion.

VII. RETINAL ARTERY OCCLUSION

•Etiology•
Occlusion may result from embolism (carotid artery disease; cardiac valve disease), inflammatory endarteritis (temporal arteritis), or atherosclerotic changes.

•Clinical Presentation•
Patients present with a sudden, painless unilateral loss of vision or visual field deficit.

•Evaluation•
1) Exam reveals a unilateral loss of vision or visual field; the pupillary exam may reveal a relative afferent pupillary defect.
2) The fundoscopic exam may demonstrate boxcarring of the retinal vessels, or a cherry red spot of the macula (representing ischemia of the entire posterior retina).
3) Perform a complete cardiovascular exam (evaluate for the etiology of the occlusion); perform a neurologic exam.
4) Consider obtaining ESR if temporal arteritis is suspected.

•Treatment•
1) Treatment attempts to increase retinal perfusion, increase oxygen delivery to the retina, and decrease intraocular pressure (which may then dislodge the embolus and move it 'downstream'). Establish IV and place patient on monitor.
2) Globe massage for 10-15 seconds with rapid release of pressure causes reflex dilation of the retinal arterioles and may dislodge the clot (may repeat 2-3 times; it is contraindicated if the patient has had eye surgery within 1 month).
3) Paper bag breathing (increases CO_2, which dilates the retinal arterioles).
4) Carbogen (95% O_2 and 5% CO_2) inhalation for 10 minutes every 2h; CO_2 dilates the retinal arterioles, and O_2 increases oxygen delivery.
5) IV or po acetazolamide (Diamox) 500 mg decreases aqueous humor

secretion, thereby reducing intraocular pressure.

6) Consider mannitol 1 gm/kg over 45 minutes to decrease intraocular pressure.

7) Administer timolol 0.5% topical solution, 1 drop every 30 minutes for 2 doses; it reduces aqueous humor production, thereby decreasing intraocular pressure.

8) Consider topical pilocarpine 2-4% (2% is used in patients with light-colored eyes, and 4% is used in patients with dark-colored eyes) every 15 minutes until pupillary constriction is achieved; pupillary constriction facilitates aqueous humor outflow.

9) Arrange an emergent ophthalmology referral for possible paracentesis of the anterior chamber, which may decrease intraocular pressure and move the embolus further downstream.

10) Thrombolytics via the ophthalmic artery within 4-6h of visual loss may be of benefit.

11) Hyperbaric oxygen therapy within 2-12h of symptoms may be beneficial.

12) Admit patient; arrange for further investigation of the etiology of the occlusion (e.g., ECG, echocardiogram, carotid Doppler exam).

VIII. RETINAL DETACHMENT

•**General**•

1) Retinal detachment is a separation of the retina from the underlying retinal pigment epithelium or choroid.

2) It may be associated with trauma, metabolic disorders, vascular disease, or vitreous disease.

•**Clinical Presentation**•

1) Patients may present with flashes, floaters, or a visual field loss described as a curtain or shadow; it may be described as wavy vision. Until proven otherwise, the sudden onset of flashes and floaters is retinal detachment.

2) Flashes may also be caused by traction of the vitreous. Floaters, if acute, may also represent vitreous detachment or a retinal tear with impending detachment. Vitreous detachment usually does not have a visual field loss, but may progress to retinal detachment. The sudden

onset of hundreds of tiny dark spots progressing to cobwebs before the eye may indicate a vitreous hemorrhage. Refer patients to ophthalmology within 24h.

3) Flashes that zigzag across the visual field that may last up to 30 minutes and may have a transient visual loss suggest migraines; symptoms may not be followed by a headache.

•Evaluation•

Perform a complete eye exam (including fundoscopic), and check visual acuity. Billowing of the retina may be observed on eye exam.

•Treatment•

Arrange an emergent referral for an indirect eye exam; the patient may require surgery.

IX. SCLERITIS

•General•

1) It is uncommon.
2) Episcleritis presents with an acute onset of eye redness (usually in a limited area of the sclera) and often a dull ache, with normal vision.
3) Scleritis presents with gradual onset of severe pain with photophobia, possibly with mildly decreased vision; it is more diffuse than episcleritis.
4) Scleritis is often associated with systemic disease (e.g. connective tissue disease).

•Evaluation•

1) Perform a complete eye exam, including slit lamp exam and visual acuity.
2) Differentiate from conjunctivitis as scleritis/episcleritis usually involves only a section of the eye, and is associated with pain and not with discharge.

•Treatment•

Arrange a prompt ophthalmology referral. Treatment involves cycloplegics, topical steroids, and pain control. Episcleritis usually improves with topical vasoconstrictors.

X. TRAUMA

A. Globe Rupture

1) Suspect an open (ruptured) globe if a patient presents with a laceration or puncture wound that extends through the eyelid. An open globe may also occur with blunt trauma.

2) Visual acuity is often markedly decreased, but normal acuity is possible.

3) The patient may have hemorrhagic chemosis, hyphema, iris injury (irregular pupil) or vitreous hemorrhage. Ptosis suggests levator palpebrae injury, traumatic Horner's syndrome, or a 3rd or 7th nerve defect. An afferent pupillary defect suggests optic nerve or retinal injury. Also, the iris may be injured, resulting in traumatic miosis or mydriasis (traumatic mydriasis can be distinguished from an afferent pupillary defect, as the pupil in traumatic mydriasis will be poorly reactive to direct and contralateral light exposure, while an afferent pupillary defect allows the pupil to have a normal consensual light reflex).

4) Signs of corneal lacerations may include an irregular pupil, a shallow anterior chamber, decreased intraocular pressure (although measurement of intraocular pressure is contraindicated), and a positive Seidel test (leakage of the fluorescein-stained aqueous humor from the globe).

5) If the foreign body is radiopaque, consider A-P and lateral plain films for diagnosis; if there is a high suspicion but negative plain films, consider CT.

6) If an intraocular foreign body or open globe is suspected, administer ceftazidime 1 gm plus vancomycin 1 gm (alternatively, consider ciprofloxacin), apply metal shield for protection (alternatively, use the bottom of a Styrofoam cup), administer sedation, antiemetics, and analgesics as necessary, and arrange an immediate ophthalmology consult. Any foreign body within the globe should be removed by an ophthalmologist.

B. Lid Lacerations

1) Partial thickness lacerations not involving the lid margin may be repaired in the ED.

2) Lid margin lacerations should be treated by an ophthalmologist.

3) Medial lid lacerations should be evaluated for potential injury to the nasolacrimal system; lacerations to the medial third of the lid should

be repaired by an ophthalmologist.

4) Upper lid lacerations parallel to the lid margin may involve the levator muscle and should also be repaired by an ophthalmologist.

5) Evaluate for possible penetrating globe injury.

C. Orbital Fractures

1) Blow out fractures usually result from a blow to the anterior orbit, and may present with enophthalmos, edema, chemosis, anesthesia, facial flattening, or a "step-off" deformity with bony tenderness.

2) Medial wall fractures may cause orbital emphysema (if the sinus cavity has been violated); medial and floor fractures may be complicated by extraocular muscle entrapment and are manifested by gaze restriction and diplopia (obtain an ophthalmology consult). Orbital rim fractures usually occur from a direct blow to the rim.

3) Ptosis suggests levator palpebrae injury, traumatic Horner's syndrome, or a 3rd or 7th nerve defect. An afferent pupillary defect suggests optic nerve or retinal injury. Also, the iris may be injured, resulting in traumatic miosis or mydriasis (traumatic mydriasis can be distinguished from an afferent pupillary defect as the pupil in traumatic mydriasis will be poorly reactive to direct and contralateral light exposure, while an afferent pupillary defect allows the pupil to have a normal consensual light reflex).

4) Perform a complete exam of lid, cornea, globe, fundus, vision, and extraocular muscles. X-ray views include Caldwell's and Waters' views (a maxillary sinus air-fluid level may indicate an inferior orbital fracture); CT is the preferred imaging test.

5) Any necessary repairs are often done electively, although the presence of muscle entrapment or enophthalmos mandates immediate ophthalmology consultation. Patients with orbital fractures are usually given prophylactic antibiotics, ice packs, decongestants and close follow-up.

XI. UVEITIS (Iritis)

•General•

1) The uveal tract is composed of the iris, ciliary body, and choroid; inflammation is usually confined to the iris and the anterior chamber.

2) Uveitis may be associated with minor trauma, autoimmune disorders or ulcerative colitis.

•Clinical Presentation•

Patients may present with unilateral blurred vision, ocular pain, conjunctival injection, watery discharge, and photophobia. Patients may complain of a deep pain which is worsened with accommodation. Ciliary muscle spasm may cause miosis.

•Diagnosis•

1) Perform a consensual light reflex (cover the red eye, and shine light into the unaffected eye); if pain is induced in the red eye, it is strongly suggestive of uveitis.

2) On slit lamp exam, cell and flare are seen; there is 360° perilimbal injection. Exclude other corneal pathology with the slit lamp exam.

3) Intraocular pressure may be normal or slightly increased. Check visual acuity.

•Treatment•

1) Administer topical steroids prednisolone 1% (Pred Forte) 1 drop every 1-6h; do not prescribe topical steroids without an ophthalmology consult. Exclude herpes keratitis before prescribing topical steroids.

2) Administer oral NSAIDs.

3) Administer a cycloplegic (homatropine or scopolamine).

4) Arrange a prompt ophthalmology referral.

CHAPTER 19
ORTHOPEDICS

I. ANKLE

•Anatomy•
1) The lateral ligaments include the anterior talofibular (most commonly sprained), calcaneofibular, and posterior talofibular; the medial ligament is the deltoid complex (which accounts for 10% of all ankle injuries).
2) Bony stability is achieved by the interposition of the talus between the tibia (medially) and the fibula (laterally).

•Evaluation•
1) Document any tenderness, ecchymosis, deformity, or swelling of the proximal fibula, medial ankle, lateral ankle, navicular, or base of 5th metatarsal.
2) Check for ligamental stability and check for an intact Achilles tendon.
3) Document the neurovascular status.
4) <u>Ottawa rules</u>: Obtain x-ray if bony tenderness at posterior edge or tip of the lateral or medial malleolus, or with inability to bear weight both immediately and in the ED (sensitivity= 100%, specificity= 49%).

X-Ray
1) Get A-P, lateral, and mortise views.
2) On the A-P view, the distal fibula and tibia should overlap by 1 cm.
3) On the mortise view, the joint space should appear symmetrical; >4 mm widening between the medial malleolus and the talus indicates diastasis and likely rupture of the deltoid complex.

•Injuries•
1) Achilles Tendon Rupture
It is identified with loss of plantar flexion and a positive Thompson test (absence of plantar flexion against gravity when the patient is prone, knee is at 90 degrees and calf is squeezed). There may be a palpable defect in the Achilles tendon. Document the neurovascular status and any associated ankle or foot injury.

2) Fractures

a) If the ankle is thought of as a closed ring surrounding the talus, then the stability of the ankle is lost when there are two disruptions in the ring; so if two separate anatomic sections are disrupted (e.g. if lateral fracture and medial (deltoid) ligamental disruption), or if the fracture is displaced, then it is unstable and likely needs surgery. Single disruptions are usually stable.

b) If the fibula is fractured above the mortise, assume torn syndesmotic ligaments and an unstable injury. Fractures below the mortise are usually stable.

c) Types of fractures include:

Bimalleolar (involving 2 elements of the ankle ring) and trimalleolar (involving the medial, lateral, and posterior malleoli) fractures- These are unstable and require urgent orthopedic evaluation and usually surgery.

Fibular shaft fractures- These are treated symptomatically (if isolated) and may be splinted for relief.

Lateral malleolus fractures- Fractures above the level of the mortise are unstable, and should be referred; fractures below the mortise are usually stable.

Maisonneuve fracture- It is an oblique proximal fibular fracture with disruption of the interosseous membrane and tibiofibular ligament, along with medial malleolus fracture or deltoid ligament rupture; it usually requires surgery.

Pilon fractures- These are fractures of the distal tibial metaphysis, and are associated with disruption of the talar dome. They usually result from axial loading forces, such as a fall. Urgent orthopedic evaluation is required.

Tibial shaft fractures- These often require an emergent consult; consider admission for observation for possible compartment syndrome if significant fracture.

3) Sprain

Grade I sprain is stretching of the ligament; Grade II is partial tear of the ligament with mild to moderate joint instability; Grade III is a complete rupture of the ligament with moderate to severe joint instability.

•Treatment•

1) Achilles Tendon Rupture
Treatment includes splinting in plantar flexion and prompt referral.

2) Fracture
    a) Stable fractures require a posterior splint, elevation, ice, avoidance of weight bearing and close orthopedic follow-up.

    b) Unstable fractures usually require orthopedic consultation and reduction.

3) Sprain
    a) For minor injuries, prescribe rest, ice, compression, elevation and NSAIDs. Consider splint and crutches.

    b) 3rd degree and severe 2nd degree sprains require a splint, crutches, and orthopedic referral. Splint with ankle at 90 degrees to the leg.

II. FOOT

•Anatomy•
The hindpart of the foot consists of the calcaneus and talus; the midpart consists of the navicular, cuboid, and the three cuneiforms; the forepart of the foot consists of the metatarsals and phalanges.

•Evaluation•
1) Document any swelling, ecchymosis, deformity or tenderness.

2) Document the neurovascular status.

3) <u>Ottawa rules</u>: Obtain x-ray if bony tenderness at base of 5th metatarsal or navicular, or if patient is unable to bear weight immediately and in the ED (sensitivity=100%, specificity=49%).

<u>X-Ray</u>- Obtain AP, lateral, and oblique views.

•Injuries/Treatment•
1) Avulsion fracture of the base of the 5th metatarsal
    a) This is usually an acute inversion injury caused by contraction of the peroneus brevis tendon. An avulsion of the base of the 5th metatarsal can be differentiated from an epiphyseal plate because the fracture line is transverse, while the epiphyseal plate is usually oblique or longitudinal.

    b) If not displaced, treat with a compression dressing and weight bearing as tolerated; if displaced, treat with a short-leg splint and crutches.

2) Calcaneal fracture

    a) This usually results from a fall from a height; there are often associated injuries (lumbar compression fractures or thoracic aortic rupture).

    b) Fractures not involving the articular surface are treated with splint, ice, elevation, non-weight bearing, and close orthopedic follow-up; intra-articular fractures may require open reduction and internal fixation.

3) Jones fracture

    a) This is a fracture through the proximal diaphysis of the 5th metatarsal (not the base).

    b) Treat with 6-8 weeks non-weight bearing cast and close orthopedic follow-up. There is a high incidence of non-union.

4) LisFranc's tarsometatarsal fracture/dislocation

    a) The 2nd metatarsal is the focal point of the tarsal metatarsal joint, so a fracture of the base of the 2nd metatarsal usually implies a disrupted joint. Patients present with midfoot pain, swelling, and difficulty bearing weight.

    b) On X-ray, the most consistent relationship in the normal foot is alignment of the medial edge of the base of the 2nd metatarsal with the medial edge of the 2nd cuneiform on the A-P or oblique view; on the oblique view, the lateral border of the 3rd metatarsal should form a straight line with the lateral border of the lateral cuneiform. If dislocated, these relationships are disrupted.

    c) Treatment options include casting or surgery.

5) Metatarsal fracture- If not displaced, treat with a short-leg cast and non-weight bearing; if displaced (especially if 1st metatarsal fracture), arrange for close orthopedic follow-up for possible open reduction and internal fixation.

6) Phalangeal fracture- Reduce, apply buddy tape with cotton between toes x 2-3 weeks; consider cast shoe. Comminuted fractures of the great toe require a posterior splint.

7) Talus Fracture

    a) Chip fractures require immobilization (splint in the neutral position, except if there is a posterior facet chip, which should be splinted in 15 degrees of equinus); large fragments may require surgical excision.

b) Fractures of the neck or body may result in avascular necrosis and need immobilization and prompt orthopedic referral.

III. FOREARM

•Anatomy•

1) The forearm consists of 2 parallel bones (the radius and ulna) that are bound together at the wrist and elbow by joint capsules. Radioulnar ligaments, an interconnecting fibrous interosseous membrane, and surrounding muscle groups help maintain stability.

2) The radial nerve supplies the wrist extension muscles, and then divides into the posterior interosseous nerve and the superficial sensory branch. The posterior interosseous nerve supplies motor innervation to the finger extensors; test by extending the wrist and fingers simultaneously.

3) The median nerve gives off the anterior interosseous nerve, which supplies motor innervation to the finger flexors except the flexor superficialis; test by having the patient make the "OK" sign, and abduct the thumb against resistance. The remainder of the median nerve supplies sensation to the radial palm and thenar muscles.

4) The ulnar nerve supplies the other intrinsic muscles of the hand (test by abducting the fingers against resistance).

•Evaluation•

1) Document any swelling, ecchymosis, deformity or tenderness.

2) Document the neurovascular status.

3) Obtain x-ray.

X-ray

1) On the A-P view, the radial styloid should extend 1 cm distal to the ulnar styloid and point laterally.

2) The radial head should align with the capitellum in all views; on the lateral view, a line through the center of the radius should pass through the center of the capitellum.

3) On the lateral view, the radiocarpal joint normally has 11° of palmar angulation; the A-P view normally shows 15-30° of ulnar angulation of the radiocarpal joint.

•Fractures•

1) Barton Fracture- The fracture involves the dorsal rim of the articular surface of the distal radius.

2) Colles Fracture
   a) It is a distal radius fracture with volar angulation (dorsal displacement of the distal radius); the ulnar styloid is fractured through its base in 60% of Colles fractures.
   b) Reduce with finger traps for traction, hematoma block, and manipulation; immobilize with wrist in 15 degrees of flexion and 15 degrees of ulnar deviation. Arrange urgent referral; emergent referral if there is radioulnar joint involvement.

3) Galeazzi Fracture- A radial shaft fracture with subluxation or dislocation of the distal radioulnar joint; these fractures often require admission for open reduction and internal fixation.

4) Hutchinson Fracture- A fracture of the distal radial styloid; it is unstable because it supports the carpal bones.

5) Monteggia Fracture- An ulnar fracture (proximal 1/3) with radial head dislocation; these fractures often require admission for open reduction and internal fixation.

6) Nightstick Fracture- An isolated ulnar fracture; it may require open reduction and internal fixation if it is significantly displaced or angulated.

7) Smith Fracture- (A reversed Colles fracture); it is a distal radius fracture with volar displacement of the distal radius.

•Treatment•

1) Reduce fracture or obtain consult.

2) Immobilize in posterior mold or sugar-tong splint.

3) Ice, elevation, sling.

4) Pain medication.

5) Arrange close orthopedic follow-up.

6) If there is significant displacement of the fracture, consider admission for potential compartment syndrome.

7) <u>Fractures that usually require emergent referral-</u> Displaced olecranon and radial head epiphyseal fractures with angulation >15 degrees usually require admission and reduction under general anesthesia. Displaced coracoid process fractures, proximal displaced or nondisplaced radial shaft fractures, displaced midshaft radial fractures, Galeazzi fractures, Monteggia fractures, and Colle's fractures (if the radioulnar joint is involved) require emergent referral.

IV. HAND

•Anatomy•

1) The flexor digitorum superficialis (FDS) tendons bifurcate near the base of each proximal phalanx and surround the flexor digitorum profundus (FDP) before inserting on the middle phalanx; the FDP inserts on the base of the distal phalanx. The FDP is tested by flexing the DIP against resistance; the FDS is tested by flexing the PIP with other fingers held in extension.

2) There is a cartilaginous volar plate at the base of the middle phalanx, which may be displaced in intra-articular fractures.

3) The extensor expansion extends each finger; it divides into a central slip that attaches to the dorsal middle phalanx and 2 lateral bands that join with tendons of the intrinsic muscles and attach to the base of the distal phalanx. Test by making fist and pointing affected finger.

•Nerves•

1) The ulnar nerve innervates the flexor carpi ulnaris, the ulnar half of the FDP, the hypothenar and intraosseous muscles, and is sensory to the ring and small finger; test motor function with finger adduction/abduction.

2) The median nerve innervates the flexor carpi radialis, FDS, radial half of FDP, flexor pollicis longus and is sensory to the volar aspect of the 1st, 2nd, 3rd and half of 4th digits; test motor function by opposing the thumb and index finger.

3) The radius nerve innervates most extensors and is sensory to the dorsal aspect of the 1st, 2nd, 3rd and half of 4th digits up to the PIP; test motor function by extending the wrist.

•Evaluation•

1) Document any swelling, ecchymosis, deformity or tenderness.

2) Document the neurovascular status.

3) Consider x-ray.

•Injuries/Treatment•

1) **Amputations**

a) Good candidates for replantation are thumb, multiple digits, partial hand, wrist or forearm, individual digits distal to the insertion of the FDS, or any amputated part in a child.

b) Finger-tip amputations in which the bone and tendon are not exposed may be treated with healing by second intention, which produces results at least as good as skin grafting, especially in children.

c) <u>For transport of an amputated part</u>, irrigate the cut surface with saline, wrap in moist saline gauze, place in a specimen cup, and place the cup in a bed of ice or ice water.

2) Dislocations

a) If dorsal dislocation (i.e., distal part is dislocated dorsally), splint in 15-20 degrees of flexion; if volar dislocation, splint in full extension.

b) A PIP joint may be difficult to reduce because of volar plate entrapment and may require surgery. Check for collateral ligament injury.

c) MCP joints are often unreducible because the metacarpal buttonholes between the flexors and lumbricals.

3) Fractures

Distal Phalanx

a) Treat closed tuft fractures with a hairpin splint for 2-4 weeks.

b) A fracture involving >25% of the articular surface may require surgery; administer antibiotics if the bone is exposed.

Middle/Proximal Phalanx

a) Rotational malalignment is never acceptable. Check for rotation by observing if all fingers point toward the scaphoid when flexed; also, the planes of the fingernails should be parallel when compared with the finger of the uninjured hand. Also, if the phalanx is rotated, the x-ray shows asymmetry in the diameter of the phalangeal fragments.

b) If not rotated and not displaced, treat with an ulnar/radial gutter splint.

c) If the fracture is unstable (displaced or rotated), splint in the safe position (MCP joint in 70 degrees of flexion, IP joints in 10-20 degrees of flexion, thumb in palmar abduction, and wrist in 15 degrees of extension).

d) Most intra-articular and spiral fractures require surgery.

e) Avulsion fractures of the base of the middle phalanx require fixation if the fracture is on the extensor surface (they result in boutonniere deformities), lateral surface, or if there is involvement of >15% of the volar surface.

Metacarpals

a) If metacarpal head fracture, treat with immobilization and early referral.

b) A neck fracture of the ring or small finger (boxer's fracture) can allow up to 25 degrees of angulation; index and middle fingers should have <10 degrees of angulation. Treat with gutter splint and referral.

c) A shaft fracture should have no rotation. In the 1st metacarpal, 20-30 degrees of angular deformity can be accepted.

d) *Bennet's fracture* is an intra-articular fracture of the volar base of the 1st metacarpal with subluxation of the MC joint. Treat with thumb spica splint and referral for possible open reduction and internal fixation.

e) *Rolando fracture* is a 1st metacarpal Y-shaped fracture involving the joint surface; it has a poor prognosis. Treat with thumb spica splint and referral for possible open reduction and internal fixation.

4) Infection

Felon

a) It is an infection of the pulp of the fingertip.

b) Treat with a longitudinal incision begun 0.5 cm distal to the DIP and 0.5 cm lateral to the nail with extension to the free edge of the nail; the incision should be deep across the entire pad, just palmar to the bone. Make the incision along the ulnar aspect of the 2nd through 4th digits and radial aspects of the 1st and fifth digits. Use caution, as lateral incisions may damage neurovascular structures. Or, consider a volar midline incision if it is the location of maximal swelling (but this may cause future pad problems). The incision should not cross the DIP (to prevent contracture).

c) Administer antibiotics (dicloxacillin or cephalexin).

Tenosynovitis

a) Patients present with tenderness along the course of the flexor tendon, symmetrical swelling of the finger, pain with passive extension, and a flexed posture of the finger.

b) There is no tenosynovium on the dorsal surface (except at the wrist). Therefore, tenosynovitis in this region is usually inflammatory.

c) Treat in the first 24-48h with IV antibiotics, splint, elevation and close observation; if presentation after 48h, consider irrigation and surgical incision and drainage. Consider surgical incision and drainage for all tenosynovitis.

5) Ligament Injuries
Gamekeepers Thumb

a) Gamekeeper's thumb is an ulnar collateral ligament injury after an abduction stress (e.g. skiing). This injury is frequently missed.

b) If >20 degrees of ulnar ligament instability is demonstrated compared to the normal side, surgery may be required. There may be an avulsion fracture of the base of the proximal phalanx.

c) Treat with a thumb spica or glove cast. It may require surgery, as the ligament may become entrapped under the adductor pollicis.

6) Nail Injuries

a) If there is blood under the nail, a laceration is present. If the nail and nail border are intact, trephination alone will prevent infection and cosmetic defect (i.e., nail removal is not necessary), regardless of whether a fracture is present.

b) If the nail is out of its base, remove the nail, repair any nail bed laceration, and either replace the nail or place adaptic gauze over the nail bed (this protects the nail and acts as a splint to allow new nail growth).

7) Tendon Injuries
Mallet Finger

a) A mallet finger is a disruption distal to the insertion of the central slip of the extensor mechanism at the base of the distal phalanx or an avulsion of the bone on which the tendon inserts.

b) If there is no articular involvement, treat by splinting only the DIP in mild hyperextension for 6-8 weeks. If dislocated or >1/3 articular involvement, treat with surgery.

Flexor Tendons
  a) All injuries should be surgically repaired within 48-72h (immediately if vascular compromise).
  b) Splint from the distal elbow with wrist neutral, MCP flexed to 90 degrees and PIP and DIP at 10 degrees. Elevate. Administer antibiotics.

Extensor Tendons
  a) Closure of extensor tendon lacerations may be delayed for 1 week.
  b) Splint with wrist in 20 degrees of extension, 0 degrees at MCP and PIP.

8) Trigger Finger
  a) A nodule forms on the tendon and gets caught on the sheath during flexion, causing the finger to stay flexed. It is common in rheumatoid arthritis.
  b) It may resolve on its own or with steroid injection.

V. HUMERUS/ELBOW

•Anatomy•
1) The proximal humerus consists of 4 parts: the articular surface, the greater and lesser tuberosities, and the humeral shaft.
2) The distal humerus consists of two columns of bone terminating in the condyles; the trochlea is the articular surface of the medial condyle and the capitellum is the articular surface of the lateral condyle. The humerus articulates with the proximal ulna and radius.
3) The wrist flexors originate from the medial epicondyle and the extensors originate from the lateral epicondyle.

•Evaluation•
1) Document any swelling, ecchymosis, deformity or tenderness.
2) Document the neurovascular status; humeral shaft fractures are associated with radial nerve injury.
3) Obtain x-ray. Humerus x-rays should include AP, lateral, and axillary views.

X-ray
1) The normal elbow x-ray may show a narrow anterior fat pad; with fracture, an intra-articular hemorrhage may displace fat into an ab-

normal posterior fat pad and may form the "sail" sign of the anterior fat pad.

2) On the lateral view, a line from the anterior surface of the humeral shaft bisects the posterior two-thirds of the capitellum (it is displaced with supracondylar fractures). In any view, a line from the long axis of the radius always passes the through the capitellum.

•Injuries/Treatment•

1) Condylar Fracture

If the fracture is not displaced, treat with immobilization of the flexed elbow in supination if the lateral condyle is fractured, and in pronation if the medial condyle is fractured. Obtain an urgent orthopedic consult.

2) Distal Supracondylar Fracture (proximal to the epicondyles)

a) The lateral x-ray shows the condyles anterior to the humerus. It is often seen in children younger than 15 years who present with the arm immobilized and the elbow at 90 degrees.

b) If it is non-displaced with < 20 degrees posterior angulation, treat with a posterior long arm splint with the elbow in over 90 degrees of flexion and obtain an emergent consultation.

c) If displaced, angulated, or if there is significant soft-tissue swelling, an immediate orthopedic referral is necessary (the brachial artery may be injured, causing a compartment syndrome). Attempt reduction only if there is vascular compromise.

d) Consider admitting all patients (whether displaced or not), as delayed swelling and neurovascular compromise are frequently seen.

3) Elbow Dislocation

a) The great majority dislocate posteriorly, usually from a fall on an extended, abducted arm.

b) Reduce posterior dislocations with distal traction and downward pressure to the proximal forearm; the elbow is brought into flexion and posterior pressure applied to the distal humerus. The elbow is then flexed to 90-120 degrees (after assuring full, passive range of motion) and immobilized. Only attempt reduction if there is vascular compromise or a significant delay in referral.

c) Reduce anterior dislocations with distal traction on the wrist and posterior pressure on the proximal forearm; avoid elbow hyperextension. (Do not attempt to reduce an anterior dislocation unless orthopedic referral is significantly delayed).

4) Humerus Fracture

    a) If midshaft fracture, treat with sling ± sugar tong; have patient remain upright to help dependency reduction (check for radial nerve injury- e.g. wrist drop).

    b) If proximal fracture without displacement and minimal angulation, treat with sling and swathe. If displaced or angulated (>45 degrees) proximal fracture, surgery may be necessary; 3 and 4 part fractures often require surgery.

    c) Any fracture involving the anatomic neck or the articular surface may compromise blood flow and result in avascular necrosis, which needs prompt referral.

5) Olecranon Fracture

    a) The lateral x-ray best demonstrates fractures.

    b) Apply a posterior long arm splint with the elbow in 70° of flexion and the forearm neutral.

6) Radial Head Fracture

    a) The lateral x-ray best demonstrates fractures; a posterior fat pad or a displaced anterior fat pad (sail sign) may indicate a hemarthrosis and fracture.

    b) If non-displaced, place arm in sling. If displaced, apply a posterior long arm splint, with the elbow in 90° of flexion and the forearm in full supination. Arrange orthopedic referral.

VI. KNEE

•Anatomy•

1) The knee joint is comprised of the tibiofemoral articulation and the patellofemoral joint. The medial and lateral cartilaginous menisci are located between the tibia and femur.

2) Outside the knee joint itself, the medial collateral ligament (MCL) and lateral collateral ligament (LCL) provide stability. Within the knee joint, the anterior cruciate ligament (ACL) and posterior cruciate ligament (PCL) prevent excessive anteroposterior translation.

3) The extensor apparatus (consisting primarily of the quadriceps muscles) stabilizes the patella.

4) The neurovascular structures are located in the popliteal fossa.

•Physical Findings•

1) Check for patellar ballottement; palpate the MCL, LCL, joint lines, popliteal fossa, and distal pulses.
2) Check for collateral ligament stability by applying a varus and valgus stress with the knee in extension and also in 30 degrees of flexion; if the knee is lax in extension, there is possible injury to the ACL or PCL in addition to the collateral ligament.
3) Check the ACL with the Lachman test (which is more sensitive than the drawer test): with 15-20 degrees of flexion, move the posterior aspect of the proximal tibia anteriorly, and document any laxity (compare to the uninjured knee).
4) A PCL injury may cause a posterior sag of the tibia when the knee is flexed to 90 degrees.
5) To test the meniscus, hyperflex the knee and then internally and externally rotate the knee while extending the knee; feel for a crunch or grind (McMurray Test). A meniscal injury may cause limited range of motion.
6) Check the extensor mechanism by having the patient raise a straight leg against gravity or extend the flexed knee.
7) A valgus or varus deformity may indicate a depressed tibial fracture.
8) An acute hemarthrosis is caused by an ACL tear 70% of the time, a meniscal tear 10%, and an osteochondral fracture 5%.

•Evaluation•

1) Document any swelling, ecchymosis, deformity, tenderness, or ligament instability.
2) Document the neurovascular status.
3) Consider x-ray (some advocate only filming patients with direct knee trauma).

Ottawa rules: Obtain an x-ray if patellar or fibular head tenderness; inability to bear weight both immediately and for 4 steps in ED; unable to flex knee to 90 degrees; or age >55 years.

<u>X-ray</u>

1) Obtain A-P, lateral, oblique, and patellar views. Consider tibial plateau views.
2) An effusion is detected by widening of the thin soft-tissue density between the quadriceps and femur of >5 mm on the lateral view and

represents the suprapatellar extension of blood in the joint.

3) An avulsion fracture of the lateral tibial condyle may indicate an anterior cruciate ligament tear; an avulsion of the medial tibial plateau may indicate a posterior cruciate ligament or medial meniscus tear.

•Injuries/Treatment•

1) Fracture

a) Treat tibial plateau, condylar or tibial subcondylar fractures with a long-leg splint; if the fracture is displaced or depressed >8 mm, it may need surgery. Tibial tuberosity avulsions often require surgery.

b) Proximal fibular fractures are associated with serious knee injury; if isolated, treat symptomatically, as the fibula supports no weight.

2) Knee Dislocation

a) If there is any vascular compromise, immediately reduce the knee with longitudinal traction. Place a long leg posterior splint and obtain an emergent orthopedic consult.

b) Popliteal artery injury occurs in 35%-45% of all knee dislocations; a normal pulse does not exclude significant vascular injury. Coexistent peroneal nerve injury occurs in 25%-35%; check sensation of the great toe and 1st web space, and evaluate the patient's ability to dorsiflex the foot.

c) Consider obtaining an angiogram of all knee dislocations, if 3 out of 4 ligaments are torn, if any suspicion of vascular injury, or if any neurologic injury (it is sometimes difficult to differentiate nerve injury from vascular injury). The vessel must be repaired within 6-8h to maintain viability.

3) Ligament/Meniscal Injury

a) The ACL is the most commonly injured ligament, often due to twisting (e.g. catching a tip while skiing); a pop is often heard, or the knee gives way. If popping or cracking is reported, 50% will have ACL damage. Symptoms may be minimal; posterolateral knee pain and immediate swelling are often seen. A complete ligament tear may be immediately painful, then painless; pain of a partial tear may persist. The patient may have a small avulsion fracture of the lateral tibial condyle.

    b) MCL injury is much more common than LCL and more likely to cause joint instability; it is usually associated with trauma to the side of the knee (e.g. side tackle during football). The patient may have tenderness along the ligament.

    c) A meniscal injury may be from twisting with the foot planted and may cause tenderness in the joint line; the patient may have painful locking of the joint on either full flexion or extension, and may have snapping or clicking after activity. Pain with meniscus injury is worse with weight bearing.

    d) Treat ligament/meniscal injury with immobilization, avoidance of weight bearing, ice and elevation; consider aspiration of hemarthrosis for comfort. Arrange orthopedic referral.

4) Patellar Injury

    a) Dislocation almost always occurs laterally; reduce by extending the knee and moving the patella medially.

    b) If fracture, check the extensor mechanism (assure patient is able to extend the knee without displacing the fracture). If the extensor mechanism is not intact (the patient is unable to raise the extended leg off the bed), if the fracture separates with knee extension, or if the fracture is displaced >4 mm, obtain an orthopedic consult (surgery is usually required).

    c) If not displaced and the extensor mechanism is intact, treat with a long-leg posterior splint.

5) Tendon Injury

Quadriceps Tendon- Rupture usually occurs in the elderly after violent contraction of the quadriceps; patients are unable to extend the knee from a flexed position and the patella migrates distally. A defect is felt in the suprapatellar region. Check x-ray for a patellar fracture. If complete rupture, immobilize the knee; treatment is surgical.

Patellar Tendon- Rupture usually occurs in athletes after violent contraction of the quadriceps; a defect is felt inferior to the patella and the patient has a high riding patella and an inability to extend the knee. Check x-ray for patellar fracture. Treatment is surgical; immobilize the knee.

VII. LOW BACK PAIN/RADICULOPATHY

•General•

1) Low back pain has multiple etiologies, including musculoskeletal, infection, malignancy, and systemic diseases. Musculoskeletal etiologies include muscle strain and nerve root impingement.

2) Nerve root impingement is characterized by radicular pain below the knee with associated paresthesias and possible neurologic deficits. Impingement can be caused by a herniated disc, the cauda equina syndrome, spinal degeneration, and spinal stenosis.

•Nerves•

1) L3-L4 root involvement produces paresthesias in the anterolateral thigh and anteromedial leg with weak knee extensors and a weak patellar reflex. Test motor function by having patient squat and rise.

2) L4-L5 causes paresthesias in the lateral leg and 1st toe web space with weak dorsiflexion of the foot. Test motor function by having the patient walk on his heels.

3) L5 produces the greatest weakness in the extensor hallucis longus.

4) L5-S1 causes paresthesias in the posterior thigh, posterior and lateral foot, and lateral toes with weak foot plantar flexion and a weak Achilles tendon reflex. Test motor function by having patient walk on toes.

•Clinical Presentation•

1) A strain of the paraspinous muscles is typically precipitated by a sudden movement or by lifting a heavy object. The pain worsens with muscle contraction or if the muscle is stretched; pain is relieved with rest.

2) Paresthesias and pain below the knees suggest nerve or disk involvement.

3) If pain is continuous and unrelated to activity, consider epidural abscess or viscerogenic pain.

4) <u>Warning signs</u> include recent trauma, prolonged steroid use, immunosuppression, age over 70 years, history of cancer, recent infection or surgical procedure, severe or progressive motor or sensory deficits, bowel or bladder dysfunction, abdominal pain or mass, temperature >100° F, IV drug use, pain not relieved by rest, or weight loss.

•Specific Syndromes•

1) Herniated Disk

    a) As the spinal discs degenerate, propulsion (herniation) of the nucleus through the annulus fibrosus may occur. It usually occurs in the lumbosacral area.

    b) If the nucleus moves posterolaterally or posteriorly into the extradural space, compression of the nerve root causes sciatica (see anatomy above); posterior protrusion may compress the cord or cauda equina. 80% of lumbosacral herniations affect the L5 or S1 roots.

2) Cauda Equina Syndrome

    a) It is caused by compression of the cauda equina from massive central disk herniation.

    b) Patients present with bilateral sciatica, saddle numbness, parasympathetic nerve deficiencies (urinary retention or incontinence), loss of anal sphincter tone, and extremity weakness (usually bilateral). Ankle jerks are usually absent.

•Differential Diagnosis•

The differential includes AAA, cancer, hyperparathyroidism, osteoporosis, diskitis, abscess, osteomyelitis, nephrolithiasis, spondyloarthropathies, and the cauda equina syndrome.

•Evaluation•

1) Check the neurovascular status (document strength and reflexes).

2) Document any abdominal tenderness or mass and any spinal point tenderness (infection may or may not produce point tenderness). Consider checking sphincter tone.

3) Straight leg raising will cause pain if there is nerve root impingement; the nerve root does not move until 30-40 degrees of elevation. Back pain without leg pain is not a positive test. Pain in the affected leg when the asymptomatic leg is lifted strongly suggests a true radiculopathy.

4) An x-ray is indicated only if suspected infection, persistent pain (4 weeks duration), trauma, or if disk symptoms (pain below the knees or positive straight leg raising).

5) Plain films only detect gross abnormalities of malignancy; changes are not seen in lytic skeletal metastases until 30% of the bone has been resorbed. A bone scan is sensitive but not specific for bony metastases.

6) Obtain an MRI if suspected cauda equina syndrome, infection, rapidly progressing neurologic deficit, or cord compression.

7) Consider labs if an infectious etiology is suspected (ESR is elevated in >90% of infectious low back pain; WBC is elevated in 50%).

•Treatment•

*For presumed muscle strain or nerve impingement symptoms that are not progressing.

1) NSAIDs.

2) Consider narcotics, muscle relaxants (e.g., cyclobenzaprine) or benzodiazepines.

3) Rest (prolonged rest is not recommended), with early mobilization; follow-up.

4) If the patient has a true radiculopathy, consider steroids and arrange close follow up.

VIII. PEDIATRICS

A. Fractures

1) <u>General</u>- Children generally do not get sprains; when a child has growth plate tenderness with a negative x-ray, assume a growth plate injury and immobilize the injured part (ligaments are stronger than growth plates).

2) <u>Carpal bones</u>- Fractures or dislocations are rare. Splint in the safe position, and arrange prompt referral.

3) <u>Greenstick Fracture</u>- It is an incomplete angulated fracture of a long bone; a fracture of the cortex occurs on the convex side but only a bend in the cortex occurs on the concave side.

4) <u>Salter-Harris Classification</u>
   a) Type I is a fracture through the epiphyseal plate with displacement of the epiphysis (there may only be widening of the radiolucent growth plate).
   b) Type II is a fracture through the epiphyseal plate plus a triangular fracture of the metaphysis.
   c) Type III is a fracture through the epiphyseal plate and epiphysis.
   d) Type IV is the same as type III, but there is also a fracture through the adjacent metaphysis.

e) Type V is a crush injury of the epiphysis (it may not be seen on x-ray).

5) Supracondylar (Humeral) Fracture (proximal to the epicondyles)

a) The lateral x-ray shows the condyles anterior to the humerus. It is often seen in children younger than 15 years who present with the arm immobilized and the elbow at 90 degrees.

b) If it is non-displaced with < 20 degrees posterior angulation, treat with a posterior long arm splint with the elbow in over 90 degrees of flexion and obtain an emergent consultation.

c) If displaced, angulated, or if there is significant soft-tissue swelling, an immediate orthopedic referral is necessary (the brachial artery may be injured, causing a compartment syndrome). Attempt reduction only if there is vascular compromise.

d) Consider admitting all patients (whether displaced or not), as delayed swelling and neurovascular compromise are frequently seen.

6) Toddler Fracture- It is a spiral fracture of the tibia. Splint and arrange prompt referral.

7) Torus Fracture- It is a buckling of the cortex (it is an incomplete fracture; the opposite cortex must be intact).

B. Legg-Calve-Perthes Disease

1) It is an idiopathic avascular necrosis of the capital femoral epiphysis of the femoral head; it is usually seen in children 3-12 years old who may complain of hip or groin pain or limp. The child is afebrile; there is usually no trauma.

2) The hip exam reveals limited abduction and internal rotation. The x-ray initially shows widening of the joint space; later films may show an increased density of the femoral head.

3) Treat with non-weight bearing and orthopedic referral.

C. Osgood-Schlatter Disease

1) Osgood-Schlatter is a traction apophysitis of the tibial tubercle; it is usually a benign process that occurs in adolescents. It is often bilateral. Physical activity may result in repetitive stress on the tibial tubercle (transmitted from the patellar tendon). Patients present with pain and swelling of the tibial tubercle, worsened by climbing or kneeling.

2) X-ray may show an irregular ossification of the tibial tuberosity and calcification of the patellar tendon.

3) Treatment includes ice, NSAIDs, avoidance of activities that cause discomfort, and orthopedic referral.

D. Radial Head Subluxation (nursemaid's elbow)

1) It is seen in children 1-3 years old; it usually occurs after the child was pulled by the hand. It is caused by an acute interposition of the annular ligament in the radiocapitellar joint.

2) Patients present with partial pronation and slight flexion at the elbow; the patient resists passive pronation/supination.

3) To reduce, begin with the child's elbow in extension and pronation, and reduce with rapid sequential downward pressure on the radial head by the physician's thumb, then passive full supination and passive full flexion; a click is often heard with reduction. If multiple attempts are unsuccessful, consider x-rays.

E. Septic Arthritis

1) It usually occurs in children under age 4 years, most often due to hematogenous spread from Staph, Strep, or H. flu. infection. Children usually present with a limp or refusal to ambulate, along with monoarticular pain; the patient may have a fever.

2) In patients with a septic hip, the exam shows a severely limited range of motion; the hip is flexed, abducted, and externally rotated to allow for the greatest volume in the joint.

3) Check x-ray; consider CT. Labs usually show an increased WBC and ESR. Needle aspiration of the hip should be done by a surgeon. Check blood cultures.

4) Septic arthritis requires admission and IV antibiotics (consider nafcillin or clindamycin).

F. Slipped Capital Femoral Epiphysis

1) It usually occurs in obese males 12-15 years old. If chronic, the child complains of a dull pain in the groin referred to the anteromedial thigh and knee, which is worse with activity. The child walks with an antalgic gait with the leg in external rotation.

2) If acute, there is a sudden, severe pain and an inability to bear weight.

The exam demonstrates leg shortening and marked external rotation of the thigh; do not have the patient ambulate.

3) Medial slips are noted on A-P x-ray views, while posterior slips are seen on frogleg views. On the A-P view, a line along the lateral (superior) aspect of the femoral neck should transect the lateral quarter of the femoral epiphysis; a slipped epiphysis will not be transected or less so than the unaffected hip.

4) Admit all patients for surgery; the patient should be non weight-bearing.

G. Transient Synovitis

1) The peak incidence is 5-6 years, but it can be seen from 18 months to 12 years. Patients usually present with a gradual limp or inability to ambulate; 50% have minor trauma or illness.

2) ESR and WBC are usually normal.

3) It is a diagnosis of exclusion, so usually admit the patient and arrange orthopedic evaluation and possible aspiration of the hip.

IX. PELVIS/HIP

•Anatomy•

The pelvis forms a ring, and consists of the coccyx, sacrum, and the bilateral ilium, ischium, and pubis. The pelvis is very vascular, and also contains the lower urinary and GI tracts. Nerves descend from the lumbar and sacral plexuses.

•Evaluation•

1) Evaluate the pelvis and hips for any deformity, tenderness, or rotation. Evaluate for associated abdominal, urethral, or other genitourinary injuries. Document the neurovascular exam.

2) Obtain any appropriate pelvis or hip x-rays.

3) Displaced hip fractures usually present with a shortened, externally rotated extremity.

4) Tenderness with gentle compression of the ileac wings may indicate a pelvic fracture (do not "rock" the pelvis, as this may increase hemorrhage).

5) Destot's sign (a hematoma above the inguinal ligament or perineum) may indicate a pelvic fracture.

X-Ray

1) Obtain an A-P view of the pelvis and routine hip views.
2) Inlet views demonstrate A-P displacement of the fracture; outlet views show sacral fractures or superior/inferior displacement.
3) Obtain Judet views if there is a suspicion of an acetabular fracture.
4) Closely examine the sacro-ileac joint for widening, and examine the inferior pubic borders for asymmetry. If the symphysis pubis is >10 mm in a child or >8 mm in an adult, it may be dislocated.

Classification of Traumatic Pelvic Fractures

I: A fracture of individual bones without a break in the ring (e.g., avulsions; horizontal sacral fracture; ileal wing fracture; single pubis or ischial ramus fracture).

II: A single break in the ring (nondisplaced ipsilateral rami fractures; nondisplaced ilium body fracture near the sacroiliac joint; vertical sacral fracture).

III: A double break in the ring; these fractures are unstable (bilateral double rami fractures; fracture dislocation of the pubis; double vertical fractures; open book pelvis; multiple displaced fractures).

IV: Acetabular fractures.

•Injuries•

1) Pelvis Fracture

a) Isolated rami fractures are stable; ipsilateral superior and inferior rami fractures are usually stable. Double breaks are unstable. Displacement >0.5 cm of any ring fracture is unstable and may require blood replacement.

b) Acetabular fractures cause pain when the sole of the foot is percussed, and are associated with hip dislocations (obtain Judet x-ray views).

c) Associated genitourinary injuries are common. There is an association between pelvic fractures and injury to the thoracic aorta.

d) Unstable fractures: If there is blood at the meatus, obtain a retrograde urethrogram/cystogram; if there is gross hematuria, obtain an IVP. Fractures that disrupt the ring generally require a cystourethrogram. Consider CT to evaluate for associated injuries. If female, consider performing a vaginal exam. Check CBC, type and screen, and urinalysis.

2) Hip Fracture

a) Hip fractures involve the proximal femur, and are classified based on the location of the fracture.

b) Femoral head fractures are usually associated with hip dislocations. Other fractures include femoral neck, intertrochanteric, trochanteric, and subtrochanteric fractures. Subtrochanteric fractures are associated with metastases.

c) If the fracture is non-displaced, signs and symptoms may be minimal; if displaced, the leg is usually shortened and externally rotated.

3) Hip Dislocation

a) A posterior dislocation is 10-20 times more common than an anterior dislocation. Dislocation usually results from a direct blow to the flexed knee (dashboard dislocation) and is often associated with an acetabular fracture.

b) The patient presents with the affected leg shortened, flexed, and adducted; the internally rotated femoral head may be palpable in the buttock.

c) On A-P x-ray, the femoral head appears smaller and is seen superolateral to the acetabulum. Get two x-ray views to rule out fracture.

•Treatment•

1) Class I and II pelvic fractures

These fractures are treated symptomatically with restricted ambulation, progressing to weight bearing.

2) Unstable pelvic fractures

Stabilize the fracture. These fractures may result in significant blood loss; most commonly, the source of bleeding is venous, but to control bleeding consider arterial embolization in addition to stabilization of the fracture (stable fractures with continued bleeding will not benefit from an external fixator).

3) Hip/Femur fractures

a) Femoral head fractures are treated with immobilization, analgesics, and admission for possible arthroplasty.

b) Femoral neck (or subcapital) fractures may result in avascular necrosis and require emergent consult for possible open reduction internal fixation (ORIF).

c) Intertrochanteric fractures require admission for possible ORIF.

d) Nondisplaced greater or lesser trochanter fractures are treated with bed rest followed by crutch walking (displaced fractures may require ORIF).

e) Subtrochanteric fractures require ORIF.

f) Femoral shaft fractures require traction splint with emergent referral and admission for IM rod (treat associated blood loss; fat embolism is a possible complication). Distal femur fractures may be treated with cast or ORIF.

g) If the x-ray is negative, but the patient has pain with internal and external rotation of the affected leg (or if the patient is unable to ambulate), consider admission and MRI, bone scan, or CT.

4) Hip Dislocation

Reduction is best accomplished by an orthopedist. If necessary, reduce the hip by sedating the patient and having an assistant stabilize the pelvis; then, flex the hip and knee to 90 degrees, and apply axial traction. If reduction is successful, immobilize the legs in slight abduction with a pillow between the legs.

X. SHOULDER

•Anatomy•

The shoulder consists of the sternoclavicular joint, the acromioclavicular joint, the glenohumeral joint, and the scapulothoracic articulation. The shoulder is stabilized by multiple ligaments; the rotator cuff surrounds the glenohumeral joint.

•Evaluation•

1) Document any swelling, ecchymosis, deformity or tenderness. Document the range of motion.

2) Document the neurovascular status.

3) If possible fracture or dislocation, obtain x-ray. Shoulder x-rays should include AP, lateral, and axillary views.

X-ray

1) The A-P view of a normal shoulder shows the humeral head overlapping the posterior rim of the glenoid fossa; the true A-P view is perpendicular to the plane of the scapula and eliminates the overlap with the glenoid.

2) Of the orthogonal views, the axillary view is preferred (it is shot into the axilla); the transthoracic lateral is least useful. If the patient is unable to abduct the arm, obtain a Y-view, which is shot from the opposite shoulder with elevation of the opposite shoulder; the scapula is seen as a Y (the coracoid and acromion form the upper limbs of the Y). In a normal shoulder, the humeral head is at the center of the Y, over the glenoid fossa.

•Injuries•

1) Dislocations

Acromioclavicular (AC) joint

   a) Check x-ray; consider stress radiographs with patient holding a 10lb weight.

   b) Type I separation is a sprain of the AC ligament. Type II is a disruption of the ligaments with a widened joint space. Type III is a complete disruption of the ligaments with a widened joint space and an increase in the coracoclavicular distance.

Anterior Shoulder Dislocation

   a) Anterior dislocations occur in 95% of dislocations, posterior 2-3%; the rest are inferior and superior. An anterior dislocation can be, in order of frequency, subcoracoid, subglenoid, subclavicular or intrathoracic (the location is demonstrated on x-ray).

   b) If anterior dislocation, the patient presents with the arm in slight abduction and external rotation, loss of the normal deltoid contour, a full anterior area (the humeral head may be palpable), and a prominent acromion. The patient resists internal rotation and abduction. It is often caused by a fall on an abducted, externally rotated arm.

   c) 8-10% of dislocations have an associated nerve injury (usually neuropraxia); examine axillary nerve sensation by testing with pinprick over the deltoid. Document the neurovascular status.

Posterior Shoulder Dislocation

   a) It often occurs after a seizure. The patient presents with the arm adducted and internally rotated; attempted abduction and external rotation are extremely painful. The posterior shoulder appears full, and the humeral head may be palpable beneath the acromion.

   b) The A-P x-ray view shows the humeral head profiled in internal rotation and appears as a "light bulb"; also, the anterior half of the glenoid fossa is missing the smooth elliptical shadow normally seen from superimposition of the humeral head on the glenoid fossa. On the Y-view, the humeral head is in a posterior position.

Luxatio Erecta (Inferior Shoulder Dislocation)

   a) It is caused by a hyperabduction force, which forces the humeral head out inferiorly.

   b) The patient presents with the humerus fully abducted, elbow flexed, and the hand behind the head.

2) Fractures

Clavicle- Class A fractures involve the middle third of the clavicle; Class B involve the distal third; Class C fractures involve the medial third.

Hill-Sachs- It is a compression fracture of the posterolateral aspect of the humeral head; it is often seen with anterior dislocations.

•Treatment•

A) Dislocations

1) Acromioclavicular (AC) Joint

Treat with sling; a type III separation may require surgery.

2) Anterior Shoulder Dislocation

Shoulder reduction often requires significant sedation and analgesia; consider IV conscious sedation protocol with fentanyl and midazolam. Another option is intra-articular lidocaine/bupivacaine. Consider ortho-pedic consultation for any dislocation with an associated fracture. Methods of reduction include:

   a) Traction/countertraction- With the patient supine and semirecumbent, loop a sheet under the injured axilla and around both the patient's torso and an assistant's waist on the opposite side of the injury. Loop a second sheet over the patient's flexed arm on the injured side at the antecubital space, then around your waist. Apply in-line traction on the injured arm by leaning away from the patient, and use your hands to manipulate the shoulder joint; have the assistant apply countertraction. A lateral force may be applied by a second sheet along the upper humerus with lateral traction.

b) <u>Modified Kocher</u>- With the patient supine, the dislocated arm is slowly adducted and the elbow flexed to 90°; the arm is then slowly externally rotated.

c) <u>Hennepin maneuver</u>- With the patient seated at 45°, support the elbow while gently rotating the arm to 90 degrees outward. Then, if not yet reduced, slowly elevate the arm into abduction.

d) <u>Stimson</u>- Have the patient lay prone with the dislocated arm hanging over the edge of the table with a 10-15 lb weight for 20-30 minutes. Attempt to manipulate the inferior part of the scapula medially.

e) <u>Milch</u>- With the patient supine, slowly abduct and externally rotate the arm to the overhead position and then apply traction with the elbow in extension; manipulate the humeral head with your other hand.

f) <u>Have the patient elevate arm</u> 10-20 degrees in forward flexion and slight abduction; forward flexion is continued until the arm is directly overhead. Abduction then is increased and outward traction is applied.

g) <u>With the patient supine</u>, the arm is slowly adducted to the side, the elbow is flexed to 90 degrees, and slow external rotation is applied.

h) <u>Hippocratic method</u>- It is effective if only one person is available to reduce the shoulder. Use your foot to apply countertraction, placing the heel between the anterior and posterior folds of the axilla (on the chest wall, not in the axilla); apply traction with internal and external rotation.

<u>Post-Reduction Care</u>- Document the neurovascular status. Always get pre- and post-reduction films to document any prior fracture and proper reduction (the reduction can be lost after leaving the ED). Immobilize the arm in adduction and internal rotation. Younger patients should be immobilized for 3 weeks before beginning range of motion exercises; immobilize older patients for only 1-2 weeks to avoid shoulder stiffness. Arrange orthopedic follow-up.

3) Posterior Shoulder Dislocation

a) Reduce with axial traction on the adducted arm and anterior pressure on the humeral head.

  b) After reduction, apply a sling or shoulder immobilizer for 3 weeks. The patient should not attempt abduction/external rotation for 6 weeks, but should perform early range of motion exercises. Arrange orthopedic follow-up.

4) Luxatio Erecta (Inferior Shoulder Dislocation)

Reduce with upward and outward traction in line with the humerus. Apply sling. Arrange orthopedic follow-up. Obtain immediate arteriography if there is any indication of vascular compromise.

B) Fractures

Clavicle- Treat with sling ± swathe; closed reductions are rarely maintained.

XI. WRIST

•Anatomy•

1) The carpal bones have a proximal and distal row. The proximal row, starting radially, consists of the scaphoid, lunate, triquetrum, and pisiform; the distal row consists of the trapezium, trapezoid, capitate, and hamate.

2) The proximal carpal row articulates proximally with the distal radius; the ulna does not articulate directly with the proximal wrist bones, but is separated from the triquetrum by a triangular fibrocartilage. The distal row of wrist bones articulates with the 5 metacarpals.

•Evaluation•

1) Document any swelling, ecchymosis, deformity or tenderness. Document the range of motion.

2) Document the neurovascular status.

3) If possible fracture or dislocation, obtain an x-ray.

<u>X-ray</u>

1) The carpal bones are separated by a uniform 2 mm joint space in the anterior view. On the A-P view, the radial styloid should extend 1 cm distal to the ulnar styloid and point laterally.

2) The long axis of the lunate and capitate form an angle within 10 degrees of each other. The central axis of the scaphoid forms a 30-60 degree angle to the long axis of the lunate.

3) On the lateral view, a long axis through the distal radius, lunate, capitate and 3rd metacarpal should form a straight line; the concavity of the radius and lunate and the convexity of the capitate form 3 Cs.

4) On the lateral view, the radiocarpal joint normally has 11° of palmar angulation; the A-P view normally shows 15-30° of ulnar angulation of the radiocarpal joint.

•Physical Findings•

1) The scaphoid is located in the snuffbox, which is on the radial aspect of the dorsal wrist, with the radial styloid forming the base of the triangle.

2) Lister's tubercle is a bony prominence of the dorsal distal radius, distal to which is an indentation that marks the location of the capitate (if the wrist is flexed, the lunate becomes palpable in this region, at the base of the index metacarpal).

3) The pisiform is palpated at the base of the hypothenar eminence; the hook of the hamate is distal and radial to the pisiform. The triquetrum is volar and just distal to the ulnar styloid.

•Injuries/Specific Treatment•

1) Barton Fracture- The fracture involves the dorsal rim of the articular surface of the distal radius. Treat with splint and prompt referral.

2) Colles Fracture

    a) It is a distal radius fracture with volar angulation (dorsal displacement of the distal radius); the ulnar styloid is fractured through its base in 60% of Colles fractures.

    b) Reduce with finger traps for traction, hematoma block, and manipulation; immobilize with wrist in 15 degrees of flexion and 15 degrees of ulnar deviation. Arrange urgent referral; emergent referral if there is radioulnar joint involvement.

3) DeQuervain's Tenosynovitis- Patients present with pain over the radial styloid; pain is exacerbated with the thumb inside the palm and the wrist in ulnar deviation. Treat with thumb spica and NSAIDs.

4) Hutchinson Fracture- It is a fracture of the distal radial styloid; this fracture is unstable because it supports carpal bones. Treat with splint and prompt referral.

5) Lunate/Perilunate Dislocation

a) The mechanism is usually a fall onto an outstretched hand.

b) On the lateral x-ray, 2 lines drawn on the volar and dorsal radius act as boundaries. If the capitate lies outside these lines, it is a perilunate dislocation; if the lunate lies outside, the lunate is dislocated. On the lateral x-ray, a dislocated lunate shows the "teacup" sign.

c) On the A-P view, the space between the capitate and lunate is obliterated, and a dislocated lunate appears triangular instead of the normal quadrangular. On the A-P view, a disrupted radiocarpal arc suggests a lunate dislocation; a disrupted midcarpal arc suggests a perilunate dislocation.

d) Reduce with traction and apply your thumb to the dorsum of the wrist. Apply a dorsal splint and arrange prompt orthopedic follow-up. If there is a widely displaced fracture, it may need a pin; consider immediate orthopedic consult for reduction.

6) Scaphoid Fracture

a) If no fracture is seen on x-ray, a clinical fracture is evidenced by at least one of following: 1) localized snuffbox tenderness (the patient must retract hand with pain); 2) pain with axial compression of the thumb, or 3) forced pronation causes patient to stop pronating.

b) Treat with thumb spica and referral. Proximal fractures have a higher incidence of necrosis.

7) Scapholunate Dissociation- On the A-P view, the space between the scaphoid and lunate is >3-5 mm. Treat with splint and referral.

8) Smith Fracture- (A reversed Colles fracture). It is a distal radius fracture with volar displacement of the distal radius; the typical mechanism is a direct blow to the dorsum of the wrist. Treat with reduction, splint, and referral.

•Treatment•

1) If there is a carpal bone fracture or dislocation, immobilize the wrist (the MCP joints are lax in extension and taut in flexion, so splint with the MCP joints in 90 degrees of flexion to prevent ligament shortening).

2) Ice, elevation, and prompt orthopedic follow-up.

CHAPTER 20
PEDIATRICS

I. Pediatric ALS; Pediatric Resuscitation Supplies and Vital Signs- see Appendix

II. ANESTHESIA

A. Analgesia/Sedation

1) **Hypnotics**
A) Chloral Hydrate
  a) The dose is 50-100 mg/kg po/pr (max 1 gm) with onset 40 minutes, duration 1-3h.
  b) Chloral hydrate does not provide analgesia; it is best for sedation during diagnostic tests. Avoid in children with liver disease.
  c) Chloral hydrate has poor predictability of onset and duration of action, and is not a first line drug.

B) Ketamine
  a) The dose is 2-4 mg/kg IM with onset 5 min, duration 10-20 min; or 1-2 mg/kg IV with onset 1-2 min, duration 5-10 min.
  b) Ketamine produces a dissociative analgesia/sedation in which spontaneous respiratory and airway reflexes are maintained; patients are aware of stimuli, but unconcerned.
  c) Ketamine stimulates salivary secretions, so consider administration of atropine 0.01 mg/kg (max 0.5 mg) or glycopyrrolate 0.01 mg/kg (max 0.2 mg) prior to administering ketamine. Fasting is preferred prior to administration, but not required.
  d) Ketamine may increase intracranial pressure, blood pressure, and intraocular pressure; it is a positive inotrope. Avoid if head injury or possible open globe injury. There is potential for laryngospasm, so **don't use in the presence of a URI**.
  e) Recovery from ketamine sedation may be associated with hallucinations or nightmares (emergence reactions). Administration of midazolam (Versed) 0.05-0.1 mg/kg decreases the incidence of emergence reactions. Avoid ketamine if the patient is younger than

3 months or older than 10 years, or if the patient has a psychiatric history (these patients have an increased incidence of emergence reactions).

2) Sedatives

*Benzodiazepines do not provide analgesia; if the procedure is painful, administer with a narcotic.

- **A)** <u>Diazepam (Valium)</u>: 0.05-0.2 mg/kg IV (titrated to max 0.4 mg/kg), with onset 3 minutes, duration 1-2h; if given pr, the dose is 0.5 mg/kg, with onset 30-60 minutes, duration 1-2h. Diazepam can be given po, but not IM.
- **B)** <u>Lorazepam (Ativan)</u>: 0.05-0.1 mg/kg IV/IM (max 2 mg); it is more potent and is faster-acting than diazepam. Peak effect if given IV is 2-3 min.
- **C)** <u>Midazolam (Versed)</u>: 0.05-0.1 mg/kg IV/IM (max 0.7 mg/kg); onset 2 minutes; duration 30 minutes; it can be given sl/pr/intra-nasally 0.2-0.4 mg/kg with onset 10-15 minutes, duration 45 minutes. Midazolam provides amnesia.

3) Sedative Analgesics (narcotics)

- **A)** <u>Codeine</u>: 1 mg/kg po (max 60 mg). It is available as a liquid.
- **B)** <u>Fentanyl</u>: 1-2 mcg/kg IV, repeat q2-3 minutes (max 3 mcg/kg). Onset is 1-2 minutes; duration is 20-30 minutes. If given too rapidly, it may cause chest wall rigidity or bradycardia. Awareness usually is maintained. There are minimal cardiovascular effects; mild respiratory depression may occur.
- **C)** <u>Hydrocodone</u>: 0.2 mg/kg po (max 7.5 mg). It is available as a liquid.
- **D)** <u>Meperidine (Demerol)</u>: 1-2 mg/kg IV/IM (max 100 mg) with onset 15-30 minutes, duration 2-3h. Meperidine is poorly titratable, causes histamine release, is a myocardial depressant, and causes CNS excitability.
- **E)** <u>Morphine</u>: 0.1-0.2 mg/kg IV/IM/po, titrate to effect (max 10 mg). Onset is 5 minutes IV, 20-60 minutes IM; duration is 4h. Morphine may cause hypotension and histamine release.

4) Combinations

- **A)** <u>Ketamine and Versed</u>: ketamine 2-4 mg/kg (max 300 mg), midazolam 0.05 mg/kg (max 3.5 mg), and atropine 0.01 mg/kg (minimum 0.1 mg; max 0.4 mg) administered IM; onset 2-5 minutes, duration 15-20 minutes.

B) <u>Fentanyl and Midazolam</u>: Start with midazolam 0.1 mg/kg IV over 30 seconds; in 3 minutes, administer fentanyl 1 ug/kg IV over 30 seconds; may repeat fentanyl x 2.

5) Reversal Agents

A) <u>Narcan</u>- 0.1 mg/kg IV/IM (max 2 mg) reverses narcotics.

B) <u>Flumazenil</u>- 0.01 mg/kg IV (may repeat every 1 min - max 1 mg) reverses benzodiazepines.

6) Precautions

Use pulse oximetry; have suction, bag-valve mask, and intubation/reversal medications ready. Discharge when baseline mental status returns, normal vital signs, normal ambulation for age, and able to take liquids.

B. Rapid Sequence Intubation (RSI)

•General•

1) Intubation is indicated in patients who are unable to protect their airway, or are unable to maintain adequate oxygenation and ventilation. Intubate before hypoxia and acidosis have occurred.

2) Children have relatively large tongues and redundant soft tissues, which may obstruct the airway; initial interventions should include opening the airway and clearing any obstruction. Children younger than 6 months are obligate nose breathers.

3) In children, the larynx is located more anterior and cephalad than in adults. Also, the trachea is very short, with the narrowest portion of the airway in the subglottic area.

•Equipment•

1) Laryngoscope blade, either curved or straight (straight is preferred in infants and small children). Check to ensure a functioning light.

2) Endotracheal tubes (ETT); have several different sizes of tubes ready (see Appendix, Resuscitation Supplies for ETT sizes). Consider applying a lubricating agent to the end of the ETT. Do not use cuffed endotracheal tubes if younger than 8 years (tracheal rings are easily damaged); the narrow subglottic area acts as a physiologic cuff.

3) Bag-valve mask attached to high-flow oxygen.

4) Suction.

5) Prepare optional methods for intubation if the patient has a difficult airway. Do not perform a surgical cricothyroidotomy in children younger than 8-12 years; a needle cricothyroidotomy with jet insufflation is the preferred surgical approach.

•Procedure•

1) Preoxygenate with 100% oxygen. Establish IV. Prepare equipment and medications. Have suction ready and place the patient on a cardiac monitor and pulse oximetry. Check the laryngoscope light and endotracheal tube (ETT) cuff. Place older patients in the sniffing position; for infants, place a roll under the shoulders. Use the Sellick maneuver (cricoid pressure), but use with caution in the very young, as it may compress and damage the trachea; release the cricoid if vomiting occurs (to prevent esophageal rupture).

2) Premedicate

   a) Consider fentanyl 2-10 mcg/kg (onset 1 min, lasts 30 minutes); opioids have sedative and analgesic effects and blunt increases in heart rate and blood pressure (but may increase intracranial pressure).

   b) Consider atropine 0.02 mg/kg IV (max 1 mg, min 0.1 mg); administer 1-2 minutes before intubation if younger than 1 year, if 4-5 years old and succinylcholine is used, if older than 5 years and receiving a second dose of succinylcholine, or if any bradycardia (children have a pronounced vagal response to succinylcholine and vagal stimulation).

   c) Consider lidocaine 1.5 mg/kg IV push, especially if head injury (it decreases the cough and gag response and blunts the release of catecholamines and thus blunts the intracranial pressure response to intubation).

   d) Consider giving a defasciculating dose of Vecuronium (0.02 mg/kg IV push) or succinylcholine (0.1 mg/kg IV); defasciculation blocks increased intracranial pressure; *do not defasciculate if patient is younger than 5 years.*

   e) Wait 3 minutes after giving medications.

3) Sedate

Sedation options for different clinical situations:

Normotensive: Thiopental or Etomidate or Midazolam.

Hypotension without head injury: Etomidate or Ketamine or 1/2 dose Midazolam.

Head injury without hypotension: Thiopental.

Head injury with hypotension: Etomidate or decreased dose of thiopental.

Status asthmaticus: Ketamine or Midazolam.

Status epilepticus: Thiopental or Midazolam.

Sedative Options/Doses

Diazepam 0.25-0.5 mg/kg- onset 2-4 min, duration 40 min; has minimal effect on intracranial pressure and blood pressure.

Etomidate 0.2-0.4 mg/kg- onset 1 min, duration 2-3 min; minimal effect on intracranial pressure, intraocular pressure, and blood pressure. May cause adrenal suppression.

Fentanyl 2-10 ug/kg- onset 1 min, lasts 30 min; little hemodynamic effect; may cause chest wall rigidity and increased ICP.

Ketamine 1-2 mg/kg- onset 1-2 min, duration 10 min; bronchodilates; increases intracranial pressure, intraocular pressure, and secretions; will not usually cause hypotension. Use with asthma. Premedicate with atropine. Do not give if cardiac disease.

Methohexital 1-1.5 mg/kg- onset 10 sec, duration 15 min; decreases blood pressure.

Midazolam 0.1-0.4 mg/kg- onset 1-2 min, duration 30 min; minimal effect on intracranial pressure and blood pressure.

Thiopental 2-5 mg/kg- onset 30 sec, duration 15 min; decreases intracranial pressure and blood pressure; increases bronchospasm. Use with status epilepticus, but avoid in asthma because it may cause histamine release.

4) Paralyze- short-acting agent (depolarizing agent (succinylcholine) or rocuronium).

Succinylcholine 1-1.5 mg/kg (1-3 mg/kg if <10 kg)- onset 30 sec, duration 5 min; increases intracranial pressure, intraocular pressure; may cause bradycardia or hypokalemia. May be given IM.

Rocuronium 1 mg/kg- onset 60 sec, duration 30 min; may use instead of succinylcholine.

5) Placement. Pass the endotracheal tube; apply cricoid pressure. Placement is best confirmed with direct visualization of the tube passing through the vocal cords. If patient becomes bradycardic during placement, administer atropine. Endotracheal tube insertion depth is 3 times the internal diameter of the endotracheal tube.

6) After Intubation- Confirm ETT placement by observing bilateral chest rise with each ventilation and listening for equal breath sounds in the bilateral anterior chest and bilateral mid-axillary line; also, listen over the epigastrium for air entering the stomach. Consider secondary confirmation with an end-tidal CO_2 detector or bulb aspiration device. Secure ETT. Obtain CXR to verify correct depth of ETT (it should be approximately 2 cm above the carina). Attach ETT to ventilator with appropriate settings (start with tidal volume 10 cc/kg; I:E ratio 1:2; PEEP 2-4; 100% FIO2). Oral or NG tubes should generally be inserted after the airway has been secured.

7) Paralyze- long acting agent (non-depolarizing agents).

Vecuronium 0.1 mg/kg (or 0.2 mg/kg for RSI, with onset 90 sec)- onset 2-3 min, duration 40 min; few cardiovascular effects; low risk for histamine release.

Pancuronium 0.1 mg/kg- onset 2-5 min, duration 60 min; may cause histamine release.

*Non-depolarizing agents can be reversed with 0.5-1 mg/kg IV edrophonium.

8) Long-term sedation- consider diazepam and morphine.

III. ASTHMA

*See Chapter 23

IV. CARDIOVASCULAR

Abbreviations: AS (aortic stenosis); ASD (atrial septal defect); CA (coarctation of aorta); CHF (congestive heart failure); CM (cardiomyopathy); PDA (patent ductus arteriosus); SVT (supraventricular tachycardia); TGA (transposition of the great arteries); TOF (tetralogy of Fallot); VSD (ventricular septal defect).

A. Congenital Heart Disease

•Etiology•
*Congenital heart disease often produces a shunt. The etiology of the

abnormality is often distinguished on the basis of the direction of the shunt.

1) **Left to Right (L-R) Shunt (*acyanotic*)**- Patients present with CHF and increased pulmonary blood flow (especially after pulmonary vascular resistance drops, usually at the 4th to 8th week of life). It is seen with VSD, ASD, TGA, CA, SVT, and PDA.

2) **Right to Left (R-L) Shunt (*cyanotic*)**- Patients present with central cyanosis that does not improve with 100% oxygen; there is decreased pulmonary blood flow. It is seen with TOF, TGA, tricuspid atresia.

•Clinical Presentation•

1) In R-L shunt, the patient is often cyanotic, hypoxemic and tachycardic without respiratory distress (i.e., no retractions).

2) In L-R shunt, the patient may be in CHF. Also, the patient may have dyspnea, sweating with feeding, hepatomegaly, cyanosis, or cardiomegaly.

3) Infants with lesions that are dependent upon a PDA usually present by day 10, at which time the ductus closes and the patient becomes symptomatic.

•Evaluation•

1) Check blood pressure in all four extremities. Check pulse oximetry. Auscultate for cardiac murmur or pulmonary rales. Check for evidence of cyanosis or accessory muscle use.

2) Obtain CXR (evaluate for increased blood flow), CBC, ECG, and ABG. Look for evidence of infection.

3) Evaluate the patient's response to oxygen.

•Treatment•

If R-L shunt

1) Establish IV. Administer oxygen. Place patient on monitor. Assess and stabilize the airway.

2) Correct any metabolic abnormality.

3) Consider prostaglandin 0.1 ug/kg/min to maintain PDA.

4) Consult pediatric cardiology and admit the patient. Surgery is usually required.

If L-R shunt

1) Establish IV. Place patient on monitor. Assess and stabilize the air-

way.

2) Administer oxygen (although a high pO2 may promote ductal closure in ductal-dependent infants: hypoplastic left heart, AS, CA).

3) Consider prostaglandin (although it may cause hypotension in infants who are not ductal-dependent, as it is a vasodilator).

4) Consider inotropy with digoxin, dobutamine, amrinone, or dopamine at 5-10 ug/kg/min (it is contraindicated in hypertrophic CM).

5) Administer furosemide 0.5 mg/kg if the patient is in CHF.

6) Consider decreasing systemic vascular resistance with nitroprusside or an ACE inhibitor (contraindicated if outflow obstruction).

7) Consult pediatric cardiology and admit the patient.

Tet Spells (Hypercyanotic Spells)

1) Tet spells are seen in patients who have an obstruction to pulmonary blood flow and the presence of an intracardiac communication (TOF, VSD with pulmonary stenosis). Tet spells are precipitated by fever, anxiety, or exercise that may cause decreased pulmonary blood flow.

2) Patients present with a sudden onset of labored breathing, cyanosis, and panic; the patient may squat to increase systemic vascular resistance (SVR) and thus decrease the R-L shunt.

3) Treat with comforting measures, having the patient assume a knee-chest position, and administering oxygen blow-by. Consider sedation with ketamine (which increases SVR) or morphine. Correct acidosis with hydration and bicarbonate (1 mEq/kg). Consider esmolol to decrease the heart rate, myocardial contractility and pulmonary outflow tract hypercontractility. Consider phenylephrine (0.01 mg/kg bolus, may repeat, drip 1-5 mcg/kg/min) to increase SVR.

B. Congestive Heart Failure

•Etiology•

*It is often aided by the age of the child:

1) Newborn with structural disease likely has severe LV outflow tract obstruction or AV valve insufficiency.

2) 2 weeks of age- CA (it occurs after duct closure).

3) 1 month of age- Patients may present in CHF if they have a large L-R shunt because after 4-8 weeks the pulmonary vascular bed matures and resistance decreases, thus increasing the L-R shunt.

4) Later presentations may be caused by SVT or myocarditis.

•Evaluation•

1) Check blood pressure in all four extremities. Check pulse oximetry. Auscultate for cardiac murmur or pulmonary rales. Check for evidence of cyanosis or accessory muscle use. The patient may present with tachypnea, tachycardia, retractions, and pulmonary rales.

2) Obtain CXR (evaluate for increased blood flow), CBC, ECG, and ABG. Look for evidence of infection (consider blood cultures).

•Treatment•

1) Establish IV. Administer oxygen (use caution, as oxygen is a pulmonary vasodilator and may increase pulmonary blood flow). Place patient on monitor. Assess and stabilize the airway.

2) Correct any metabolic abnormality.

3) Consider prostaglandin if the patient is dependent on PDA.

4) If hypotensive, consider dopamine (although it is contraindicated in hypertrophic CM).

5) Consider furosemide 0.5-1.0 mg/kg.

6) Consult pediatric cardiology and admit the patient.

C. Supraventricular Tachyarrhythmias

•Etiology•

WPW is the most common form of SVT in children, followed by A-V node re-entry.

•Clinical Presentation•

1) Infants present with poor feeding, tachypnea, pallor, and lethargy; syncope is very rare.

2) Usually, the heart rate is >220 bpm with <10 bpm variation.

•Treatment•

1) Establish IV. Administer oxygen. Place patient on monitor. Assess and stabilize the airway.

2) If poor perfusion, consider vagal maneuvers (see below), and attempt cardioversion with 0.5-2 J/kg; pre-treat with lidocaine 1 mg/kg if the patient is on digoxin (use sedation if possible), or immediate adenosine 0.1 mg/kg (max first dose 6 mg) rapid IVP, may double and repeat dose (max 12 mg). Adenosine slows the SA node and A-V node;

it will increase A-V nodal block (i.e., slow the ventricular response) in atrial fibrillation/flutter or re-entrant atrial tachycardia. Adenosine terminates SVT of A-V nodal re-entry, sinus node re-entry, and A-V re-entry involving an accessory pathway.

3) If persistent PSVT, consider amiodarone 5 mg/kg IV over 20-60 minutes; or procainamide 15 mg/kg IV over 30-60 min.

3) Otherwise, attempt vagal maneuvers, which include an ice bag to the forehead and nostrils for 20 seconds x 3; rectal thermometer; if old enough, have patient blow on his thumb or perform other Valsalva maneuver. Ocular pressure is contraindicated. Vagal maneuvers stimulate the vagus nerve and increase the AV block, slowing and potentially terminating an arrhythmia.

4) If adequate perfusion, consider vagal maneuvers (as above). Consider adenosine 0.1 mg/kg (max first dose 6 mg) rapid IVP, may double and repeat dose (max 12 mg). Consider cardioversion with 0.5-2 J/kg (use sedation if possible).

5) If no hemodynamic compromise, consider digoxin (if not WPW); or verapamil or propranolol (if older than 1 year); or procainamide 3-6 mg/kg over 5 minutes. If younger than 1 year, or if CHF, wide complex tachycardia, or hypotension, avoid verapamil and propranolol as these drugs may precipitate cardiovascular collapse. Consider esmolol, amiodarone, or overdrive pacing.

5) Identify and treat possible causes: hypoxemia, hypovolemia, hyperthermia, hyper/hypokalemia, metabolic disorders, cardiac tamponade, pneumothorax, overdose, and pulmonary embolism.

V. CONSTIPATION

•Etiology•

Constipation may be associated with maternal drugs, congenital GI anomalies, cystic fibrosis, Hirschsprung's disease, poor dietary intake, anal fissure, or (if acute and associated with lethargy and poor feeding) botulism.

•Evaluation•

Evaluate the abdomen and perianal area. Consider performing a rectal exam. Evaluate for precipitants (dehydration). Consider abdominal films.

•Treatment•

1) If mild symptoms, increase fluids and add bulk; consider 4 oz. prune juice/grape juice with each meal.

2) If younger than 6 months, consider a glycerin suppository. If older than 2 yrs, consider Fleets enema; lactulose 5-10 ml bid; milk of magnesia; or Metamucil.

VI. CYANOSIS

•Definition•

1) Central cyanosis is defined as tongue, mucous membrane and peripheral skin involvement and indicates $\geq$ 5 mg of reduced Hgb.

2) Peripheral cyanosis is blue discoloration limited to the extremities.

•Etiology•

1) Etiologies include cyanotic heart disease, arrhythmia, inborn metabolic errors, pneumonia, respiratory foreign body, polycythemia, shock, sepsis, seizures, reflux, and methemoglobinemia.

2) **Breath Holding**- It is not volitional. There is usually a prodrome of injury, fright, or crying; the patient may have brief tonic/clonic activity. Check Q-T interval on the ECG. There is a benign prognosis.

•Evaluation•

1) Perform cardiac, skin, and lung exams.

2) Check pulse oximetry, CXR, ECG, ABG, and CBC.

3) Check RSV titers and consider pertussis.

•Treatment•

1) Establish IV. Administer oxygen. Place patient on monitor. Assess and stabilize the airway.

2) Specific treatment depends on the etiology.

•Disposition•

In general, admit all patients who present with cyanosis or a history of cyanosis.

VII. DERMATOLOGY

A. Candida Diaper Dermatitis

•Diagnosis•

1) The diaper area shows beefy red erythema with small satellite papules and discrete margins, usually involving the intertriginous areas. Any diaper rash present longer than 72h is likely to be secondarily infected with Candida.

2) In contrast, contact dermatitis is limited to convex surfaces, spares creases and has no satellite lesions; atopic dermatitis almost always involves other areas; psoriasis is recalcitrant to therapy and has discrete borders; and seborrhea has discrete borders with greasy scales on the scalp, axillae, and groin.

3) Consider impetigo and syphilis.

•**Treatment**•

1) Recommend frequent diaper changes; avoid excessive cleansing.

2) Administer topical antifungals (clotrimazole, miconazole, or ketoconazole) after each diaper change. Administer 1% hydrocortisone cream twice/day and Desitin.

3) Discontinue baby wipes, which may contain alcohol (use moist cotton balls) and expose the diaper area to as much open air as possible.

4) Consider barrier creams such as zinc oxide paste or petroleum jelly to minimize skin contact with feces and urine.

B. Seborrheic Dermatitis

•**Diagnosis**•

Patients present with greasy, yellow, flaky, scaly patches on the scalp, behind the ears, over the face, or in the diaper area.

•**Treatment** •

1) On cradle cap, use a soft toothbrush with slightly warmed mineral oil to remove larger scales.

2) Selenium sulfide shampoo.

3) Consider a topical steroid/antifungal if severe dermatitis.

C. Tinea Capitis

•**Diagnosis**•

A fungal culture is mandatory. A Wood's lamp may sometimes be helpful in diagnosis, as certain fungal species fluoresce a yellow-green. The patient may have lymphadenopathy in the posterior auricular and cervical chains. Tinea capitis has multiple forms:

Dandruff-like tinea- mild dandruff scale with or without erythema.

Black dot tinea- areas of alopecia and scale with some hairs broken off at the scalp, resembling black dots.

Kerion- large, boggy masses, frequently red and devoid of hair.

•Treatment•

1) Treat with terbinafine (Lamisil) 250 mg/d po for 4 weeks. Alternatively, consider griseofulvin 15-20 mg/kg/d with fatty meal for 8 weeks; lab monitoring of LFTs is unnecessary if the patient is healthy, asymptomatic, and the treatment is less than 8 weeks.

2) If a kerion is present, consider prednisone.

3) Selenium sulfide or ketoconazole shampoo twice/week.

4) If lesions are not weeping, it is probably OK to return to school.

D. Tinea Corporis (ringworm)

•Diagnosis•

1) It is a fungal infection of non-hairy skin.

2) Red patches spread outward, developing into annular lesions, usually with a sharp border and a healing center.

•Treatment•

1) Limited skin infections can be treated with topical antifungal preparations such as miconazole 2% or clotrimazole 1% or ketoconazole 2% applied tid.

2) Resolution should be achieved in 1-3 weeks, and therapy continued for another 2 weeks.

VIII. GASTROENTERITIS

•Etiology•

1) Etiologies include viral pathogens (rotavirus, Norwalk virus, adenovirus), bacteria, parasites, foodborne pathogens, drugs, or inflammatory bowel disease.

2) In children, diarrhea can be a presenting sign of appendicitis.

3) If the patient is younger than 3 months old and presents with bloody diarrhea, consider salmonella (which may need an evaluation for meningitis).

•Evaluation•

1) Assess the patient's hydration status, the amount of vomiting and diarrhea, and the frequency of urination. Assess skin turgor, mucous membranes, and vital signs.
2) Document any weight loss, abdominal pain, or fevers.
3) Check stool cultures in all neonates with diarrhea, and in children with bloody stools or severe diarrhea. Consider the ELISA test for rotavirus.
4) Consider checking electrolytes.

•Treatment•

1) If the patient is severely dehydrated, establish IV and administer saline.
2) If the patient is mildly to moderately dehydrated, consider oral rehydration therapy (ORT) 1 tsp or syringe (5 ml) every 1-5 minutes; larger boluses cause gastric distention and vomiting (see fluid choice below). ORT is 90% effective for mild-to-moderate dehydration. Involve the parents when attempting ORT.
3) Reassess hourly. Do not administer antidiarrheal agents. If the child worsens, administer IV fluids.
4) Early refeeding with age-appropriate foods containing complex carbohydrates will lessen stool losses and aid mucosal repair- e.g. rice, wheat, potatoes, bread, breast milk, and chicken. Milk is usually well tolerated.
5) <u>Fluid Choice</u>
   a) Pedialyte and Infalyte are the best options.
   b) Coupled transport is the principle of ORT, linking glucose to Na, which is effective even with the inflammation of enteritis. For maximal transport, the fluid should be a 1:1 ratio of carbohydrates: Na; it should be iso-osmolar or hypo-osmolar to reduce the risk of osmotic diarrhea. Juice has too many carbohydrates and may worsen diarrhea; sports drinks have insufficient sodium.
   c) Do not give water.

IX. HEMOLYTIC-UREMIC SYNDROME

•General•

1) It occurs when microthrombi occlude arterioles, mostly in the kidneys. The peak incidence is 6 months – 4 years.

2) It often follows a prodrome of diarrhea (especially E. coli) or URI.

3) Diagnostic criteria include acute renal failure, thrombocytopenia and microangiopathic hemolytic anemia.

•Clinical Presentation•

Patients may present with abdominal pain, vomiting, diarrhea, hypertension, oliguria, seizures, or coma.

•Evaluation•

1) Check CBC, platelets, electrolytes, BUN/Cr, PT/PTT, and urinalysis.

2) Labs usually demonstrate a microangiopathic hemolytic anemia, decreased platelets, and a markedly elevated BUN/Cr. PT/PTT are usually normal.

3) Urinalysis usually shows RBCs and proteinuria.

•Treatment•

1) Supportive therapy, including early dialysis and antihypertenisve therapy as needed..

2) Up to 90% of patients regain normal renal function.

X. HENOCH-SCHONLEIN PURPURA

•General•

1) Henoch-Schonlein purpura is a self-limited vasculitis involving primarily small vessels; it is mediated by immune complexes. It may be precipitated by various infectious and noninfectious stimuli.

2) There is an excellent prognosis.

•Clinical Presentation•

1) Patients may present with a purpuric, tender dermatovasculitis with a propensity for the lower trunk, buttocks, and lower extremities.

2) The vasculitis may involve the glomeruli, which may cause hematuria.

3) Involvement of the bowel wall causes colicky abdominal pain and may cause melena/hematochezia; 8% of patients have a massive GI bleed or intussusception.

4) Migratory periarthritis is common.

•Evaluation•

Check urinalysis, BUN/Cr, CBC, platelet count (there is usually no thrombocytopenia), PT/PTT, and stool guaiac.

•Differential Diagnosis•

The differential includes Rocky Mountain spotted fever, bacterial endocarditis, reactive arthritis, meningococcemia, and lupus.

•Treatment•

Treatment is supportive.

XI. INFECTIOUS DISEASE

A. The Febrile Child (Without a Source)

(Data obtained from guidelines detailed in Annals of Emergency Medicine, and Pediatrics.)

•General•

1) <u>Definition of Fever</u>- Temperature >38°C/100.4°F rectally (some use cut-off of 38.5°C/101.5°F) without a source. (Tympanic thermometry is not recommended for young children). For each 1°C temperature increase, there is an increase of 10 bpm in heart rate and 2.5 breaths/min.

2) <u>Definition of Low Risk</u>- The patient is considered low-risk if previously healthy, full-term, fully immunized with no focal infection (except otitis media) and negative lab evaluation (defined as WBC 5000-15,000, bands <15, normal urinalysis, and <5 WBCs in stool if diarrhea is present).

3) **Admit all toxic-appearing children for a sepsis evaluation and parenteral antibiotics**. If the child is well appearing, the following is a guideline for deciding which diagnostic tests will aid in the diagnosis of occult bacteremia in febrile children without a source. Occult bacteremia places the child at a higher risk for serious bacterial infection and should be treated with parenteral antibiotics.

4) <u>Occult Bacteremia- Some Statistics:</u>
   a) The incidence of bacteremia in a febrile child is the same with or without a focus of infection, which is 2.8% in well-appearing children 3 months –36 months with a temperature ≥39°C. 6 month-18 month old infants are at the greatest risk for occult bacteremia. The predominant organism causing occult bacteremia is S. pneumoniae, which is much less invasive than H. influenza or N. men-

ingitides, and is more likely to clear spontaneously; H. influenza vaccination has greatly decreased the incidence of H. influenza bacteremia.

b) A temperature <38.9°C has a negative predictive value for occult bacteremia of 99%.

c) If WBC is >15,000, the probability of bacteremia is 10-15%; if >20,000, the probability is 20%. A normal WBC has a negative predictive value of 99%.

d) Bacteremia occurs in 80% of meningitis, 10% of pneumonia and 1.5% of otitis media.

e) If the patient has occult bacteremia, the risk of meningitis if no antibiotics are given is 9.8%. If oral antibiotics are given, the risk of meningitis is 8.2%; with parenteral antibiotics, the risk is 0.3%.

•Evaluation•

The approach is determined by the age of the child.

1) Check vital signs and pulse oximetry; perform a complete physical exam.

2) If child is younger than 28days of age and temperature >38°C:
Perform a full septic work-up (CBC, urinalysis, CXR, blood and urine culture, LP), administer parenteral antibiotics and admit.

3) If child is 28-90 days of age and temperature >38°C:
Consider a full septic work-up (CBC, urinalysis, CXR, blood and urine culture, LP). If the work-up is negative and the patient is non-toxic and low risk, consider outpatient treatment with IM ceftriaxone 50 mg/kg and follow-up within 24h. (Another option is to check urine and blood cultures, and careful observation). Admit if high-risk.

4) If child is 3 months-36 months of age:
If temp <39°C (102.2°F): No work-up is necessary. Administer acetaminophen; advise follow-up if the child worsens or if the fever persists > 48h.

If temp ≥39°C: Obtain urine culture if male and younger than 6 months or female and younger than 2 years. Obtain CXR if dyspnea, tachypnea, rales, or decreased breath sounds. Obtain blood cultures (optional if WBC <15,000 and normal bands). Consider empiric antibiotics; administer acetaminophen. (If there is a source of fever, a full work-up is probably still necessary).

5) One large study suggested that patients 2-3 years old with temperature <39.5°C have a very low risk of bacteremia (0.7%) and do not merit lab evaluation or antibiotics. Patients 2-3 years old with temperature >39.5°C and patients 3 months -24 months with temperature >39°C have a risk of bacteremia of 2.6% and the evaluation should include a WBC; if the absolute neutrophil count (ANC) is >10,000 (ANC is more predictive than total WBC or band count), these patients have an 8.2% risk of bacteremia, so blood cultures and antibiotics should be considered to reduce the risk of serious bacterial infection.

6) Multiple studies show that a CXR is unnecessary in the absence of pulmonary findings. However, one study showed that a significant percentage of patients with a temperature >39°C and WBC >20,000 had occult pneumonia even in the absence of respiratory findings (even if there was another minor focus of infection).

7) Up to 50% of patients with a normal urinalysis may have a culture proven UTI. Most UTIs in boys occur in those who are uncircumcised. Pyuria is often present in febrile children without a UTI; 5-10% of febrile children have proteinuria.

•Treatment•

1) Antibiotics- infants: ceftriaxone 50 mg/kg/d q24 (up to 1 gm) or cefotaxime 50 mg/kg IV (infants may have difficulty metabolizing ceftriaxone); ± ampicillin 100 mg/kg. If older than 3 months, administer ceftriaxone 75-100 mg/kg/d q24h.

2) Antipyretics include acetaminophen (elixirs have concentrations of 120 mg/5 cc and 250 mg/5 cc); the dose is 15-20 mg/kg q4-6h (fever falls in 30 minutes, nadir at 3h). Or, ibuprofen (elixir concentration is 100 mg/5 cc); the dose is 10 mg/kg q4-6h.

3) The American Academy of Pediatrics recommends vancomycin be started as empiric treatment for probable bacterial meningitis or if the patient is critically ill with other invasive infection, as there is increasing resistance to pneumococcus. Some recommend acyclovir for all septic infants younger than 3 weeks, as herpes may be difficult to distinguish from a bacterial infection.

4) Otitis media does not rule out coexisting serious bacterial infection; 20% of patients with meningitis have evidence of otitis. Afebrile neo-

nates with otitis may be treated as outpatients if well-appearing and close follow-up is arranged.

5) <u>Follow-up</u> – Arrange close follow-up for all discharged patients. If blood cultures are positive at 24h for occult bacteremia with S. pneumoniae and the child is afebrile and well at 24h follow-up, then the child may be managed with amoxicillin as an outpatient; admit all others. If the urine culture is positive and there is a persistent fever at 24h, admit for evaluation and antibiotics (if the child is well-appearing and afebrile, consider oral antibiotics).

•Disposition•

Admit all toxic-appearing children. In general, admit all neonates younger than 28 d. In other children, if well-appearing and a negative evaluation, outpatient treatment and close follow-up is appropriate.

B. Bronchiolitis

•General•

1) Bronchiolitis is a viralinfection of the bronchioles.
2) Respiratory syncytial virus (RSV) is the most common etiology (it usually occurs from November to March); other etiologies include parainfluenza and Mycoplasma.
3) It is usually seen in children younger than 2 years.

•Clinical Presentation•

Patients may present with rhinorrhea, cough, dyspnea, wheezing, tachypnea, and ± fever. Patients may also present with respiratory failure.

•Evaluation•

1) Check pulse oximetry. Document the lung exam and any presence of retractions.
2) A CXR may demonstrate bilateral hyperlucency with increased A-P diameter and flat diaphragms; there are often scattered regions of subsegmental atelectasis.
3) Lab evaluation is generally unnecessary. Antigen tests of nasal washings may detect RSV.

•Treatment•

1) Administer oxygen and hydration.

2) Consider nebulized epinephrine, especially if severe symptoms.
3) Consider albuterol nebulizer treatment.
4) Consider a macrolide if Mycoplasma is prevalent.
5) Consider ribavarin in high-risk children with RSV.
6) There has been no demonstrated benefit of steroids, but some recommend prednisone 1-2 mg/kg/d x 5 days (especially if there is a history of reactive airway disease).
7) There is no good evidence supporting the routine use of ribavarin, steroids, or antibiotics.

•Disposition•
Consider admission if respiratory distress, apnea, prematurity, age under 2 months, underlying cardiopulmonary disease, or pulse oximetry <94% after treatment.

C. Conjunctivitis (newborn)

•Clinical Presentation•
1) Chlamydia often presents at 3-6 weeks of life with a coexisting URI; patients usually have a mild inflammation/serosanguinous discharge.
2) Gonorrhea may present at 2-5 days of life with a serosanguinous discharge that becomes thick and purulent with eyelid edema and chemosis

•Evaluation•
Obtain a conjunctival scraping for Chlamydia and gonorrhea culture, and perform a fluorescein stain to evaluate for herpes.

•Treatment•
1) If Chlamydia: erythromycin po 40 mg/kg/d divided qid x 14d (systemic treatment is needed because of the risk of pneumonia) plus topical antibiotics.
2) If gonorrhea: ceftriaxone 25-50 mg/kg/d divided q12h x 7d plus frequent irrigation and topical antibiotics and urgent referral.
3) If herpes: acyclovir 30 mg/kg/d divided q8h x 14d and topical vidarabine.
4) Warm compresses and q1-2h ophthalmic irrigation with saline.

D. Croup (laryngotracheobronchitis)

•General•

1) Croup is a viral infection of the upper airway, usually caused by parain-fluenza type 1.

2) It generally occurs in children 6 months- 3 years.

•Clinical Presentation•

1) There is usually a 2-3 day history of a URI and a gradually worsening cough, especially at night; by the 3rd or 4th day, the child has a barking cough, stridor (usually biphasic), hoarseness and dyspnea. Fever may be present.

2) The patient is usually non-toxic appearing, but may present with severe respiratory distress.

•Evaluation•

1) Document the lung exam, and any presence of retractions or stridor. Document pulse oximetry. Lab evaluation is generally unnecessary.

2) Consider soft tissue neck films. If mild, the films are usually normal; if more severe, the lateral may show a normal epiglottis, and the A-P may show a narrowed tracheal air column (a "steeple" sign instead of the normal square shoulders of the subglottic area).

3) Consider foreign body and epiglottitis.

•Treatment•

1) Administer cool mist, oxygen, hydration, and acetaminophen.

2) Consider aerosolized racemic epinephrine (0.25-0.50 cc of 2.25% solution in 2 cc NS; half-life 1-2h) if severe symptoms, stridor at rest, or no improvement with mist. Racemic epinephrine consists of a mixture of the D and L isomers of epinephrine (it is used because the D isomer has less alpha effects than the L isomer that is used for all other indications). However, regular nebulized epinephrine (1 cc of the 1:1000 concentration) is less expensive and equally effective. If epinephrine is given, administer dexamethasone 0.6 mg/kg (max 8 mg) IM/po within 30 minutes of epinephrine and observe for at least 2-3h. The rebound effect of epinephrine (stridor worsens after epinephrine wears off) was overstated; administration of epinephrine does not mandate hospitalization.

3) Consider dexamethasone 0.6 mg/kg (max 8 mg) IM/po in all patients. Prednisone is probably an acceptable alternative to dexamethasone, but has a shorter half-life.

4) 2 mg nebulized budesonide (a steroid) may be beneficial in the treatment of croup.

•Disposition•

1) If the patient is stable with mild obstruction and no stridor or retractions, consider discharge after a 2-4h observation.

2) Admit if toxic-appearing, significant stridor or retractions at rest, hypoxia, hypercarbia, no improvement with epinephrine, or if worsening symptoms 2-3h after epinephrine.

E. Epiglottitis (Supraglottitis)

•General•

1) Epiglottitis is usually caused by H. influenzae, and most often occurs in children 2-7 years old. The HIB vaccine has led to a decrease in the incidence of epiglottitis.

2) Inflammation of the supraglottic structures may lead to respiratory compromise.

•Clinical Presentation•

1) Patients may present with fever, sore throat and a muffled voice, progressing to drooling, stridor, and respiratory compromise; symptoms progress rapidly.

2) The child appears toxic and often sits in the tripod position with neck extended.

•Evaluation•

1) Do not attempt to directly visualize the epiglottis until preparations are made for intubation. Check pulse oximetry.

2) Soft tissue lateral neck x-rays may show an enlarged epiglottis (the "thumbprint" sign) with obliteration of the vallecula. When obtaining x-rays, the patient should be monitored and accompanied by personnel capable of securing the airway.

3) CBC and blood culture should be obtained only after the airway has been secured.

•Treatment•

1) Allow the patient to be as comfortable as possible. Do not perform procedures unless the airway has been secured. Administer blow-by oxygen.

2) All patients need to have the airway secured. The preferred method is fiberoptic nasotracheal intubation. Ideally, intubation should occur in the operating room, as a tracheostomy may need to be performed.

3) In the emergent situation, if orotracheal intubation is unsuccessful, consider needle cricothyroidotomy.

4) Establish IV.

5) Administer antibiotics- ceftriaxone 75-100 mg /kg/d IV q12h-24h; or cefuroxime 100-150 mg/kg/d IV tid.

F. Erythema Infectiosum (Fifth disease)

•General•

1) Patients present with prodromal viral symptoms (fever, headache, sore throat) for up to 1 week, then have a 1 week symptom-free period, then develop a "slapped cheek" rash, followed by a maculopapular rash with a lacy, reticular pattern on the trunk and extremities.

2) It is caused by the human parvovirus B19.

•Treatment•

Treatment is symptomatic.

G. Hand, foot and mouth disease

•Etiology•

It is usually caused by Coxsackie virus; it is usually seen in summer and fall.

•Clinical Presentation•

Patients present with fever, anorexia, malaise, lymphadenopathy, coryza, oral ulcers (occasionally vesicular) and vesiculopapular lesions on the dorsum of the hands and feet (the lesions may also be on the palms and soles).

•Treatment•

Treatment is supportive.

H. Impetigo

•General•

1) Etiology is usually Streptococcus; it usually occurs after an insect bite, abrasion or eczema.

2) Acute post-streptococcal glomerulonephritis may follow a skin infection.

•Clinical Presentation•

1) The first sign is a pruritic vesicle that becomes pustular followed by a discharge that produces a crusty lesion. Infection is confined to the epidermis. There are no systemic manifestations (fever). Attempt to distinguish impetigo from herpes simplex infection.

•Treatment•

1) Topical mupirocin for limited disease is as effective as oral antibiotics.

2) If more severe, consider dicloxacillin 12.5-25 mg/kg/d divided q6h x 10d; cephalexin 25-50 mg/kg/d divided q8h; or clindamycin 20-30 mg/kg/d divided q6h.

I. Kawasaki Disease

•General•

Kawasaki disease is a self-limited vasculitis; it is more common in Asians.

•Diagnosis•

1) Diagnosis requires fever for at least 5 days, plus the presence of four of the following: bilateral conjunctival injection, mucosal changes (fissured lips, strawberry tongue), edema/erythema of hands/feet (with desquamation in the convalescent stage), nonvesicular rash and cervical lymphadenopathy.

2) Patients may also have sterile pyuria. 50% of patients develop myocarditis in the first 3 weeks; 25% of untreated patients develop coronary arteritis/aneurysm.

3) Obtain an echocardiogram.

•Treatment•

1) Aspirin 80-100 mg/kg/d po divided qid x 14d, then 3-5 mg/kg po qd for 6-8 weeks.

2) IgG 2 gm/kg over 10-12h.

J. Lymphadenitis

•Etiology•
It is usually from S. aureus or Streptococcus, but may be mycobacterial. It may also be due to malignancy, cat scratch disease, TB, or infected thyroglossal or brachial cleft cysts.

•Diagnosis•
1) Patients present with an enlarged, red, edematous lymph node, usually cervical.
2) Differentiate from cervical lymphadenopathy, which is nonsuppurative, caused by a viral infection or adjacent bacterial infection, and is usually not red or fluctuant.
3) If fluctuant, aspirate lymph node and send culture; place PPD.

•Treatment•
1) If systemic symptoms, admit for IV nafcillin.
2) Otherwise, administer dicloxacillin 12.5-25 mg/kg/d divided q8h or clindamycin 20-30 mg/kg/d divided q6h.

K. Measles (Rubeola)

•Clinical Presentation•
1) Patients present with fever >101°F, generalized rash for $\geq$ 3 days and one or more of: cough, coryza or conjunctivitis.
2) Measles is extremely infectious (it is spread by respiratory droplets); viral shedding continues for 3-4 days after the rash appears.

•Diagnosis•
1) The measles rash often begins at the hairline and spreads caudally; it is maculopapular, erythematous, and involves the palms and soles.
2) Koplik spots (white spots on red buccal mucosa) are pathognomonic.
3) Check pulse oximetry and consider CXR, as pulmonary infiltrates are seen in 20-60% of patients.

•Treatment•
Treatment is supportive.

L. Meningitis/Sepsis

•Etiology•
1) <u>Neonate</u>- Group B streptococcus, E. coli, Listeria.
2) <u>5-12 weeks of age</u>- Group B streptococcus, E.coli, Listeria, S.

pneumoniae, H flu.

3) <u>13 weeks - 6 years of age</u>- N. meningitis, S. pneumoniae, TB, H flu.

4) <u>Head trauma, post neurosurgical procedure</u>- Pseudomonas, enterobacteriacae, S. aureus.

5) <u>CSF shunts</u>- S. epidermidis.

6) H. flu has almost been eliminated due to the effective vaccine and the herd effect of immunization, in which even infants who have not had the vaccine are unlikely to contract H flu because of the diminished reservoir pool.

7) Infants often develop bacteremia (and subsequent seeding of the meninges) from bacteria found in the GI tract- Group B streptococcus, E. coli.

•Clinical Presentation•

1) Infants or young children may present with decreased activity, fever, poor feeding, lethargy, bulging fontanel, hypothermia, inconsolability, shock, or paradoxical irritability (the child is quiet at rest but cries when picked up because movement causes meningeal irritation).

2) Older children may localize symptoms to the CNS- headache, fever, lethargy, and nuchal rigidity.

•Evaluation•

1) Perform a full septic workup, including CBC, urinalysis, CXR, blood cultures, and LP.

2) A head CT is unnecessary prior to LP if there is no evidence of increased intracranial pressure, focal CNS signs, or papilledema.

CSF

1) <u>Normal CSF</u> has 0-5 WBCs, 0-15% PMNs, glucose 45-65 mg/dL, protein 20-45 mg/dL.

2) <u>Bacterial meningitis</u> shows >1000 WBCs, 90% PMNs. CSF glucose <40 mg/dL or CSF glucose/blood glucose ratio <0.3-0.5 suggests bacterial infection, as does protein >150-170 mg/dL. However, some patients with bacterial meningitis have a predominance of lymphocytes on the initial CSF and only mild changes in glucose/protein. In some cases, the CSF may initially be normal.

3) <u>Viral meningitis</u> shows 100-1000 WBCs, <50% PMNs, glucose 45-65 mg/dL (normal), protein 50-100 mg/dL (slightly elevated); PMNs predominate in the first 48h and lymphocytes predominate thereaf-

ter. There are no bacteria.

4) Cryptococcal antigen is more sensitive than India Ink; consider in AIDS patients.

5) In a traumatic LP, there are approximately 1000 RBCs for every 1-2 WBCs. Also, a traumatic LP usually clears. Or:

Number of WBCs introduced/cc = [(Peripheral WBC) x (CSF RBCs)]/ (Peripheral RBCs).

6) A Gram stain has a 60-90% sensitivity.

7) If the patient is clinically ill but has a normal CSF, consider sepsis (meningococcemia) or early meningitis.

•Treatment•

1) Establish IV. Monitor fluid balance. Monitor patient for signs of increased intracranial pressure and seizures. If meningitis is strongly considered or the child is severely ill, start antibiotics immediately and admit the patient.

2) If newborn, administer cefotaxime 50 mg/kg IV ± ampicillin 100 mg/kg (infants may have difficulty metabolizing ceftriaxone).

3) If patient is older than 1 month, administer ceftriaxone 100 mg/kg/d divided q12-24h or cefotaxime 75 mg/kg/d IV q8h.

4) The American Academy of Pediatrics recommends vancomycin (15 mg/kg; max 500 mg) be started as empiric treatment for probable bacterial meningitis because of the increasing incidence of resistant pneumococcus.

5) If herpes is suspected, administer acyclovir 30 mg/kg/d IV divided q8h (some recommend acyclovir for all septic infants younger than 3 weeks, as it may be difficult to distinguish herpes from a bacterial infection).

6) If older than 3 months, and bacterial meningitis is suspected, consider dexamethasone 0.15 mg/kg q6h IV x 4d; the effect is maximized if given 10 minutes before the first dose of antibiotics (it inhibits inflammatory mediators in the CNS but may decrease the CNS penetration of vancomycin; use with caution if herpes is suspected). Dexamethasone may decrease the incidence of hearing loss in meningitis due to H. flu and Streptococcus.

7) Prophylaxis

If Neisseria: prophylax all household members or close contacts to oral secretions with rifampin 20 mg/kg/d (max 600 mg/d) q12h x 2d. Or, administer ceftriaxone 250 mg IM once if older than 12 years, or 125 mg IM once if younger than 12 years. Or, administer ciprofloxacin 500 mg once if older than 18 years.

If H. flu: Prophylax household members only if ≥1 child <4 years old in the household; use rifampin 20 mg/kg single daily dose x 4d.

If Streptococcus, prophylaxis is not indicated.

M. Mononucleosis

•Etiology•
Epstein-Barr virus (EBV) is the etiology in 80% of mononucleosis; other etiologies include CMV.

•Clinical Presentation•
1) It is usually a subclinical infection, especially in childhood. Adolescents may have an acute onset of pharyngitis (palatal petechiae occur in 50%), bilateral posterior and anterior cervical lymphadenopathy, splenomegaly, fever, and fatigue.
2) The patient may have bilateral periorbital edema. A rash may be present. There usually are minimal GI and URI symptoms.

•Diagnosis•
1) CBC usually demonstrates a leukocytosis, with at least 50% lymphocytes and ≥10% atypical lymphocytes; there is usually a mild thrombocytopenia. LFTs are usually moderately elevated.
2) Other lab tests include the heterophile antibody (it is present in 40-60% of patients in the first week of illness, and in 80-90% by the 3rd or 4th week), or antibodies to specific EBV antigens. The Monospot is an improved variation on the heterophile test. The Monospot only identifies the Epstein-Barr virus; it may be falsely negative in the first few days of acute disease, and young children may have falsely negative results.

•Treatment•
1) Supportive therapy.
2) Avoid contact sports (to avoid splenic injury).
3) Consider steroids if severe pharyngeal swelling.
4) Do not prescribe ampicillin or amoxicillin, as 95% of patients will develop a rash.

N. Omphalitis

•Diagnosis•
Erythema around the umbilicus in neonates suggests omphalitis, which may quickly develop into peritonitis, a liver abscess, or sepsis. A full septic work-up is usually required (especially if febrile).

•Treatment•
Ampicillin 100-200 mg/kg/d IV divided q4h plus gentamicin 5 mg/kg/d divided q12h in first week of life and 7.5 mg/kg/d divided q8h thereafter.

O. Orbital/Periorbital Cellulitis

* See Chapter 18

P. Osteomyelitis

•Etiology•
1) It may be secondary to hematogenous seeding, or contiguous spread from local infection. S. aureus is the most common pathogen; H. influenzae is another important pathogen.
2) Consider Salmonella in patients with sickle cell disease; consider pseudomonas in patients with puncture wounds to the foot.

•Clinical Presentation•
Patients may have pain, local signs of inflammation, and fever.

•Evaluation•
1) Check x-ray, blood cultures, CBC, and ESR; consider bone scan.
2) Definitive diagnosis is made by culturing pathogens from bone.

•Treatment•
Nafcillin 100 mg/kg/d q6h or vancomycin 10 mg/kg/dose q8h.

Q. Otitis Media

•General•
1) Otitis media results from intrinsic eustachian tube dysfunction or dysfunction secondary to obstruction by hyperplastic adenoidal tissue; viral or allergic responses predispose to bacterial infections.
2) Common pathogens include S. pneumoniae, H. influenzae, and M. catarrhalis.

3) The presence of otitis media does not rule out serious bacterial infection; 20% of patients with meningitis also have evidence of otitis.

4) Well-appearing febrile children with otitis have the same rate of occult bacteremia as well-appearing children with fever of unknown origin.

5) Potential complications include hearing loss, mastoiditis, cholesteatoma, and tympanic membrane perforation.

6) Bullous Myringitis- Patients present with intense ear pain, low-grade temperature, and hearing loss. The tympanic membrane has watery, herpetic blebs and is slightly purple. The etiology is usually viral, but may be Mycoplasma. Treat with topical analgesia, and consider antibiotics.

7) Otitis Media with Effusion- It is a chronic infection lasting >2 weeks, usually secondary to acute otitis. Clinically, it is an asymptomatic middle ear effusion. If it has been present >3 months, consider steroids.

8) The Draining Ear- If it is a perforated otitis, treatment is the same as for regular otitis. If chronic perforation, treat with topical antibiotic drops (they are not contraindicated in perforations), and oral antibiotics if resistant to topical treatment. Consider cholesteatoma.

•Diagnosis•

1) The normal tympanic membrane is concave, translucent, pearly grey and easily mobile with air insufflation; a light reflex is usually visible.

2) If infected, the tympanic membrane is opaque, hyperemic, sometimes bulging, immobile and without easily discernible bony landmarks.

3) Most consider some associated symptoms (fever, pain) necessary for the diagnosis.

•Treatment•

1) The initial antibiotic choice is often amoxicillin 40 mg/kg/d divided tid x 10d (if high risk for penicillin-resistant pneumococcal infection, consider 80-90 mg/kg/d). If treatment failure, consider Augmentin, oral cefuroxime, or a 3-day course of IM ceftriaxone. S. pneumoniae is becoming increasingly resistant to penicillin and macrolides.

2) Other options, depending on local resistance, initial response, and cost, include Bactrim 8-10 mg/kg/d divided bid x 10d; Augmentin 40 mg/kg/d divided tid x 10d; azithromycin 10 mg/kg/d on day 1, then 5 mg/kg qd on days 2-5; loracarbef 15-30 mg/kg/d divided bid (if over 6 mos); Ceftin (cefuroxime) 30 mg/kg/d divided bid; Pediazole 50 mg/kg/d divided q6 x 10d; or ceftriaxone 50 mg/kg IM x 1.

3) Topical antibiotics are possibly toxic to the cochlea if the tympanic membrane is perforated; they can be used, but with caution.

4) For pain, administer acetaminophen, ibuprofen or Auralgan drops (if the tympanic membrane is not perforated).

5) To remove wax, use Colace drops with cotton for 10-20 minutes, and lavage with warm water.

6) Antihistamines and decongestants are not recommended.

7) Some, especially in Europe, advocate withholding antibiotics and watching for complications, as 81% of cases spontaneously resolve; however, most advocate antibiotics to avoid long-term complications.

R. Pharyngitis

* See Chapter 13

S. Pityriasis Rosea

•Etiology•
The etiology is probably viral.

•Clinical Presentation•
1) Patients present with a 2-6 cm herald patch (a red, raised lesion usually on the chest or back) followed 1-2 weeks later by widespread, symmetrical, pink or salmon-colored oval maculopapular lesions, sometimes with a "Christmas tree" pattern on the back.

2) The rash may last 3-8 weeks.

•Treatment•
Treatment is symptomatic, and healing is complete; steroid creams and antihistamines may relieve pruritis.

T. Pneumonia

•Etiology•
Neonates- Group B Streptococcus, gram-negative enteric pathogens, viruses, S. pneumoniae.

<u>Infants</u>- Viruses (respiratory syncytial virus, parainfluenza, adenovirus); atypical organisms (Chlamydia); B. pertussis; bacterial pathogens (S. pneumoniae, H. flu).

<u>Young Children</u>- Viruses (similar to infants); S. pneumoniae; Myco-plasma.

<u>Older Children</u>- Viruses; S. pneumoniae; Mycoplasma, Chlamydia.

•Clinical Presentation•

1) Neonates present with tachypnea, grunting, lethargy, nonspecific complaints (poor feeding, irritability), and possible fever or hypothermia; cough is unusual.

2) Infants present with cough, URI symptoms, respiratory difficulty, poor feeding, and possible fever.

3) Older children may have cough, URI symptoms, fever, and constitutional symptoms (sore throat, headache, and diarrhea).

•Evaluation•

1) Look for signs of respiratory distress (tachypnea, grunting, nasal flaring, and retractions). Grunting usually localizes disease to the lower respiratory tract, but may also occur in patients with non-respiratory conditions. Auscultate for focal rales, wheezing, and decreased breath sounds.

2) Check pulse oximetry; consider CXR. Consider CBC and blood cultures (although one study showed blood cultures are not usually positive, and probably not necessary).

•Diagnosis• (for specific pathogens)

1) **Group B Strep (GBS)**- GBS is seen in neonates, usually within several hours of delivery, but may be delayed several days. Patients present with respiratory difficulty ± fever and diffuse crackles. The CXR often shows a "ground glass" appearance with air bronchograms. GBS often progresses to sepsis, and a full sepsis work-up is required. Treat with ampicillin 100 mg/kg and gentamicin 2.5 mg/kg (these two agents have synergism against GBS).

2) **Bronchiolitis**- See <u>Pediatrics; Bronchiolitis.</u>

3) **Chlamydia**- It is usually seen at 1-4 months of age, with a peak at 4-6 weeks. Children usually present with rhinorrhea, tachypnea, and may have the classic staccato cough; the patient is usually afebrile.

Conjunctivitis is seen in 50% of patients. In adolescents, it is insidious in onset and a concurrent sore throat is often present. WBC is usually minimally elevated; there may be eosinophilia. The CXR shows hyperaeration and increased interstitial markings. Treat with macrolides.

4) **Mycoplasma**- It is most common in school age children. There are two distinct patterns: 1) acute nonproductive cough, fever, and myalgias. The CXR may show segmental consolidation; an effusion may be seen; and 2) an indolent course of malaise, lethargy, and dyspnea; most patients do not have a cough. The CXR shows a bilateral reticulonodular pattern. Treat with macrolides.

5) **Pertussis**- Pertussis peaks in late summer/early fall. Paroxysmal coughing is nearly universal and children usually go into paroxysms with stimulation or gag. Many patients have no whoop. Patients may have conjunctival injection, coryza, or fever. If younger than 6 months, admit to rule out potential apnea. Treat with erythromycin.

•Treatment•
1) Administer oxygen as needed; consider albuterol nebulizer.
2) In an acutely ill neonate, treat as septic with ampicillin and an aminoglycoside (or monotherapy with cefotaxime).
3) If older than 3 months and well appearing, treat with amoxicillin or Augmentin (40 mg/kg/d divided tid) or Pediazole 50 mg/kg/d divided tid or azithromycin. Beta-lactams may be the optimal choice in children < 5 years of age, as atypical pathogens are less common in this age group.
4) Otherwise, administer cefuroxime 150 mg/kg/d IV divided q8h or cefotaxime; consider vancomycin.

U. Retropharyngeal/Peritonsillar Abscess

•Diagnosis•
Retropharyngeal Abscess
1) It is usually a disease of young children, as the retropharyngeal lymph nodes atrophy at age 5. Infectious spread is a serious risk, and can result in airway obstruction, mediastinitis, or erosion into the carotid artery.
2) Patients present with fever, odynophagia, neck swelling, drooling and

torticollis.

3) The lateral neck x-ray is 88% sensitive and may demonstrate air-fluid levels or soft tissue swelling anterior to the cervical vertebral bodies (normal soft tissue should be less than 7 mm anterior to C2 and less than 14 mm anterior to C6; or, less than 1/2 the width of the vertebral body). CT is a more accurate imaging method. Check CBC and blood cultures. Consider CXR.

Peritonsillar Abscess

1) It is primarily a disease of young adults. Bacteria include Group A beta hemolytic streptococci, S. viridans, and anaerobes. Bacterial infection of the tonsils can spread to the peritonsillar space between the tonsillar capsule and the superior constrictor muscle of the pharynx. This may progress to an abscess (presumably preceded by a cellulitis).

2) Patients present with unilateral dysphagia, trismus, fever, and a displaced uvula secondary to tonsillar swelling. Patients usually have a coexistent bilateral exudative tonsillitis, with fever, odynophagia, and tender adenopathy.

3) Severe complications include airway compromise, deep space infections of the neck, and mediastinitis.

•Treatment •

1) Assess and stabilize the airway. Administer IV fluids.

2) Antibiotic options include PCN G 100,000-400,000 U/kg/d divided q6h (max 24 m/d); clindamycin 20-40 mg/kg/d divided q8h plus gentamicin; or third generation cephalosporin plus a penicillinase-resistant PCN.

3) Arrange an urgent ENT consult.

V. Roseola

•Etiology•

The etiology is human herpesvirus type 6; it occurs between 6 months and 3 years of age.

•Clinical Presentation•

The patient is febrile and usually irritable, but otherwise well; the initial fever is 102°-106°F. The fever lasts 3-4 days with an abrupt defervescence followed by a maculopapular rash on the trunk, extremities, and face.

•Treatment•

Treatment is symptomatic.

W. Sinusitis

* See Chapter 13

X. Urinary Tract Infection (UTI)/Pyelonephritis

•Etiology•

1) In neonates, UTI is presumed to result from hematogenous spread. After the neonatal period, UTIs generally result from an ascending infection from perineal contaminants (E. coli, Klebsiella, Proteus).
2) Urinary tract abnormalities, immunologic or systemic disease, and prematurity may predispose to infection

•Clinical Presentation•

1) Neonates may present with fever, hypothermia, poor feeding, jaundice, or lethargy; infants may also have foul-smelling urine.
2) Older children may have fever, vomiting, abdominal pain, flank pain, dysuria and urinary frequency.
3) Children with pyelonephritis are often toxic-appearing with fever, nausea and vomiting.

•Evaluation•

1) Check urinalysis and culture; consider checking CBC, BUN/Cr and blood culture.
2) Evaluate hydration status; document any abdominal or flank pain.

Urinalysis

1) Urine is infected if it shows 5-10 WBCs plus ≥ 1 bacteria; or the presence of leukocyte esterase and nitrites. Esterase and nitrites are indirect evidence of pyuria and bacteriuria (esterases result from the breakdown of WBCs, and nitrates are converted to nitrites by gram-negative organisms). Nitrites become positive if bacteria act on nitrate for >6h (thus, the first morning void is the most sensitive). Urinary frequency dilutes the number of WBCs. Send urine culture, even if specimen is inconclusive.
2) If the patient is old enough, a clean catch urine specimen is appropri-

ate. Otherwise, a straight catheter specimen or suprapubic aspiration should be obtained. A bag specimen if useful only if negative; the bag should be removed immediately after the specimen is obtained.

•Treatment•

1) Toxic appearing or dehydrated children or febrile infants younger than 3 months should be admitted for parenteral therapy.

2) If uncomplicated cystitis, oral therapy may be appropriate. Consider amoxicillin 30-50 mg/kg/d po divided q8h; or Augmentin 50 mg/kg/d q8h; or cefixime 8 mg/kg/d q12h; or, if over 2 months old, Bactrim 5-10 mg/kg/d (based on trimethoprim) po divided q8h.

3) For outpatient treatment of mild upper tract infection, consider ceftriaxone 50-75 mg/kg/d IV or IM; or gentamicin 2.5 mg/kg IV or IM followed by Bactrim.

4) For inpatient treatment, administer ampicillin 200 mg/kg/d IV divided q6h and gentamicin 2.5 mg/kg/dose q12h in the first week of life and q8h thereafter; or, cefotaxime 100-200 mg/kg/d q8h; or, ceftriaxone 75 mg/kg/d q6-8h.

5) Early treatment of UTIs may decrease the risk of renal damage. Appropriate follow-up may include radiographic evaluation (e.g., voiding cystourethrogram or renal cortical scan) to evaluate for possible structural or functional etiologies of UTI.

Y. Varicella (Chicken Pox)

•General•

1) The etiology is varicella-zoster virus (a herpes virus).

2) It is usually a benign, self-limited infection spread by direct contact or inhalation of secretions. Incubation period is 10-21 days. The patient is contagious 1-2 days before the rash appears, and until all lesions have crusted.

•Clinical Presentation•

1) Patients present with fever, malaise, and rash. The usual lesions are vesicles on an erythematous base; lesions are initially papules and then progress to vesicles and then pustules before crusting over.

2) Generally, there are lesions in various stages of development. The rash is pruritic, and usually first appears on the face, then the trunk.

Complications

1) Complications are rare in immunocompetent children, but may include varicella pneumonia, encephalitis, acute cerebellar ataxia, and skin superinfection; scarring is probably secondary to scratching.

2) Immunocompromised children are at risk for developing progressive varicella.

•Treatment•

1) Prescribe an antihistamine for pruritis.

2) Local care with oatmeal baths (Aveeno) and calamine lotion.

3) Acetaminophen.

4) If varicella pneumonia or encephalitis, or if child is immunocompromised, administer acyclovir 80 mg/kg/d po in 4 divided doses for 5 days or 30 mg/kg/d IV divided q8h.

5) In high-risk patients who have been exposed to varicella, consider Varicella Immune Globulin 125 U/10kg body weight.

XII. INTUSSUSCEPTION

•General•

1) Intussusception is the telescoping of one segment of the bowel into an adjacent segment; the most common location is the terminal ileum. It is the most common cause of bowel obstruction in children younger than 2 years; it usually occurs between 4 and 12 months.

2) In intussusception, venous obstruction produces congestion and edema of the bowel wall, eventually causing ischemia; mucus and hemorrhage cause "currant jelly" stools. There may be a "lead point" (enlarged lymphoid tissue, Meckel's diverticulum, polyp, or lymphosarcoma) that precipitates the intussusception.

•Clinical Presentation•

1) Patients present with a sudden onset of severe colicky abdominal pain every 15-30 minutes; infants often draw up their legs. Nausea and vomiting are rare in the first few hours, but develop after 6-12h.

2) Initially, the child appears well between attacks; the child may later become lethargic. Alternating colic and lethargy strongly suggests intussusception.

•Evaluation•

1) Check CBC, electrolytes. Obtain abdominal x-rays.

2) Almost all patients are hemoccult positive; 50% have "currant jelly" stools. A "sausage mass" may be palpable in the abdomen.

3) Abdominal films may show dilated small bowel loops, absence of air distal to the obstruction, and a soft tissue mass, usually in the right lower quadrant (but the films may be non-diagnostic). Consider abdominal ultrasound, which may demonstrate a "bulls eye".

4) An air or barium enema is diagnostic and reduces the intussusception in 75% of patients (arrange surgery back up in case of perforation during the procedure). Enema is contraindicated in the presence of perforation or shock unresponsive to IV fluids.

•Treatment•

1) Administer IV fluid resuscitation as necessary. Consider bowel decompression with nasogastric tube.

2) Surgical reduction is indicated if the enema is unsuccessful.

3) Admit for 24h even if reduced by enema, as up to 25% recur.

XIII. JAUNDICE

•General•

1) Newborns have hepatic insufficiency which usually resolves by 4-6 weeks of life. Normal neonates have an average bilirubin of 6 mg/dL.

2) Prolonged unconjugated hyperbilirubinemia may result in kernicterus, which may manifest as lethargy, poor feeding, or seizures.

•Etiology•

Elevated indirect (unconjugated) bilirubin- It is due to an increased bilirubin load, usually from hemolysis (consider blood group incompatibility, autoimmune hemolytic anemia, G6PD, or sepsis), or a defect in the ability of hepatocytes to take up and conjugate bilirubin.

Elevated direct (conjugated) bilirubin- It is due to a decrease in the ability of the liver to excrete conjugated bilirubin; consider hepatitis, cholestasis, cystic fibrosis, sepsis, inborn errors of metabolism, inflammation, or a mass lesion. Conjugated hyperbilirubinemia is abnormal and requires further evaluation.

Physiologic jaundice- It is from the breakdown of RBCs, which peaks at 5-6 mg/dL on day 2-4 of life, returning to <2 mg/dL by day 5-7 of life.

Breast-feeding jaundice- It starts on day 3-4 of life, and peaks at 10-

27 mg/dL by the 3rd week of life.

•Evaluation•

If there is significant hyperbilirubinemia and symptoms of illness, obtain direct and indirect bilirubin, Hgb, reticulocyte count, Coombs test, and a smear for hemolysis. Direct bilirubin should be < 15% of total bilirubin. Consider LFTs and evaluation for infection.

•Treatment/Disposition•

1) Treatment depends on the etiology, age, appearance, and bilirubin level. Possible treatment options include phototherapy and exchange transfusion. Treat the underlying disorder (e.g., sepsis).

2) Admit if ill appearance, anemic, if bilirubin is approaching transfusion levels (20 mg/dL), if conjugated hyperbilirubinemia, or if pathologic hyperbilirubinemia.

XIV. METABOLIC

Estimated Maintenance Fluid Requirements

1) For patients under 10 kg, administer 4 cc/kg/h or 100 cc/kg/d

2) For patients 10-20 kg, administer 40 cc/kg/h plus 2 cc/kg/h for every kg over 10 kg. Or, over 24h administer 1000 cc plus 50 cc/kg/d for each kg over 10 kg.

3) For patients over 20 kg, administer 60 cc/kg/d plus 1 cc/kg/h for every kg over 10 kg. Or, over 24h administer 1500 cc plus 20 cc/kg/d for each kg over 20 kg.

4) In infants, administer 0.25 normal saline; in small children, administer 0.45 normal saline.

5) If hypoglycemic, do not administer D25 if younger than 6 months, as it may sclerose the veins and cause rebound hypoglycemia; administer 0.5 g/kg of D10. If older than 6 months, administer D25 at 0.25-1.0 g/kg (1-4 cc/kg).

XV. REYE'S SYNDROME

•General•

1) Reye's syndrome is an acute noninflammatory encephalopathy associated with hepatic failure.

2) It often follows a viral illness (most commonly influenza or varicella infection), and is associated with aspirin use during the illness.

•Clinical Presentation•

1) The patient is usually 5-14 years old. A prodromal illness is followed by a recovery phase with persistent vomiting.

2) Neurologic changes then develop, which may include lethargy, seizures, and coma. Jaundice typically does not occur.

•Evaluation•

1) Check CBC, electrolytes, BUN/Cr, glucose, LFTs, and ammonia level. Check head CT, LP.

2) The ammonia level is >1.5 x normal; the transaminases ALT, AST are > 3 x normal. Bilirubin is usually less than 3 mg/dL; glucose is often decreased. PT/PTT may be elevated; BUN/Cr may be increased. Head CT is usually normal, but may show cerebral edema. CSF shows less than 9 WBCs.

3) A liver biopsy will demonstrate characteristic changes. Consider a metabolic work up to investigate possible inborn errors of metabolism.

•Treatment•

1) Supportive measures.

2) Correct electrolyte and fluid abnormalities.

3) Correct elevated ammonia with sodium phenylacetate/sodium benzoate or lactulose.

4) Treat any elevation in intracranial pressure (e.g., intubation, sedation, and mannitol).

XVI. SEIZURES

A. Seizures

•Classification•

1) Generalized Seizures

Generalized seizures are characterized by synchronous involvement of both hemispheres; consciousness is almost always impaired. Types of generalized seizures include:

a) <u>Absence/petit mal seizures</u>- brief episodes of loss of consciousness that may appear as staring or lip smacking. There is no aura or postical period. It generally occurs in patients less than 20 years old.

b) <u>Atonic seizures</u>- drop attacks with sudden loss of muscle tone and brief or no loss of consciousness.

c) <u>Clonic seizures</u>- continuous rhythmic jerking motions (alternating contraction and relaxation of the flexor muscles) with altered consciousness.

d) <u>Myoclonic seizures</u>- brief muscular contractions with jerking of extremities; there is no altered mental status.

e) <u>Tonic seizures</u>- stiffening of muscles (continuous muscle contraction) with altered consciousness.

f) <u>Tonic-clonic/grand mal seizures</u>- sudden loss of consciousness, followed by rhythmic jerking; the seizure is followed by a postical period.

2) Partial/focal Seizures

Partial seizures arise from a focus of brain activity; they may remain focal or spread and progress to a generalized seizure. The presence of an aura implies a focal seizure (which may generalize); postical (Todd's) paralysis also suggests a focal onset. Types of partial seizures include:

a) <u>Simple seizures</u>- it may have motor, sensory, or autonomic components; there is no impairment of consciousness.

b) <u>Complex partial seizures</u>- consciousness or mentation is affected, sometimes producing hallucinations, automatisms, or affective disorders.

•Etiology•

1) Neonates, children- etiologies include birth trauma (subarachnoid or intraventricular hemorrhage), hypoxia, meningitis, CNS malformations, phenylketonuria, metabolic derangements, febrile seizures, and toxins.

2) Adolescents, young adults- etiologies include stroke (vascular tumor causing embolism or infarction), substance abuse, noncompliance, withdrawal, or trauma.

•Diagnosis•

1) Seizures have an abrupt onset and termination, are usually not pro-

voked by environmental stimuli, have purposeless movements, usually last 1-2 minutes, and are stereotyped.
2) Patients have lack of recall.
3) Except for petit mal or simple partial seizures, seizures are followed by post-ictal confusion.
4) In neonates, true seizures are unlikely to be initiated or worsened by stimulation, activity should not stop with gentle restraint, and seizures should be associated with autonomic changes.

•**Evaluation**•
1) Perform a complete neurologic and cardiac exam. Evaluate for signs of trauma (especially cervical spine injury). Check for signs of meningitis (fever, nuchal rigidity or petechiae); check for a bulging fontanel in infants. Attempt to exclude trauma, infection, metabolic abnormalities, intoxication and space occupying lesions.
2) In patients with a previous seizure history who present with a typical seizure (and the patient has had a full recovery), check medication levels; other tests are unnecessary.
3) Obtain a head CT if atypical seizure, status epilepticus, abnormal CNS exam, persistent altered mental status, protracted headache, history of malignancy, recent head injury, on anticoagulants, or HIV positive. Consider electrolytes, calcium, toxicology screen, and glucose. Consider ABG, ECG, and urinalysis.
4) Perform an LP if meningitis is suspected.
5) If first-time seizure- If not related to trauma, hypoglycemia, or alcohol or drug use, consider CBC, electrolytes, calcium, magnesium, urinalysis, toxicology screen, head CT (with and without contrast), and LP. Arrange an outpatient EEG.

•**Treatment**• (for status epilepticus)
1) Establish IV access. While administering medications, assess and stabilize the airway, breathing, and circulation. Check glucose. Administer 100% oxygen, monitor the patient and suction secretions. Administer D5NS. Immobilize the cervical spine if trauma is suspected.
2) Administer 25% glucose 2 ml/kg IV if hypoglycemic. Consider naloxone 0.1 mg/kg IV if narcotic overdose. Consider pyridoxine 50-100

mg if suspected INH overdose.

3) Administer lorazepam (Ativan) 0.05- 0.1 mg/kg IV (over 2 minutes, repeat x 2, max 0.2 mg/kg) or diazepam (Valium) 0.2- 0.5 mg/kg IV (1 mg/min, repeat x 3, max 5 mg if younger than 2 years, 10 mg if older than 2 years). Use Valium with extreme caution in infants (it interferes with bilirubin binding). Valium has a faster onset but shorter effective half-life than Ativan; respiratory depression and decreased blood pressure are related to the speed of administration. Do not administer Valium through an endotracheal tube or IM.

4) If seizure continues, administer phenytoin (Dilantin) 18-20 mg/kg IV (1 mg/kg/min, max 1000 mg). Fosphenytoin can be given in equivalent doses, up to 150 mg/min IV; if necessary, fosphenytoin may be given IM. In neonates, use phenobarbital before Dilantin.

5) If seizure continues, administer phenobarbital 10-20 mg/kg IV (max 400 mg) at a rate of 1 mg/kg/min.

6) If unable to establish IV, consider IM midazolam (Versed) 0.2 mg/kg IM, onset 10 minutes; or diazepam (Valium) 0.5 mg/kg PR, onset 20 minutes; consider intranasal Versed. Consider Klonopin 0.3 mg/kg NG (max 10 mg); or Depakote 60 mg/kg PR.

7) If seizure continues, consider general anesthesia with pentobarbital 5-10 mg/kg IV or midazolam (Versed) 0.2 mg/kg IV. The patient must be intubated, and if long-acting paralytics are used, continuous EEG monitoring should be employed to evaluate for persistent seizures.

8) If meningitis is strongly suspected, administer antibiotics.

9) Absence seizure status is treated in a similar manner; consider administering ethosuximide, valproic acid, or clonazepam after administering benzodiazepines.

10) Admit to ICU.

•Disposition•

1) If first-time seizure and the evaluation and physical exam are normal, it is usually acceptable to discharge the patient with close follow-up.

2) Consider anticonvulsants based on the risk of recurrence. The risk of recurrence after a first unprovoked nonfebrile seizure is 27-40%; it is 60% if there is a previous remote CNS infection, head trauma, stroke or abnormal EEG. Therefore, patients with a remote CNS disturbance should be considered for anticonvulsants; it is unclear if prophylactic

anti-seizure medications are beneficial for idiopathic seizures.
3) If the patient is discharged, avoid swimming, driving, and hazardous tools.

B. Febrile Seizures

•General•

1) Febrile seizures usually occur in children 6 months -5 years old.
2) A complex febrile seizure is defined as lasting >15 minutes, more than one febrile seizure in 24h, or a focal seizure.
3) Most patients have a temperature >39°C, but some may seize at temperatures as low as 37.7°C. A single febrile seizure slightly increases the risk of epilepsy.
4) There is no higher risk of occult bacteremia in children with febrile seizures, as compared to children with similar temperatures who have not had a seizure; it is unusual for bacterial meningitis to present with only a febrile seizure in a child older than 18 months.
5) Shigella gastroenteritis has been associated with febrile seizures.
6) Risk factors for recurrence include seizures at lower temperatures, complex febrile seizures, seizures at a younger age, and family history of seizures. If simple seizure, 30-40% recur, and 50% of recurrences are within 6 months.

•Evaluation•

1) Check glucose in all children. Perform an LP in all children with febrile seizures who have petechiae, nuchal rigidity, continued seizure activity, persistent drowsiness, focal CNS deficits, are difficult to assess or are already on antibiotics.
2) However, if the child is >18 months and appears well, an LP is probably unnecessary (but consider checking glucose, CBC, and urinalysis to evaluate for a source of the fever). The AAP recommends that an LP should be strongly considered for the first febrile seizure if the patient is younger than 12 months; older children should be judged individually. The AAP does not recommend an EEG, head CT, or blood studies.

•Treatment•

1) Treat the fever.
2) If seizing, administer benzodiazepines.

3) Prophylaxis is usually not required.

XVII. SICKLE CELL DISEASE

*See Chapter 12

XVIII. STRIDOR

•**Etiology**• (Based on anatomic location)

1) <u>Supraglottic Airway</u> (defined as from the nose to the vocal cords; stridor is mostly inspiratory, as the airway collapses from the negative inspiratory pressure; patients may have drooling and a muffled voice)- consider epiglottitis, retropharyngeal abscess.

2) <u>Glottic and Subglottic Airway</u> (from the vocal cords to the proximal trachea; stridor may be inspiratory or both inspiratory and expiratory, as this part of the airway is not easily collapsible)- consider croup, laryngomalacia, and vocal cord paralysis.

3) <u>Intrathoracic Airway</u> (stridor is mostly expiratory, as elevated intrathoracic pressure during expiration may cause airway collapse)- consider asthma, foreign bodies, congenital disorders.

•**Etiology**• (Based on quality of stridor)

1) <u>Sonorous, snoring</u>- consider nasal problems or foreign body.

2) <u>Muffled voice</u>- consider pharyngeal etiology from tonsillar hypertrophy. If febrile, consider tonsillitis, epiglottitis, or peritonsillar abscess.

3) <u>High-pitched inspiratory, hoarse</u>- consider laryngeal etiology from subglottic stenosis (especially if previous intubation), vocal cord paralysis, or congenital disorder. If febrile, consider croup, epiglottitis, or retropharyngeal abscess. Stridor worsening with cry suggests laryngomalacia.

4) <u>Inspiratory and expiratory</u>- consider tracheal etiology from a foreign body if acute; consider tracheal mass.

5) <u>Expiratory wheeze</u>- consider bronchial etiology from asthma; or consider foreign body, especially if the wheeze is asymmetrical.

•**Evaluation/Treatment**•

1) Check pulse oximetry. Consider soft tissue neck films or CXR.

2) Stabilize the airway.

3) Further evaluation/treatment is dictated by the underlying etiology.

CHAPTER 21
PSYCHIATRY

I. PANIC DISORDER

•Diagnosis• - Criteria for diagnosis include:
1) An unexpected sudden onset of fear or discomfort, usually not triggered by stressful events; symptoms typically peak within 10 minutes.
2) Four attacks within 1 month.
3) Four of the following symptoms are present during the attack: shortness of breath, dizziness, palpitations, shaking, nausea, sweating, chest pain, or fear of dying.
4) Symptoms usually last 20-60 minutes and resolve spontaneously. The chest pain is usually sharp and stabbing.

•Evaluation•
1) Consider an evaluation to exclude a medical etiology for the symptoms.
2) Patients have a significant risk of suicide; document the presence or absence of suicidal ideation.

•Treatment•
1) Consider administering benzodiazepines: alprazolam (Xanax) 0.25-0.5 mg po tid.
2) Long-term medications may include selective serotonin reuptake inhibitors (Zoloft is perhaps the most effective). These are generally not prescribed in the emergency department.
3) Arrange mental health follow-up.

II. PSYCHOSIS

•Definition•
Psychosis results in thought process disturbances and loss of reality testing, which often manifests as hallucinations, delusions, or bizarre speech.

•Evaluation•

1) Attempt to differentiate between an acute brain syndrome (suggested by an acute onset with disorientation or impairment of memory), drug-induced psychosis, and psychiatric disorders (which usually present with an onset over weeks to months without impairment of memory or orientation). Perform a complete physical exam, including an evaluation of vital signs (especially temperature).

2) If the diagnosis is unclear (especially in patients without a prior psychiatric history), consider checking toxicology screen, ECG, CBC, glucose, electrolytes, LFTs, BUN/Cr, and head CT.

•Treatment•

1) If acute agitation, consider haloperidol (Haldol) 5-10 mg IM or 5 mg IV. (Use caution, as Haldol may lower the seizure threshold, has anticholinergic effects, should not be used with cocaine, and may cause dystonic reactions).

2) Droperidol (Inapsine) 2.5 mg IM/IV is associated with QT interval prolongation and Torsades de Pointes, and should only be administered if an ECG demonstrates no QT interval prolongation and other options have proved ineffective.

3) Consider lorazepam (Ativan) 2 mg IM.

4) If acute brain syndrome or toxic/metabolic disorders have been excluded, arrange the appropriate psychiatric consultation and disposition.

CHAPTER 22

RENAL

I. ACUTE RENAL FAILURE

•Etiology•

Prerenal- may be from CHF, renal artery stenosis, or hypovolemia (typically, the BUN/Cr ratio is >10:1, urinary Na is <20 mEq, and FeNa is <1%).

Intrinsic Renal Disease- may be from glomerular disease, Henoch-Schonlein purpura, lupus, or glomerulonephritis (which presents with RBC casts, proteinuria, and hematuria). Interstitial disease is usually secondary to drugs (including penicillin, NSAIDs, and diuretics). Acute tubular necrosis may be secondary to renal ischemia, nephrotoxic agents, or rhabdomyolysis.

Post-renal- it is from obstruction (tubular obstruction from crystals; ureteral obstruction from calculi or tumor; or urethral obstruction from prostatic hypertrophy, tumor, stricture, or obstructed catheter).

•Evaluation•
1) Check CBC, electrolytes (hyperkalemia and hypocalcemia are common), BUN/Cr, and a microscopic urinalysis.
2) A normal urinary sediment is consistent with prerenal and post-renal etiologies of renal failure. RBC casts indicate glomerulonephritis. WBC casts indicate acute interstitial nephritis and pyelonephritis. Granular casts may indicate acute tubular necrosis, glomerulonephritis, or interstitial nephritis.
3) Check urine chemical indices (urinary sodium, creatine, and osmolarity).
4) Consider imaging studies (ultrasound, CT) to evaluate for possible obstruction. A renal biopsy may provide a definitive diagnosis.

•Treatment•
1) Correct any electrolyte or intravascular fluid abnormalities.
2) Dialysis is indicated if lethargy, severe vomiting, pulmonary edema, refractory acidosis, hyperkalemia, or pericarditis.
3) Relieve any obstruction.
4) Treat the underlying condition.

CHAPTER 23
RESPIRATORY

I. ASTHMA

•General•

1) The hallmarks of asthma are airway obstruction, airway hyperresponsiveness, and airway inflammation with edema; certain stimuli (e.g., inhaled antigens, cold, smoke, exercise, or infection) lead to increased airway reactivity, resulting in bronchoconstriction.

2) The early phase of an asthma exacerbation (smooth muscle contraction and mucosal edema) responds to albuterol; the late phase (inflammation) occurs within 2-8h, persists for 24-48h, and improves with steroids.

3) Hypoxemia occurs from ventilation/perfusion mismatches; these mismatches are secondary to uneven inflammation, constriction, and plugging. Oxygen may relieve pulmonary vasoconstriction and bronchoconstriction. The mismatch increases the work of breathing, causing retractions and fatigue.

4) Hypercarbia results from the inability to maintain minute ventilation (in asthmatics, poor oxygenation is usually not a significant problem and responds to treatment; however, ventilation may be severely impaired, thereby increasing pCO_2, especially after exhaustion). Pulsus paradoxus occurs when pulmonary hypertension causes diastolic dysfunction, leading to decreased stroke volume during inspiration vs. expiration.

5) Progressive obstruction leads to air trapping, hyperinflation, and increasing intrathoracic pressure at end-exhalation (auto-peep); this may interfere with cardiac filling and lead to bradycardia, hypotension or, when acidosis and dehydration are present, cardiac arrest.

•Evaluation•

1) Monitor the respiratory rate, accessory muscle use, the intensity of breath sounds, and the duration of the expiratory phase. Wheezing is not correlated with the severity of obstruction. Initially, most patients have expiratory wheezing, which may progress to both inspiratory

and expiratory wheezing. Wheezing may not be present if there is significantly diminished airflow.

2) Check pulse oximetry and peak expiratory flow rate (PEFR). A CXR is generally not indicated in routine asthma exacerbations; however, consider CXR if severe asthma, unexplained fever, immuncompromised patient, or suspicion of infection, pneumothorax, CHF, or foreign body. In children, a CXR with the first episode of bronchospasm is recommended (no clinical variable identifies those patients with pathology). A CBC typically demonstrates eosinophilia, but is generally not useful.

3) Assess the severity of the patient's asthma history by documenting the last hospitalization, any prior intubations, and last steroid use. Attempt to identify any precipitants of current symptoms.

4) A severe exacerbation is defined as heart rate >120 bpm; RR >30; PEFR <30%-50% of predicted or personal best, or <100; failure to improve peak flow at least 10%; pulse oximetry < 90%; or pO2 <60 mm Hg or pCO2 ≥40 mm Hg (a normal CO2 may indicate impending ventilatory failure). Altered mental status and accessory muscle use also indicate a severe exacerbation.

5) Reserve ABG for patients with exhaustion or mental status deterioration, mainly to verify a normal or increased pCO2 (if patients are ventilating well, tachypnea should result in a low pCO2).

Predicted Peak Expiratory Flow Rates (L/min) in Adult Males

Age (yr)	60 inch (height)	65 inch (height)	70 inch (height)	75 inch (height)	80 inch (height)
20	547	588	630	672	714
30	522	564	606	647	689
40	497	539	581	623	665
50	473	515	556	598	640
60	448	490	532	574	615
70	424	465	507	549	591

Predicted Peak Expiratory Flow Rates (L/min) in Adult Females

Age (yr)	55 inch (height)	60 inch (height)	65 inch (height)	70 inch (height)	75 inch (height)
20	410	439	467	495	524
30	392	421	449	477	506
40	374	403	431	459	488
50	356	385	413	441	470
60	338	367	395	423	452
70	320	349	377	405	434

Normal Peak Expiratory Flow Rates for Children

Height (inch)	Mean Peak Flow (L/min)
39	110
43	160
47	210
51	260
55	320
59	370
63	420
67	475
71	530
75	570

(Adapted from data obtained by Godfrey et. al., *Brit J Dis Chest*, 1970; 64:15.)

•Treatment•

1) Administer oxygen. Assess the need for intubation; consider non-invasive ventilation (BiPAP) as an alternative.

2) If airflow is very poor, consider epinephrine 0.3-0.5 mg of a 1:1000 solution SC (peds: 0.01 mg/kg SC, max 0.3 mg) every 20 minutes x 3 (may give regardless of age if no cardiac disease, although it has not been shown to be more effective than nebulizer treatment). Or, consider terbutaline 0.25-.5 mg SC (peds: 0.01 mg/kg SC); may repeat once after 15-30 minutes. Terbutaline may also be administered in adults as 200 mcg IV over 10 minutes, then 2-12 mcg/min.

3) **Bronchodilators**

Albuterol. It may be administered as a metered dose inhaler (MDI) with spacer, 6-8 puffs per treatment; or albuterol nebulizer treatment 2.5-5 mg (0.5 ml of 0.5% albuterol mixed with 2.5 ml normal saline) every 20 minutes or continuously (continuous nebulizer treatment is most effective if the peak flow is <200). The pediatric dose is 0.1 mg/kg as a single nebulizer treatment, or 0.3 mg/kg/h continuously. Duration of action is 4-6h. Multiple studies have shown that MDI spacers are equally effective as nebulizer treatments, unless the patient is in status asthmaticus or is uncooperative. Albuterol is a beta-agonist that effects bronchial smooth muscle relaxation; tachyphylaxis does not occur with albuterol or ipratropium.

Ipratropium. It may be administered as a metered dose inhaler, 4-8 puffs per treatment; or 0.5 mg nebulizer every 3-4h (onset 20 minutes, max effect 1-2h). The pediatric dose is 0.25-0.5 mg nebulizer. Ipratropium is an anticholinergic agent that improves vagally mediated bronchoconstriction in larger airways. When combined with albuterol and steroids, ipratropium improves outcomes.

Aminophylline 5-6 mg/kg over 20 minutes, then 0.6-0.9 mg/kg/h may be helpful in status asthmaticus; however, its use is generally not recommended.

4) **Anti-inflammatory agents**: Consider Solumedrol 60-125 mg IV (there is no evidence that dosages >60 mg are any more effective) or prednisone 60 mg. The pediatric dose is Solumedrol 2 mg/kg IV every 6h, or prednisone 1-2 mg/kg/d divided bid. NIH guidelines suggest administering steroids if there is an incomplete response to one nebu-

lizer treatment or if the patient is already taking oral or inhaled steroids; steroids should be given immediately if the patient is in moderate to severe distress. Steroids take several hours to achieve their effect; oral and IV steroids are equally effective.

5) Mg 2-4 gm IV (peds: 30-70 mg/kg) over 1h (it effects bronchodilation and smooth muscle relaxation by inhibiting cellular calcium uptake) is a safe adjunct of possible benefit in patients with severe exacerbations.

6) Heliox (a 60:40 mixture of helium:oxygen) may be beneficial in severe asthma by lowering airway resistance and decreasing the work of breathing.

7) Consider aggressive IV fluids to replace insensible losses from increased work of breathing.

8) Consider BIPAP in cooperative patients with normal mentation and normal facial anatomy. Start with inspiratory pressure 8 cm H_2O, and expiratory pressure 3 cm H_2O.

9) Episodes lasting more than several days are likely to be associated with mucosal edema and plugging, decreasing the efficacy of acute treatment.

10) Leukotriene receptor antagonists (Accolate, Ultair) or lipoxygenase inhibitors (Zyflo) may be of benefit in chronic asthma (especially if caused by aspirin).

Intubation

1) Hydrate and preoxygenate well with bag mask before intubation to reduce the risk of post-intubation arrhythmias and hypotension.

2) Perform a rapid sequence intubation with ketamine 0.2-1.5 mg/kg then 0.3-2.0 mg/kg/h and midazolam (to prevent an emergence reaction), or midazolam alone (especially if cardiac disease). Administer succinylcholine and vecuronium for paralysis. Avoid thiopental and morphine, as these agents cause histamine release.

3) Use a large endotracheal tube to facilitate airflow and secretion management.

4) Use controlled hypoventilation with RR 8-10, inspiratory/expiratory $\geq$1:3; tidal volume 5-7 ml/kg to keep peak pressure <35; no PEEP.

5) Attribute hypotension to hyperinflation (give trial of apnea) or a pneumothorax.

6) Mechanical ventilation decreases the delivery of aerosols.

•Disposition•

1) Discharge is appropriate if the PEFR has returned to 70% of the predicted or personal best and symptoms are minimal after a 30-60 minute observation period after the last nebulizer treatment. Discharge the patient on MDIs, pulse-dose steroids 60-100 mg/d (peds: 1-2 mg/kg/d) x 5-10 days (tapering is probably not necessary), and inhaled corticosteroids.

2) If the peak flow is 50-69% of the predicted or best, assess individually for suitability for discharge.

3) Admit if the peak flow is <200 or < 50% of predicted or best, if no subjective improvement, if the post-treatment peak flow is not improved by >15%, or if the patient has a pneumothorax.

II. COPD

•General•

Three disease processes overlap:

1) Asthma

Asthma results in airway inflammation with bronchoconstriction and mucus plugging.

2) Bronchitis

    a) It is characterized by inflammation, obstruction, and excessive mucus production. Bronchitis is defined as a chronic cough for at least 3 months of the year for 2 consecutive years.

    b) Irritation causes an inflammatory response that leads to fibrosis; inflammation and secretions lead to obstruction. The patient compensates for diminished oxygenation by increasing cardiac output. Also, CO_2 levels rise, which increases perfusion through a poorly ventilated lung, leading to polycythemia and cor pulmonale.

    c) The patient is a "blue bloater" with a prominent cough, normal blood pressure and often little air hunger with no hyperventilation. There is often minimal emphysema, so the CXR has normal lung volumes and slight hyperaeration of the upper lungs.

3) Emphysema

a) It is characterized by airway collapse and the progressive destruction of lung tissue caused by chronic irritants. The body responds with hyperventilation, decreased cardiac output, and decreased tissue oxygen utilization. Also, the chest cavity expands to increase lung capacity. The CXR typically demonstrates increased radiolucency and flattened diaphragms.

b) The patient becomes a cachectic "pink puffer" (increased energy demands cause malnutrition) with pursed lips and a near normal ABG.

•Differential Diagnosis•
In an acute exacerbation, consider pneumothorax, lobar atelectasis, pulmonary embolus, pneumonia, CHF, cancer, and MI.

•Evaluation•
1) Check CXR (severe pneumonia is more likely to develop with chronic bronchitis than emphysema) and pulse oximetry. Consider checking ECG, CBC, electrolytes, ABG, and pulmonary function tests.
2) Consider a cardiac evaluation.

•Treatment•
1) Assess the need for intubation. If intubated, avoid a precipitous drop in CO2 (i.e., do not hyperventilate), as it may lead to a metabolic alkalosis.
2) Consider BIPAP in the cooperative patient (start expiratory pressures at 3 cm H_2O and inspiratory pressures at 8 cm H_2O; increase inspiratory pressure by 2 to titrate to CO2; expiratory pressure levels are titrated to pO2).
3) Administer oxygen to maintain the saturation above 90%, regardless of the CO2 level (if CO2 narcosis occurs, the patient should be intubated). In normal patients, elevated CO2 levels increase the respiratory drive; COPD patients may lack this response, and instead depend on hypoxia for a respiratory stimulus. Therefore, avoid aggressive use of oxygen, as this may decrease the respiratory drive and lead to CO2 retention. [However, depression of the hypoxemic stimulus to the respiratory drive is not the only etiology of acute hypercarbia (other etiologies include increases in CO2 production, increased ventilatory dead space, and bronchospasm that leads to hypoventilation

and a shift of the hemoglobin-CO_2 binding curve termed the Haldane effect), and thus CO_2 retention can be accompanied by a normal respiratory rate.]

4) Administer bronchodilators. <u>Albuterol</u>: nebulizer treatment (2.5-5 mg q 20 min) or MDI with spacer 4-10 puffs. <u>Ipratropium</u> (Atrovent): nebulizer treatment (0.5 mg; onset 5-15 minutes, max effect 1-2h, duration 4-12h) or MDI with spacer 4-6 puffs. In general, MDIs with spacers are as effective as nebulizers.

5) Consider steroids (although there is no clear benefit to all patients with COPD; most benefit occurs in patients with coexisting asthma): Solumedrol 60-125 mg IV or prednisone 60 mg po. Oral and IV steroids are equally effective.

6) Consider antibiotics. Empiric antibiotics improve outcome (even if there is no evidence of pneumonia or only a slight change in chronic sputum quantity/character/color). Consider azithromycin, levofloxacin (for more complicated cases) or, although no atypical coverage, Bactrim.

7) If obtunded, consider terbutaline 2.5 mg SC every 30 minutes x 2.

8) Consider Mg 1-2 g IV over 15 min; it may be effective as a bronchodilator.

9) Consider Heliox (a 60:40 mixture of helium:oxygen), which may decrease the work of breathing.

10) The need for admission is determined by the underlying disease status and the response to treatment.

CHAPTER 24

RHEUMATOLOGY

I. ACUTE ARTHRITIS

•Etiology•

Etiologies of Polyarticular Arthritis include:

1) Gout and pseudogout.
2) HIV.
3) Lyme disease.
4) Lupus, polymyalgia rheumatica, rheumatic fever, and rheumatoid arthritis with acute onset.
5) Spondyloarthropathies, which include:

Ankylosing spondylitis- Patients have a chronic sacroiliitis and spondylitis, usually with some eye and heart involvement.

Enteropathic- It is usually bilateral, and associated with inflammatory bowel disease.

Psoriatic- Patients have the skin manifestations of psoriasis and chronic arthritis.

Reactive- Patients have a prominent sacroiliitis, spondylitis, and acute peripheral arthritis; there is usually a history of urethral discharge or diarrhea. It is usually from Shigella, Salmonella or Chlamydia. Treat with a 12 week course of doxycycline or erythromycin.

Reiter's- It is characterized by arthritis, conjunctivitis (instead of the uveitis seen in other reactive arthritides), and urethritis. It is the most common type of reactive arthritis and may be secondary to Shigella, Salmonella, Chlamydia, or Yersinia. Disease onset occurs 1-4 weeks after microbial exposure and presents with urethral discharge or cervicitis, fever, malaise and, late in the course, acute asymmetrical arthritis with involvement of the lower extremities and back pain. Consider checking for Chlamydia; consider stool cultures. Treat with NSAIDs.

Etiologies of Monoarticular Arthritis include:

1) Crystal-induced

2) <u>Septic/infectious</u> (gonococcal and nongonococcal disease). It usually presents with fever and joint pain. Gonorrhea and meningococcal infections have a prodromal phase; migratory arthritis and tenosynovitis predominate before the pain and swelling settle in one or more septic joints. Vesiculopustular lesions, especially on the fingers, are suggestive of gonorrhea.

3) <u>Traumatic</u>

•Diagnosis•

1) Obtain joint fluid for culture, cell count, protein, glucose, gram stain, and crystal examination; consider CBC, ESR, and urethral cultures.

2) Crystals: gout demonstrates negatively birefringent (urate) crystals, while pseudogout shows positively birefringent (calcium pyrophosphate) crystals.

3) Synovial fluid WBCs:

<u>Normal</u>: <200 WBCs with <25% PMNs.

<u>Noninflammatory (traumatic; osteoarthritis)</u>: <4000 WBCs with <25% PMNs.

<u>Inflammatory (gout, rheumatoid)</u>: 2000-50,000 WBCs with >50% PMNs.

<u>Infectious</u>: >50,000 WBCs with >50% PMNs.

•Treatment•

Treatment depends on the etiology and lab results.

II. GOUT

•General•

1) Gout is inflammation from monosodium urate crystals; pseudogout is inflammation from calcium pyrophosphate crystals. It often occurs in middle-aged men and postmenopausal women; males usually have a history of increased alcohol use, recent illness or diuretic use.

2) The disease is usually secondary to derangements in uric acid production or excretion.

•Clinical Presentation•

1) Pain and swelling most often occurs in the great toe MTP joint, tarsal joint, ankle and knee; it is most commonly monoarticular.

2) The patient may be febrile and erythema is common.

•Evaluation•

1) Consider CBC, Bun/Cr, ESR, and arthrocentesis.

2) Labs may show leukocytosis and increased ESR. Uric acid is not helpful in the acute setting.

3) The clinical exam cannot distinguish between septic arthritis and crystal-induced arthritis (synovial fluid analysis is required).

4) Diagnostic arthrocentesis should be performed for definitive diagnosis and to rule out septic arthritis. Synovial fluid should be sent for cell count, culture, gram stain, culture, and crystal analysis. In gout, the synovial fluid shows inflammatory changes, and 85% of patients with gout have monosodium urate crystals in the synovial fluid.

•Treatment•

1) Indomethacin 50 mg tid x 2d, then 25 mg tid x 3d (use with caution in the elderly or if renal disease); or sulindac 400 mg in ED then 200 mg bid. Consider other NSAIDs and narcotics.

2) If the patient is unable to take NSAIDS, consider corticosteroids. If unable to take steroids, consider IM ACTH 40-80 U. Consider joint aspiration for pain relief, and corticosteroid injection.

3) Or, although no longer in favor, colchicine 1-2 mg IV over 10 min or 0.6 mg po every hour until pain is controlled, max 4-6 mg. The IV route is preferred; rapid resolution helps distinguish from septic arthritis. It is contraindicated if hematologic, renal, or hepatic dysfunction; it is most effective if administered in the first 24h.

4) Treatment for pseudogout is the same.

5) Long-term therapy for reduction of urate concentrations should be delayed until several weeks after the last attack of gout, as it may precipitate further attacks.

CHAPTER 25
TOXICOLOGY

I. GENERAL TOXICOLOGY

A. General Approach

1) For significant ingestions, establish IV access, monitor the patient, and assess and stabilize the airway. Consider activated charcoal.

2) For significant ingestions, check ECG, electrolytes, BUN/Cr, pregnancy test if female, and urine and serum toxicology (including alcohol level and aspirin and acetaminophen levels).

3) If altered mental status, check glucose and serum osmolarity; administer naloxone 2 mg (or 0.1 mg/kg), thiamine, and glucose (D10 in children).

4) After benzodiazepines, phenobarbital is the anticonvulsant of choice in toxic seizures.

B. Interventions

1) Activated charcoal

    a) The dose is 1 g/kg. Charcoal adsorbs toxins and inhibits their absorption. The first dose is often given with a cathartic (e.g., sorbitol). Routine administration may not be indicated more than 1 hour after drug ingestion.

    b) Multiple dose activated charcoal is indicated for theophylline, phenobarbital, carbamazepine, quinine, dapsone, beta-blockers, or any drugs with enterohepatic absorption. Administer charcoal every 3-4h (use cathartics only with the first dose).

    c) Contraindications include caustic acids/alkalis, and the presence of an ileus.

    d) Substances not absorbed by activated charcoal include alcohols, strong acids/bases, iron, lithium, cyanide, pesticides, solvents, and hydrocarbons.

2) Cathartics

    a) Options include sorbitol 1 gm/kg PO; Mg citrate 4 ml/kg PO; or MgSO4 250 mg/kg PO.

    b) Cathartics may increase elimination of charcoal-bound toxins.

However, cathartics have not been shown to improve clinical outcomes; also, cathartics may cause hypovolemia and electrolyte disturbances (especially in children). If used, only administer cathartics with the first dose of charcoal.

3) Gastric Lavage

    a) Consider lavage if the patient has ingested a potentially life-threatening dose of toxin, and the lavage can be performed within 60 minutes of ingestion; also, consider lavage in hemodynamically unstable patients with an unknown ingestion.

    b) Otherwise, the risks outweigh the benefits, and lavage is discouraged.

    c) If performed, use a 36-40 F Ewald tube, and lavage until return is clear.

4) Ipecac

    a) The use of Ipecac is generally discouraged.

    b) Dose- if 6-12 months: 10 ml with 15 ml/kg H_2O; 1-12 years: 15-30 ml with 240 ml H_2O; >12 years: 30-60 ml with 240 ml H_2O. Repeat once if no emesis in 20 minutes.

    c) Contraindications include any risk of depressed mental status, caustic or hydrocarbon ingestions, age <6 months, or bleeding diathesis.

5) Whole Bowel Irrigation

The procedure is to administer polyethylene glycol 1-2 L/h (25 cc/kg/h in children) until rectal effluent is clear. It is used for substances not adsorbed by activated charcoal, especially toxic ingestions of sustained release or enteric-coated agents; consider its use in body-packers or ingestions of lead, or iron. Do not administer if ileus or obstruction.

6) Hemodialyzable Toxins

These include aminoglycosides, bromide, ethanol, ethylene glycol, isopropanol, lithium, methanol, phenobarbital, salicylates, uremia, theophylline, and barbiturates.

7) Hemoperfusable toxins

These include barbiturates, carbamazepine, disopyramide, sedatives, theophylline, and valproic acid.

C. Toxidromes

Cholinergics: SLUDGE (Salivation-Lacrimation-Urination-Defecation-GI upset-Emesis).

Anticholinergics: Hyperthermia, dry skin, mydriasis, delirium, tachycardia, urinary retention.

Sympathomimetics: Diaphoresis, mydriasis, tachycardia, hypertension, hyperthermia, seizures.

Narcotics: Miosis, hypoventilation, CNS depression, bradycardia, hypotension.

Withdrawal: Diarrhea, mydriasis, tachycardia, lacrimation, hypertension, yawning, abdominal cramps, hallucinations, seizures.

D. Differential Diagnosis from Lab Results

Anion Gap (AG): Na - (Cl + HCO3); normal is 11-13.

Osmolar Gap: Measured serum osmolarity - calculated osmolarity.

Calculated osmolarity = 2 Na + (glucose/18) + (BUN/2.8) + (ethanol/4.6) + (methanol/2.6) + ethylene glycol/5) + (acetone/5.5) + (isopropanol/5.9). The normal gap is <10.

(Obtain serum osmolarity with any unknown ingestion with altered mental status.)

Agents that cause an increased AG metabolic acidosis: Alcohol ketoacidosis, carbon monoxide, cyanide, DKA, ethylene glycol, isoniazid, lactic acidosis, methanol, paraldehyde, salicylates, theophylline, toluene, uremia.

Agents that cause a non-AG metabolic acidosis: Acetazolamide, diarrhea, hyperventilation, pancreatic fistula, renal tubular acidosis, ureterosigmoidostomy.

Agents that cause metabolic alkalosis: Aldosteronism, alkalis, diuretics, gastric drainage, vomiting.

Agents that cause an increased osmolar gap: Diuretics (mannitol), ethanol, ethylene glycol, isopropyl alcohol, methanol.

E. Differential Diagnosis from Vital Signs

Bradycardia: Anticholinesterase drugs, beta blockers, calcium channel blockers, clonidine, digoxin, ethanol or other alcohols, opiates, propafenone.

Tachycardia: Amphetamines, anticholinergics, antihistamines, cocaine, sympathomimetics, theophylline.

Hypotension: ACE inhibitors, beta blockers, calcium channel blockers, clonidine, antidepressants, ethanol or other alcohols, iron, nitrates, opiates, phenothiazines, sedative-hypnotics, theophylline.

Hypertension: Amphetamines, anticholinergics, cocaine, nicotine, PCP, sympathomimetics, thyroid supplements.

Hypothermia: Carbon monoxide, ethanol, opiates, oral hypoglycemics, sedative-hypnotics.

Hyperthermia: Amphetamines, anticholinergics, antidepressants, antihistamines, cocaine, neuroleptic malignant syndrome, nicotine, PCP, phenothiazines, salicylates, sympathomimetics, theophylline, thyroid supplements.

Bradypnea: Barbiturates, clonidine, ethanol, opiates, sedative-hypnotics.

Tachypnea: Cocaine, methanol, ethylene glycol (or any toxin induced metabolic acidosis), PCP, salicylates.

F. Differential Diagnosis from Pupil Size

Miosis: Cholinergics, clonidine, opiates, organophosphates, phenothiazines, pilocarpine sedative-hypnotics.

Mydriasis: Amphetamines, anticholinergics, antidepressants, antihistamines, cocaine, sympathomimetics.

G. Differential Diagnosis from Physical Exam

Diaphoresis: Organophosphates, PCP, salicylates, sympathomimetics.

Dry Skin: Antihistamines, anticholinergics.

Bullae: Barbiturates and other sedatives.

Flushed or Red Appearance: Anticholinergics, boric acid, carbon monoxide, cyanide, disulfram, MSG, niacin, scombroid poisoning.

Cyanosis: Aniline dyes, dapsone, ergotamine, nitrates, nitrites, or any agent that causes hypoxemia or methemoglobinemia.

H. Agents that Induce Seizures

Amphetamines, anticholinergics antidepressants, camphor, cocaine, INH, insulin, lead, lidocaine, lindane, lithium, methylxanthines (theophylline, caffeine), oral hypoglycemics, organophosphates, PCP, sympathomimetics, withdrawal (from ethanol or benzodiazepines).

I. Agents with potential toxicity after an initial asymptomatic period

Ethylene glycol, methanol, lomotil, MAOIs, mushrooms, nitrile (nail glue remover), sustained-release preparations (lithium, theophylline, calcium channel blockers), and thioridazine.

J. Agents in which one dose may be lethal in a pediatric patient

Benzocaine, calcium channel blockers, camphor, chloroquine, cyclic antidepressants, Lomotil, methylsalicylate, sulfonylureas.

K. Agents that are radioopaque

Chloral hydrate, chlorinated hydrocarbons, enteric coated agents, heavy metals (lead, arsenic, mercury) iodides, iron, potassium, psychotropics, solvents (chloroform, CCl4).

II. ACETAMINOPHEN

•General•
1) In an acute overdose, the metabolic pathways become saturated, and glutathione is depleted. This allows accumulation of the toxic acetaminophen metabolite and the production of free radicals that cause hepatocellular damage.
2) The toxic dose is 140 mg/kg (7.5 g total in adults); significant toxicity occurs if ingestion of 250 mg/kg.

•Clinical Presentation•
Stage I: 1-24h- nausea and vomiting, malaise.
Stage II: 24-48h- abdominal pain, elevated LFTs, oliguria.
Stage III: 3-4 days- peak LFTs, jaundice, hepatic encephalopathy.
Stage IV: 4 days-2 weeks- resolution or hepatic failure.

•Evaluation•
1) Check acetaminophen level, electrolytes, BUN/Cr, LFTs, aspirin level, PT/PTT, and ECG.
2) Plot the acetaminophen level on the nomogram; the nomogram is useful only for a single acute ingestion of regular (not extended release) acetaminophen.

•Treatment•
1) Establish IV access. Place patient on monitor. Administer oxygen. Assess and stabilize the airway. If altered mental status, check glu-

cose and consider administering naloxone.
2) Administer activated charcoal; the amount of N-acetylcysteine (NAC) bound by activated charcoal is negligible.
3) NAC is the antidote. Administer NAC 140 mg/kg po load, then 70 mg/kg po every 4h x 17 doses (NAC replenishes glutathione); it is very effective if given within 8h. The dose of NAC is large, so it is not necessary to increase the dose if giving activated charcoal; larger doses increase the risk of vomiting. Continue NAC until acetaminophen level=0, LFTs <1000, normal PT and patient is asymptomatic. NAC does not affect acetaminophen levels/nomogram. Administer NAC before acetaminophen levels return if a large ingestion is suspected.

Nomogram for Acute Acetaminophen Overdose

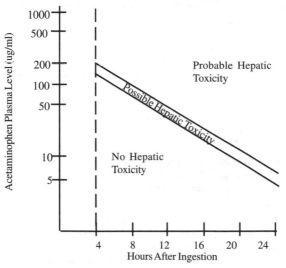

(Reproduced with permission from *Pediatrics*, Vol. 55, page 873, Figure 1, Copyright 1975.)

III. AMPHETAMINES

•General•

1) Amphetamines are a group of compounds that produce various levels of stimulation of the central and peripheral nervous systems. Amphetamines are indirect sympathomimetics; they inhibit the reuptake of catecholamines from synaptic nerve endings, increasing the concentration of neurotransmitters in the synapse.

2) Tolerance occurs through down-regulation of receptors; chronic use can result in the depletion of catecholamine stores and the "wash out" syndrome.

3) Amphetamine use may be via the oral, inhalation, or IV routes.

•Clinical Presentation•

1) The relative amounts of central and peripheral nervous system effects depend on the type of amphetamine used (e.g., methamphetamine produces significant CNS effects but only minor cardiovascular toxicity).

2) Sympathomimetic effects may include mental status changes, increased alertness, seizures, euphoria, agitation, tachycardia, hypertension, hyperthermia, diaphoresis, dry mouth, urinary retention, and mydriasis.

•Evaluation•

1) Mild amphetamine intoxication requires no lab evaluation.

2) If mental status changes or seizures, check glucose and electrolytes; consider head CT, ECG, serum osmolarity, and toxicology screen.

3) If hyperthermic, consider infectious evaluation.

4) Consider checking CPK for rhabdomyolysis. Obtain CXR and ECG if chest pain or respiratory distress.

•Treatment•

1) Establish IV access. Place patient on monitor. Administer oxygen. Assess and stabilize the airway. If altered mental status, check glucose and consider administering naloxone.

2) If acute oral ingestion, administer activated charcoal 1 gm/kg Consider cardiac monitoring.

3) If agitation, treat with benzodiazepines (lorazepam or diazepam).

4) If hypertension, treat initially with benzodiazepines. If evidence of end-organ damage, consider phentolamine 1-2 mg IV or nitroprusside. Avoid beta-blockers due to possible unopposed alpha effects.

5) If cardiac dysrhythmias: treat SVT initially with benzodiazepines; otherwise, treat dysrhythmias according to normal protocols (but avoid beta-blockers).

6) If hyperthermia, aggressively cool according to hyperthermia protocols. Consider neuromuscular paralysis. Consider haloperidol 5 mg IV/IM (although it may lower the seizure threshold and alter thermoregulation). Consider dantrolene.

•Disposition•

1) Patients with minor intoxication may be observed for 6h and discharged when toxic signs resolve.

2) Significant toxic manifestations (seizures, hypertension, hyperthermia, dysrhythmias) require admission to a monitored setting.

IV. ANTICHOLINERGICS

•General•

1) Anticholinergics competitively antagonize muscarinic acetylcholine receptors, resulting in the inhibition of cholinergic transmission.

2) Examples include atropine, benztropine, antihistamines, antiparkinsonians, antipsychotics, cyclic antidepressants, antispasmodics, and jimsonweed.

•Clinical Presentation•

Anticholinergic effects include dry skin, altered mental status, flushed skin, fever, tachycardia, and mydriasis.

•Evaluation•

1) Check toxicology screen and ECG; consider checking electrolytes, BUN/Cr.

2) If altered mental status, check glucose and serum osmolarity; consider CPK if rhabdomyolysis is suspected.

•Treatment•

1) Establish IV access. Place patient on monitor. Administer oxygen. Assess and stabilize the airway. If altered mental status, check glucose and consider administering naloxone.

2) Administer activated charcoal 1 gm/kg (GI decontamination may be beneficial for several hours after ingestion, as cholinergic blockade delays gastric emptying).

3) Physostigmine 1-2 mg IV (children 0.2-0.6 mg IV) is an acetylcholinesterase inhibitor. Consider physostigmine if significant CNS toxicity (intractable seizures or pronounced agitation) or narrow complex tachydysrhythmias resulting in hemodynamic compromise. Administer a 0.5 mg test dose over 2 minutes first (in adults), and then the remaining 1.5 mg The patient should respond within 20-30 minutes. Do not administer if a cardiac conduction abnormality is evident on ECG. Keep patients on monitor.

4) Sinus tachycardia does not require treatment in the stable patient.

5) Treat agitation and seizures with benzodiazepines. Avoid phenothiazines.

6) Treat fever with antipyretics and active cooling measures.

•Disposition•
If asymptomatic, normal mental status, and normal heart rate for 4-6h, the patient may be discharged.

V. BENZODIAZEPINES

•General•
1) Benzodiazepines are relatively safe drugs that potentiate the effects of gamma-aminobutyric acid (GABA), resulting in sedation and anxiolysis.

2) Peak serum levels of most agents occur in 1-3h. Metabolization occurs mostly in the liver.

•Clinical Presentation•
1) Patients present with sedation, confusion, dysarthria, dizziness, and unresponsiveness. Hypotension and respiratory depression can occur.

2) Coma is unusual, and should prompt a search for other etiology.

•Evaluation•
Check electrolytes, glucose, BUN/Cr, ECG, and toxicology screen.

•Treatment•
1) Establish IV access. Place patient on monitor. Administer oxygen.

Assess and stabilize the airway. If altered mental status, check glucose and consider administering naloxone.

2) Administer activated charcoal 1 gm/kg.

3) Consider flumazenil 0.1-0.2 mg IV q 1 min (max 3 gm in 1 h). Flumazenil is a selective competitive antagonist of the GABA receptor. Flumazenil may result in status epilepticus, especially if underlying seizure disorder, chronic benzodiazepine use, or co-ingestion of tricyclic antidepressants. Consider flumazenil only if the patient is unresponsive and there is no history of chronic use or seizure disorder.

•Disposition•

If the overdose is not severe, the patient may be discharged if symptoms have resolved after a 4h observation.

VI. BETA BLOCKERS

•General•

1) Beta-adrenergic receptors are classified as beta-1 or beta-2 receptors. Beta-1 receptor stimulation increases conduction through the AV node, and increases the force and rate of myocardial contraction. Beta-2 receptor stimulation dilates the smooth muscles in vessel walls, bronchi, and the GI and GU tracts.

2) Beta blockade inhibits the effects of catecholamines, thereby decreasing heart rate, blood pressure, and myocardial contractility. Beta blockade also results in bronchial constriction and the inhibition of glycogenolysis.

3) Different beta blockers have different affinities for beta-1 and beta-2 receptors. Nonselective beta blockers (especially propranolol) are the most toxic.

•Clinical Presentation•

1) Patients present with bradycardia, A-V block, and hypotension. Hypoglycemia and bronchospasm may occur. Tachycardia may occur with sotalol, pindolol, or practolol. Most patients develop symptoms within 1-2h of ingestion.

2) Seizures may occur (usually with propranolol).

•Evaluation•

1) Check ECG, glucose, electrolytes, BUN/Cr, and toxicology screen.
2) Consider cardiac enzymes if hemodynamically unstable. Consider CXR to evaluate for possible pulmonary edema.

Treatment•

1) Establish IV access. Place patient on monitor. Administer oxygen. Assess and stabilize the airway. If altered mental status, check glucose and consider administering naloxone.
2) Administer activated charcoal 1 gm/kg. Consider gastric lavage.
3) If hypotensive, administer IVNS 20-30 cc/kg.
*If persistent hypotension or bradycardia, consider:
4) Atropine 1 mg IV.
5) Glucagon 5 mg IV, then infusion, as glucagon has a half-life of 10 minutes.
6) Pacemaker.
7) Epinephrine infusion 2-100 ug/min.
8) Calcium chloride 5-10 ml IV.
9) Additional vasopressors (dobutamine).
10) Some agents (atenolol, nadolol) are reported to be dialyzable.
11) Consider amrinone 0.75 mg/kg, then infusion of 5 mcg/kg/min.
12) Consider admission to ICU.

VII. CALCIUM CHANNEL BLOCKERS

•Pathophysiology•

1) Calcium channel blockade results in vasodilation, decreased A-V node conduction, decreased S-A node discharge, and decreased cardiac contractility.
2) Sustained-release preparations may cause symptoms more than 15h after exposure.

•Clinical Presentation•

Patients present with bradycardia, A-V nodal block, hypotension, and mental status changes.

•Evaluation•

1) Check ECG, glucose, electrolytes, BUN/Cr, and toxicology screen.
2) Consider cardiac enzymes if hemodynamically unstable. Consider CXR to evaluate for possible pulmonary edema.

•Treatment•

1) Establish IV access. Place patient on monitor. Administer oxygen. Assess and stabilize the airway. If altered mental status, check glucose and consider administering naloxone.

2) Administer activated charcoal 1 gm/kg. Consider gastric lavage.

3) If hypotensive, administer IVNS 20-30 cc/kg.

*If persistent hypotension or bradycardia, consider:

4) Calcium chloride 1-4 g (5-10 ml) IV; may repeat.

5) Glucagon 5 mg IV, then infusion, as glucagon has a half-life of 10 minutes.

6) Epinephrine infusion 2-100 ug/min; or norepinephrine infusion.

7) Dopamine infusion 5-10 mcg/kg/min.

8) Consider atropine 1 mg) although heart block secondary to calcium channel blockade is usually unresponsive to atropine.

9) Consider pacemaker.

10) If refractory hypotension, some studies suggest that insulin/glucose infusions may improve cardiac output.

11) Consider admission to ICU.

VIII.   CARBON MONOXIDE (CO)

•Pathophysiology•

1) Toxicity primarily results from cellular hypoxia, and is determined (in part) by the percent of hemoglobin bound to CO. Toxicity can be classified as minimal (<15% COHgb); moderate (15-39% COHgb); or severe (40-60% COHgb); however, a single COHgb level does not always correlate well with clinical signs.

2) CO binds to Hgb with a 250-fold greater affinity than oxygen, reducing oxygen-carrying capacity and shifting the dissociation curve to the left (thereby decreasing the availability of oxygen). CO also inhibits cytochrome oxidase and causes brain lipid peroxidation.

3) The half-life of CO at room air is 250 minutes, at 100% oxygen it is 45 minutes, and at 2 atm, it is 27 minutes.

•Clinical Presentation•

1) Patients present with headache, dizziness, nausea and vomiting, malaise, lethargy, confusion, seizure, coma, and cherry red skin (one clue to the diagnosis is that others in the same dwelling often present with similar symptoms).

2) CO toxicity may result from fires, auto exhaust systems, stoves, portable heaters, and methylene chloride.

•Evaluation•

1) Check pulse oximetry, ABG, ECG, CBC, electrolytes, glucose, toxicology screen, and CXR; consider CPK and head CT (if persistent mental status changes).

2) Pulse oximetry may be falsely elevated in CO poisoning, as COHgb may be interpreted as oxygenated Hgb, thus overestimating Hgb saturation (pulse oximeters can only detect oxygenated and deoxygenated Hgb, and not any other dyshemoglobins).

3) Co-oximeters can detect methemoglobin and carboxyhemoglobin. The pO_2 of a non-co-oximeter ABG is not useful as it measures dissolved oxygen (which may remain normal) and then calculates saturation; it assumes the absence of dyshemoglobins (only a co-oximeter directly measures the oxygen saturation and the concentration of different forms of Hgb). If there is a saturation gap (a difference between the calculated saturation and the co-oximeter determined saturation), it indicates that a dyshemoglobin is present. Venous and arterial COHgb levels are equivalent.

•Treatment•

1) Establish IV access. Place patient on monitor. Administer 100% oxygen. Assess and stabilize the airway. If altered mental status, check glucose and consider administering naloxone.

2) Consider hyperbaric oxygen (HBO); call 919-684-8111 or www.diversalertnetwork.org for the nearest HBO facility. HBO dissolves enough oxygen in the blood to meet metabolic needs, even in the absence of a normal Hgb. Universal criteria for HBO have not been established. However, consider HBO if COHgb levels >20-30%. Other criteria for HBO (regardless of COHgb level) include coma, comorbid disease, persistent symptoms, focal neurological deficits, severe metabolic acidosis, any syncope, age >60 years, end-organ dysfunction (i.e., ischemic ECG changes), or if pregnant. If pregnant, consider HBO if CO level is 10-20%, as the fetus concentrates CO and CO has a longer half-life in the fetus (CO is also a teratogen in the second and third trimesters); treat 5 times longer than the time

needed to treat the mother alone. Blood CO levels may not correlate with long-term clinical effects; residual CNS effects are lessened with hyperbaric oxygen.

3) Treat acidosis with oxygen and improvement of hemodynamics; administering HCO3 will worsen the left shift of the oxygen dissociation curve.

IX. CAUSTIC INGESTIONS

•General•
1) Acids cause coagulation necrosis and superficial burns. Substances include HCl, HSO4, and HF (e.g. toilet bowl/drain cleaners and battery acids).
2) Alkali cause liquefaction necrosis and deep burns. Substances include lye, button batteries, and oven/drain cleaners (e.g. Drano, Liquid Plumber, and Easy Off).

•Clinical Presentation•
Patients may present with dysphagia, glottic edema, abdominal pain (gastric perforation), stridor, dyspnea, or bleeding.

•Evaluation•
1) Examine the oropharynx, lungs, and abdomen. Check for ocular or cutaneous burns. The initial physical exam may be unremarkable; 10-30% of patients with esophageal burns have no oropharyngeal lesions.
2) Check the pH of the ingested material, if available.
3) Consider checking CBC, electrolytes, BUN/Cr, and ABG. Consider upright CXR to rule out perforation. Acids may cause electrolyte abnormalities and metabolic acidosis.
4) Consider endoscopy.

•Treatment•
1) **Soaps/Detergents**- observe.
2) **Bleaches**- if <5% concentration, observe; if >5% concentration, treat as a corrosive ingestion.
3) **Acids/Alkalis**
   a) Establish IV access. Place patient on monitor. Administer 100% oxygen. Assess and stabilize the airway. If altered mental status,

check glucose and consider administering naloxone.

b) All patients require an endoscopy, urgently if dysphagia, drooling, or burns.

c) Induced emesis is contraindicated.

d) If ingestion of solid alkali occurred within 30 minutes of presentation, consider dilution with water or milk (250cc in adults, 3-5 cc/kg in children). Use caution, as dilution will increase the volume of gastric contents, which will increase the risk of vomiting. Avoid dilution if ingestion of liquid alkali (tissue injury is already done). Acids should not be diluted with water because of increased heat production. Neutralization with a weak acid or alkali is contraindicated because of excessive heat production.

e) Consider lavaging acid ingestions. Do not place NG tube if alkaline injury (to avoid perforation).

f) Do not administer activated charcoal (it does not adsorb caustic ingestions and obscures the endoscopy).

g) Steroids and antibiotics are not helpful in 1st degree and 3rd degree burns (no 1st degree burns and all 3rd degree burns develop strictures regardless of treatment); they are controversial in second-degree burns (give both or none).

h) Administer H-2 blockers to reduce the exposure of the esophagus to gastric contents.

X. CHOLINERGICS

•General•

1) The principal agents are pesticides, most of which are either organophosphates or carbamate compounds. Pesticides can be absorbed through the lungs, skin, and GI tract; symptoms usually occur within several hours of exposure.

2) Organophosphates irreversibly bind to acetylcholinesterase, which allows acetylcholine to accumulate in the synapse; this initially produces overstimulation from acetylcholine excess, followed by eventual exhaustion of the cholinergic system. Involvement of the autonomic ganglia and neuromuscular junction produces nicotinic effects, while involvement of the post-ganglionic parasympathetic synapses produces muscarinic effects.

3) Carbamates have a less severe toxicity (they have poor penetration of the CNS), and produce a reversible inhibition of acetylcholinesterase that lasts 6h.

•Clinical Presentation•

1) Muscarinic manifestations include salivation, lacrimation, urination, diaphoresis, miosis, GI upset, and bradycardia.
2) Nicotinic manifestations include fasciculations, weakness, and paralysis.
3) Altered mental status occurs in severe poisoning.

•Evaluation•

Check blood for RBC cholinesterase level (it should be depressed). Check ECG, CBC, electrolytes, BUN/Cr, glucose, and toxicology screen. Consider CXR.

•Treatment•

1) Using proper equipment and precautions, decontaminate the patient by removing clothing and irrigating exposed skin.
2) Establish IV access. Place patient on monitor. Administer oxygen. Assess and stabilize the airway. If altered mental status, check glucose and consider administering naloxone.
3) Consider gastric lavage and activated charcoal 1 gm/kg if acute ingestion.
4) Atropine 2-10 mg IV (children 0.2 mg/kg, minimum 0.1 mg) treats the muscarinic effects. Administration of >100 mg may be necessary; titrate to the clearing of secretions, not the heart rate or pupil size.
5) Pralidoxime (2-PAM) 1-2 gm IV, then 500 mg/h IV (the initial dose in children is 25-50 mg/kg IV) is a specific antidote for organophosphates (it reactivates acetylcholinesterase). Pralidoxime should be given if there is any muscle weakness; it is generally not needed for carbamate poisoning. Pralidoxime is most effective if given early.
6) Administer benzodiazepines for seizures.
7) Consider nebulized ipratropium 0.5 mg to dry secretions.
8) Significant exposures should be admitted to the ICU.

XI. COCAINE

•General•

1) Cocaine inhibits nerve conduction by blocking sodium channels; it also increases the release of presynaptic norepinephrine and blocks the reuptake of catecholamines and serotonin.

2) IV and inhaled cocaine has a half-life of 40-60 minutes; nasal and oral cocaine has a half-life of 60-90 minutes.

•Clinical Presentation•

1) Cocaine use results in sympathomimetic symptoms, including agitation, combativeness, hyperpyrexia, hypertension, tachycardia, seizures and, in contrast to anticholinergics, diaphoresis. Symptoms dissipate in 1-2h.

2) Crack cocaine has particulates that may cause significant pulmonary injury.

3) Cocaine, even hours to days after use, may cause ischemia of bowel, kidney, or brain.

4) <u>Cocaine Chest Pain</u>- Chronic use causes accelerated atherogenesis and thrombotic plaques; also, the sympathomimetic effects of cocaine may result in MI if there is underlying coronary disease. Consider cocaine use a strong risk factor in the decision to monitor a patient.

5) <u>Washed out syndrome</u>- Chronic binges may deplete norepinephrine and cause a profound depression in the level of consciousness; it is a diagnosis of exclusion. Consider admission to ICU for supportive care.

•Evaluation•

1) Check EGG; consider toxicology screen. Consider checking for rhabdomyolysis with CPK and urine dipstick (which would be positive for blood without hematuria).

2) If seizure, obtain head CT, as patients may have intracranial infarctions or hemorrhages.

3) If chest pain or dyspnea, consider CK-MB and CXR (especially if cocaine was inhaled). Cocaine users have common ECG variants that mimic MI (early repolarization). Ischemia has been reported hours to days after cocaine use and in the absence of acute toxicity. Consider echocardiogram or cardiac catheterization.

4) The cocaine metabolite may persist up to 3 weeks in chronic users and 24-72h after acute use.

•Treatment•

1) Establish IV access. Place patient on monitor. Administer oxygen. Assess and stabilize the airway. If altered mental status, check glucose and consider administering naloxone.

2) Administer benzodiazepines for sedation. Administer IV fluids to maintain urine output. Treat any hyperpyrexia.

3) If arrhythmia:

<u>SVT</u>: Administer oxygen and escalating doses of benzodiazepines.

<u>Stable Ventricular Tachycardia/Wide Complex Tachycardia</u>: Administer oxygen, HCO3 1-2 mEq/kg, and diazepam (Valium) 5-10 mg. If arrhythmia persists, consider lidocaine 1.0-1.5 mg/kg.

<u>Ventricular Fibrillation/Unstable Ventricular Tachycardia</u>: Use the standard ACLS protocols; limit epinephrine to 1 mg every 5-10 min. Avoid repeated lidocaine. Consider bretylium.

4) If severe hypertension:

Consider nitroprusside or phentolamine for uncontrolled hypertension; beta-blockers may lead to unopposed alpha stimulation and hypertension.

5) If chest pain:

Aspirin and nitroglycerin should be administered; beta-blockers should be avoided. If persistent pain accompanied by ST-segment deviation, consider verapamil, diltiazem or phentolamine. If persistent ST-segment elevation despite treatment, consider coronary arteriography. Use fibrinolytic therapy with caution, as these patients likely had multiple episodes of uncontrolled hypertension; also, many cocaine-related MIs may be due to spasm and not thrombus. Therefore, consider coronary arteriography before administering thrombolytics.

XII. CYANIDE

•General•

1) Cyanide causes cellular hypoxia by binding to iron on mitochondrial cytochrome oxidase and inhibiting aerobic metabolism. Cellular hypoxia leads to metabolic acidosis.

2) Cyanide is used in the extraction of gold and silver from mineral, and to recover silver from photographic materials. It is also used in the production of plastics, pigments, and dyes. Combustion of plastics, polyurethane, wool, silk, nylon, rubber and paper products can lead

to the production of cyanide gas.

•Clinical Presentation•

1) Patients may present with anxiety, dizziness, or headache, progressing to seizure and coma; there is usually no cyanosis unless respiratory arrest occurs. The patient may have a bitter almond odor. Patients may develop cherry red skin.

2) Consider cyanide poisoning in the comatose, bradycardic, acidotic patient without hypoxia on ABG or clinical cyanosis.

•Evaluation•

1) Check ABG, lactic acid, glucose, electrolytes, BUN/Cr, CBC, toxicology screen, and ECG.

2) There is no rapid cyanide test. Cyanine poisoning is suggested by a persistent metabolic acidosis with an anion gap. Also, suspect cyanide poisoning in patients with respiratory distress but normal pO2 (cyanide prevents the use of oxygen by the tissues).

•Treatment•

1) Establish IV access. Place patient on monitor. Administer oxygen. Assess and stabilize the airway. If altered mental status, check glucose and consider administering naloxone.

2) If the diagnosis is suspected clinically, administer the Cyanide Antidote Kit immediately. Place amyl nitrate 0.3 cc over the nose for 15 seconds, and then off for 15 seconds until IV access is established. Then, administer sodium nitrite 300 mg IV (adjust for anemia and children); the pediatric dose is 0.2 cc/kg. This produces a methemoglobinemia that combines with cyanide to form cyanomethemoglobin. Then give sodium thiosulfate 12.5 g IV (children 412.5 mg/kg) to form thiocyanate, which is excreted in the urine.

3) Consider activated charcoal 1 gm/kg if co-ingestion is suspected (charcoal does not adsorb cyanide). Consider gastric lavage.

4) If hypotensive, administer IVNS bolus.

5) If hemodynamically unstable or pH < 7, administer HCO3.

6) If persistent hypotension, consider vasopressors.

7) If no response to antidote, consider hyberbaric oxygen.

8) In smoke inhalation patients with possible cyanide poisoning, or for empiric treatment, sodium thiosulfate alone avoids the hypotensive

and methemoglobin effects of nitrates (the induction of methemoglobinemia is contraindicated in smoke inhalation patients who already
have carboxyhemoglobinemia).

9) Hydroxocobalamin 5 gm is an alternative to treatment with the Cyanide Antidote Kit. It forms cyanocobalamin, and is a treatment used
in Europe.

10) Never treat asymptomatic patients.

XIII. DIGOXIN

•General•

1) Digoxin inhibits Na-K ATPase, causing an increase in calcium in the
sarcoplasm, which increases contractility.

2) Digoxin also increases extracellular potassium, depresses conduction
through the A-V node, and increases atrial conduction, ectopic im-
pulses and vagal tone.

•Clinical Presentation•

1) Patients may present with anorexia, nausea and vomiting, diarrhea,
syncope, visual disturbances, headache, confusion, agitation, and psychosis. Patients may present with hemodynamic instability.

2) Toxicity may not develop for several hours after ingestion.

•Evaluation•

1) Check ECG, digoxin level, electrolytes, and BUN/Cr. In acute
ingestions, toxicity may not correlate with digoxin levels. Repeat the
digoxin levels in 2-4h to guide therapy.

2) Quinidine, verapamil, and amiodarone reduce the elimination of
digoxin; omeprazole, clarithromycin, erythromycin and tetracycline
increase the GI absorption of digoxin.

ECG

1) Digoxin toxicity has many potential ECG manifestations: PACs, PVCs,
ventricular bigeminy or trigeminy, ventricular tachycardia, accelerated junctional rhythm, PAT with 2:1 block, high levels of A-V block,
bi-directional ventricular tachycardia, slow atrial fibrillation, and regular atrial fibrillation (fibrillation with complete heart block and junctional rhythm).

2) Atrial fibrillation with rapid ventricular response is virtually never associated with digoxin toxicity.

3) Although no ECG is diagnostic, slow rhythms with impaired conduction in combination with increased automaticity of ectopic foci suggest digoxin toxicity.

•Treatment•

1) Establish IV access. Place patient on monitor. Administer oxygen. Assess and stabilize the airway. If altered mental status, check glucose and consider administering naloxone.

2) Administer activated charcoal 1 gm/kg. Consider gastric lavage.

3) Electrical cardioversion may precipitate ventricular fibrillation; use only if life threatening, hemodynamically significant arrhythmia (start with 25J).

4) Stable bradydysrhythmias, bigeminy, trigeminy, and SVT may be treated with observation and discontinuation of digoxin.

5) If symptomatic bradycardia or complete heart block, administer atropine; consider Digibind and pacer.

6) If stable ventricular tachycardia, administer Digibind. Also, consider Mg 2 gm IV, then 1-2 gm/h. Consider lidocaine 1 mg/kg, then infusion 1-4 mg/min; consider phenytoin 15 mg/kg, administered in boluses of 100 mg every 5-10 min. (Lidocaine and phenytoin suppress automaticity without depressing the SA node). Avoid procainamide as it depresses A-V node conduction. Cardioversion is relatively contraindicated, as it may precipitate asystole or ventricular fibrillation.

7) If unstable ventricular tachycardia, defibrillate with 25-50J, then 200J, then 300J. Administer Digibind. Administer Mg, lidocaine and phenytoin (as above in stable ventricular tachycardia).

8) Other indications for Digibind include: hemodynamic compromise; life threatening tachyarrhythmias or bradyarrhythmias; hyperkalemia; 6h digoxin level >10-15 ng/L; adult ingestion >10mg; or pediatric ingestion >0.3 mg/kg with serum digoxin level >5.0 ng/L.

9) If acute ingestion, the patient is likely hyperkalemic; treat as other hyperkalemics but avoid administering calcium, as it may enhance cardiac toxicity.

10) If chronic ingestion, the patient is likely hypokalemic and hypomagnesemic; replete both.

XIV. ECSTASY

•General•

1) Ecstasy (MDMA) is a hallucinogenic amphetamine that acts as a central stimulant (by increasing catecholamines at adrenergic receptors), and also has hallucinogenic properties (which may be mediated by serotonin and dopamine). Ecstasy is a designer drug popular at "raves". Ecstasy is also known as Adam, E, and XTC.

2) Ecstasy produces mood alteration (loss of inhibition and increased sensuality) and euphoria. Symptoms begin in 30-60 minutes and peak at 90 minutes; symptoms may persist for 8 hours.

•Clinical Presentation•

1) Patients may present with symptoms of sympathetic stimulation (tachycardia, hypertension, mydriasis, and diaphoresis). Patients may also have hallucinations and other CNS disturbances. Patients may have muscle rigidity (especially jaw-clenching).

2) Patients may present with dehydration, hyponatremia, hyperthermia (possibly mediated by serotonin), arrhythmias, rhabdomyolysis, DIC, or CNS abnormalities. Ecstasy may cause long-term neurotoxicity.

•Evaluation•

Measure core temperature. Consider checking electrolytes, BUN/Cr, glucose, CPK, LFTs, and ECG. Consider head CT if altered mental status or focal neurologic signs.

•Treatment•

1) Establish IV access. Place patient on monitor. Administer oxygen. Assess and stabilize the airway. If altered mental status, check glucose and consider administering naloxone.

2) If acute oral ingestion, administer activated charcoal 1 gm/kg Consider cardiac monitoring. Provide hydration; correct any electrolyte abnormalities.

3) If agitation, treat with benzodiazepines (lorazepam or diazepam).

4) If hypertension, treat initially with benzodiazepines. If there is evidence of end-organ damage, consider phentolamine 1-2 mg IV or nitroprusside. Avoid beta-blockers due to possible unopposed alpha effects.

5) If hyperthermia, treat with the usual cooling measures.

XV. ETHANOL

A. Alcohol Intoxication

•Pathophysiology•
Ethanol is metabolized by alcohol dehydrogenase and slightly by P450 (thus, drugs metabolized by P450 will have low levels in alcoholics secondary to induction of P450 enzymes).

•Evaluation•
1) Check glucose. If the diagnosis is uncertain, check ethanol level; if the ethanol level is inconsistent with the patient's level of alertness, search for an underlying disorder . Consider an evaluation for trauma, infection, and overdose.
2) The majority of alcoholics have an elevated MCV and GGT.

•Treatment•
1) Consider D5 normal saline, 1 mg folate, 100 mg thiamine IM/IV, 2 gm Mg (low Mg may cause thiamine resistance), and multivitamin. Administer thiamine before glucose, as glucose may deplete thiamine reserves.
2) Consider hemodialysis if ethanol level >600 mg/dl with severe acidosis, especially in children.

B. Alcohol Withdrawal

•Clinical Presentation•
1) Symptoms typically begin 8-24h after the last drink, and include agitation, tremors, anxiety, nausea and vomiting.
2) At 12-24h, patients have severe tremors, fever, sweating, tachycardia, hypertension, and respiratory alkalosis.
3) At 24-72h, patients may experience delirium tremens (DTs), which presents as confusion, hallucinations, and marked autonomic activity (fever, diaphoresis, and tachycardia). DTs are always accompanied by a profound hyperadrenergic state. Alcoholic hallucinations can occur without DTs

•Evaluation•

Check CBC, electrolytes, BUN/Cr, glucose, Mg, calcium, alcohol level, toxicology screen, and ECG; consider head CT.

•Treatment•

1) Establish IV access. Place patient on monitor. Administer oxygen. Assess and stabilize the airway. If altered mental status, check glucose and consider administering naloxone. Administer D5 normal saline, 1 mg folate, 100 mg thiamine IM/IV, 2 gm Mg (low Mg may cause thiamine resistance), and multivitamin.

2) Treat tremors and the sympathetic response with benzodiazepines: chlordiazepoxide (Librium) 25-100 mg po q6h; lorazepam (Ativan) 1-2 mg IV q3-4h (diazepam is less titratable and has metabolites with longer half-lives); or midazolam (Versed) 2-20 mg/h.

3) Consider phenobarbital 30-120 mg po or IV.

4) Consider clonidine 0.1-0.3 mg po q8h, which achieves a peak concentration in 60-90 minutes (transdermal application takes 2 days). Clonidine does not cause excessive hypotension or respiratory depression.

5) Consider beta-blockers.

6) If delirium tremens are refractory to benzodiazepines, consider intubation with paralytics, and sedation with barbiturates or propofol.

•Disposition•

1) Outpatient benzodiazepines are an unproven treatment. A short supply of benzodiazepines is acceptable if the patient is tremulous; significant withdrawal or abnormal vital signs requires inpatient treatment.

2) Admit patients with delirium tremens to the ICU.

C. Alcohol-related Seizures

•General•

1) Seizures may be the sole or first manifestation of withdrawal. Seizures typically occur 6-48h after a reduction in alcohol use; 30% of patients will manifest further withdrawal symptoms. If the alcohol level is >100 mg/dL, look for another source of the seizure.

2) Seizures are almost always grand mal. 10-20% of patients have ≥2 seizures. Always consider trauma/subdural hematoma. Binge drinkers are also at risk for seizures.

•Evaluation•

1) If first withdrawal seizure, check head CT. If the patient has a history of withdrawal seizures, a normal neurologic exam, and no evidence of trauma, then head CT is probably unnecessary.

2) Consider checking CBC, electrolytes, BUN/Cr, glucose, Mg, calcium, alcohol level, toxicology screen, and ECG.

•Treatment•

1) Establish IV access. Place patient on monitor. Administer oxygen. Assess and stabilize the airway. If altered mental status, check glucose and consider administering naloxone. Administer D5 normal saline, 1 mg folate, 100 mg thiamine IM/IV, 2 gm Mg (low Mg may cause thiamine resistance), and multivitamin.

2) Administer benzodiazepines. There is no role for phenytoin.

•Disposition•

If the evaluation is negative and the patient had only one seizure, consider discharge after a 4-6h observation. Admit if focal seizure or multiple seizures.

D. Alcohol-related Complications

1) **Acute Alcoholic Hepatitis**- Chronic alcohol abuse may result in inflammatory liver damage. Patients may present with nausea and vomiting, right upper quadrant pain, malaise, jaundice, coagulopathy, symptoms of portal hypertension, and possible fever. Labs reveal a moderate increase in the transaminases, with AST > ALT, and an increased bilirubin and WBC. Alcohol abuse usually results in an increased MCV; patients may be anemic, as alcohol is a marrow suppressant. Consider abdominal ultrasound to evaluate for gallbladder disease, biliary obstruction or liver abscess.

2) **Alcoholic Ketoacidosis**- It occurs in chronic alcoholics with poor nutritional intake and recent binge drinking. A decrease in carbohydrate intake depletes glycogen stores, and reduced glycogen and insulin production result in lipolyis and ketoacidosis. Patients experience vomiting and diffuse abdominal pain; this further decreases oral intake, and worsens the ketoacidosis. The intracellular effects of alcohol (excess NADH) and the mobilization of free fatty acids when glucose/glycogen stores are depleted results in an anion gap metabolic acidosis, ketonemia and a

compensatory respiratory alkalosis. Check electrolytes, glucose, and ketones; consider ABG. Alcohol levels are usually low and glucose is usually <400 mg/dL. Treat with D5 normal saline and thiamine; insulin and bicarbonate are generally not indicated.

3) Hypoglycemia- Depleted liver glycogen from malnutrition makes patients dependent on gluconeogenesis, which is inhibited by alcohol (it may not become apparent for 30h after the last ingestion of alcohol); it is clinically rare. Children are at greater risk. Do not administer glucagon (alcohol enhances the insulin response to glucagon). Administer glucose; if persistent hypoglycemia, consider ACTH insufficiency and give steroids.

4) Hypomagnesemia- Hyperlacticacidemia may enhance excretion of Mg; also, decreased oral intake may result in low Mg.

5) Lactic acidosis- It is produced from an altered redox state.

6) Pancreatitis- It may involve stimulation of pancreatic secretions; normal amylase and lipase do not exclude the diagnosis. Abdominal CT may show hemorrhage, abscess, or pseudocysts. Treat with NG tube and narcotics.

7) Wernicke's Encephalopathy- It results from thiamine deficiency. Patients present with confusion, cerebellar ataxia, and oculomotor disturbances. Treat with thiamine; some cases require up to 1000 mg thiamine in the first 12h. Administer Mg, as decreased Mg may cause thiamine resistance.

XVI. ETHYLENE GLYCOL

•General•
1) Ethylene glycol is a component of antifreeze, engine coolants, and hydraulic brake fluids. The lethal dose is 1.4 ml/kg.
2) The metabolites of ethylene glycol (glycolic acid and oxalic acid) are responsible for the toxicity of ethylene glycol.

•Clinical Presentation•
1) Symptoms usually begin 30 minutes to 12h after ingestion and initially may include inebriation and euphoria, followed by CNS depression, encephalopathy, ataxia, seizures, nausea and vomiting. Symptoms may be delayed if the patient also ingested ethanol.
2) Metabolic acidosis may develop with compensatory hyperventilation;

cardiovascular failure may result from metabolic acidosis.

3) Renal failure occurs 24-48h after ingestion, and is secondary to oxalate deposition in the kidney.

•Evaluation•

1) Check ECG, ABG, electrolytes, glucose, BUN/Cr, serum osmolarity, lactate, ketones, and ethylene glycol level (if the patient delays treatment, ethylene glycol levels may be low, but the toxic metabolite concentrations may be high).

2) Ethylene glycol poisoning is characterized by high anion and osmolal gaps (an osmolal gap >10 and a serum ethanol of 0 supports the diagnosis).

3) Check calcium, as it may precipitate, causing hypocalcemia.

4) Urine may fluoresce under the Woods lamp (manufacturers add fluorescein to antifreeze), but there may be false positives. Urine may also show calcium oxalate crystals.

5) Both ethylene glycol and methanol cause a metabolic acidosis and an elevated anion gap. However, the first metabolites are osmotically active but do not cause acidosis; subsequent metabolites cause acidosis. Thus, shortly after ingestion, the patient may have a significantly increased osmolal gap with a normal acid-base status; as the methanol or ethylene glycol is metabolized, the osmolal gap decreases, and the production of toxic acids elevates the anion gap.

•Treatment•

1) Establish IV access. Place patient on monitor. Administer oxygen. Assess and stabilize the airway. If altered mental status, check glucose and consider administering naloxone.

2) Consider gastric lavage if ingestion was within 30-45 min; activated charcoal is not beneficial if only ethylene glycol was ingested.

3) Administer IVNS (initially at a rate of 250-500 cc/h) to enhance the renal clearance of toxins.

4) If acidotic, give bicarbonate (use caution, as it may cause sodium overload and calcium deposition with resultant hypocalcemia).

5) The antidote is fomepizole (Antizol) 15 mg/kg IV over 30 min, which is a competitive inhibitor of alcohol dehydrogenase and blocks the formation of toxic metabolites. Begin treatment immediately if suspi-

cion of ethylene glycol ingestion.

6) If fomepizole is not given, administer ethanol (the loading dose of a 10% solution in dextrose is 7.6 ml/kg, then maintenance dose of 0.83 ml/kg/h if non-alcoholic and 1.96 ml/kg/h if alcoholic; keep ethanol level 100-150 mg/dL); it competes for alcohol dehydrogenase, preventing the conversion of ethylene glycol to its toxic metabolites.

7) Pyridoxine 50-100 mg IV q6h may decrease the production of toxic metabolites; it is a co-factor in ethylene glycol metabolization.

8) Administer thiamine 100 mg IV every 6h; it is a co-factor in ethylene glycol metabolization.

9) Consider dialysis for all confirmed cases (because renal failure is common), especially if level > 25 mg/dL, severe acidosis, or renal failure. (However, one study indicated that patients treated with fomepizole who do not experience metabolic acidosis, elevated creatinine, or worsening clinical status despite treatment may not need dialysis, regardless of ethylene glycol level; unmetabolized ethylene glycol should be eliminated with little potential for toxicity.)

10) Do not give folinic acid.

XVII. GAMMA-HYDROXY BUTYRATE (GHB)

•General•

1) GHB binds to GABA receptors in the brain and causes CNS depression. Clinical effects occur in 5-15 minutes; the half-life is 30 minutes. Elimination occurs through expired carbon dioxide. GHB comes in powder or liquid forms.

2) GHB was originally used as a general anesthetic, but its use was abandoned because of lack of analgesia and a tendency to cause seizure-like activity. It then became popular as a bodybuilding supplement, and as an illicit drug at "raves". It has been implicated as a date rape drug.

•Clinical Presentation•

1) Patients may present with neurologic symptoms ranging from dizziness and ataxia to coma. Coma usually resolves in 3-6h. Respiratory depression and nausea and vomiting may occur. Patients often become violent after stimulation.

2) Bradycardia and hypotension may occur.

•Evaluation•

Check ECG, electrolytes, BUN/Cr, glucose, toxicology screen, and osmolar and anion gap. Consider head CT if the diagnosis is not clear.

•Treatment•

1) Establish IV access. Place patient on monitor. Administer oxygen. Assess and stabilize the airway. If altered mental status, check glucose and consider administering naloxone.
2) If co-ingestion is suspected, consider gastric lavage and activated charcoal 1 gm/kg
3) Consider atropine if symptomatic bradycardia.
4) Treatment is generally supportive; perform intubation if airway protection is necessary.
5) If there is a reliable history of a sole ingestion of GHB, some recommend only supportive care (without intubation) and close observation, even with profound CNS depression.
6) Reversal of GHB with physostigmine is controversial.

•Disposition•

If symptoms resolve completely, and the patient is hemodynamically stable, the patient may be discharged after a 6h observation. Otherwise, admit to a monitored setting.

XVIII. IHHALANTS/OCCUPATIONAL EXPOSURE

A. Inhalants

•General•

1) Toxicity occurs from sniffing, huffing (wetting a rag and placing over mouth) or bagging glue or hydrocarbons.
2) Inhalants may cause a chemical pneumonitis, bronchospasm, pulmonary epithelium destruction, or non-cardiogenic pulmonary edema. Inhalants sensitize the heart to catecholamines; therefore, sudden activity or fright may release catecholamines and induce ventricular fibrillation/ventricular tachycardia. All solvents are simple asphyxiants and cause hypoxia. Many pesticides are combined with hydrocarbon vehicles.

3) The lower the viscosity, the greater the potential toxicity (from aspiration).

4) Substances include benzene (gasoline), toluene (airplane glue, acrylic paint), xylene (solvent), methylene chloride (paint stripper), trichloroethane (typewriter correction fluid), turpentine, nitrites, and acetone (nail polish remover).

Aliphatic hydrocarbons- lighter fluids, fuels, paint thinner, solvents.

Alkyl halides- paint stripper, solvents, spot removers, typewriter correction fluid.

Alkyl nitrites- room odorizers.

Aromatic hydrocarbons- (benzene, toluene)-glue, solvent, paint, shoe polish.

Ethers- solvents.

Ketones- glue, adhesives, solvents.

Nitrous oxide- aerosol propellants.

•Clinical Presentation•

1) Acutely, the patient presents with CNS excitation and euphoria, followed by CNS depression.

2) Patients may also present with respiratory symptoms (coughing, choking, tachypnea, or dyspnea), usually within 30 minutes of inhalation. After inhalation, symptoms usually resolve within 30 minutes, but may last 5-6h. If the patient has mouth burning or coughing, assume aspiration.

3) Toluene can present with peripheral sensorimotor neuropathy, similar to the Guillain-Barre syndrome.

•Evaluation•

Check CXR, pulse oximetry, and ECG; consider electrolytes and ABG. CXR changes manifest in 30 min-24h.

•Treatment•

1) Establish IV access. Place patient on monitor. Administer oxygen. Assess and stabilize the airway. If altered mental status, check glucose and consider administering naloxone.

2) GI decontamination is generally not indicated; however, consider activated charcoal if mixed ingestion (it is not indicated if only solvents were ingested).

3) Treatment is generally supportive. Consider albuterol nebulizer treatment.

4) If cardiac arrest, consider holding epinephrine and adding beta-blockers.

5) CHAMP toxins (camphor, halogenated hydrocarbons, aromatic hydrocarbons, metals, and pesticides) require GI decontamination. The toxicity of aliphatic hydrocarbons is related mostly to aspiration, so GI contamination is not required.

6) Methylene chloride is metabolized to carbon monoxide; consider treatment with hyperbaric oxygen.

•Disposition•

1) Observe all patients for 6h. Discharge is appropriate if the patient is asymptomatic, with a normal CXR and pulse oximetry.

2) Admit if electrolyte or acid-base abnormality, cardiopulmonary dysfunction, seizure, persistent mental status changes, or if ingestion of aliphatics and symptomatic on arrival.

B. Occupational Exposure

•General•

Simple asphyxiants- argon, CO2, ethane, helium, hydrogen, methane, nitrogen. These substances are inert.

Chemical asphyxiants- CO, HCN, hydrogen sulfide, methylene chloride. These substances interfere with oxygen delivery to tissues.

Pulmonary irritants- NH3, Cl, HCL, HF, NO2, SO2, and phosgene. These substances cause direct cellular injury.

•Evaluation•

1) Check pulse oximetry and CXR. Consider ABG with co-oximeter (for metHgb and carboxyHgb).

2) Check for corneal involvement.

•Treatment•

1) Administer oxygen and albuterol nebulizer treatments.

2) If exposure to chemical asphyxiants or pulmonary irritants, monitor the patient. Hydrogen sulfide toxicity is treated with IV sodium sulfate, which creates a methemoglobinemia.

XIX. IRON

•General•
1) Iron may be found in iron tablets, vitamins, and prenatal vitamins.
2) Iron ingestion may result in direct corrosive effects on the GI mucosa, and also cellular toxicity (impaired oxidative phosphorylation and mitochondrial dysfunction).
3) The lethal dose is 200-300 mg/kg. Generally, <20 mg/kg is nontoxic; >60 mg/kg is highly toxic.

•Clinical Presentation•
1st stage: direct corrosive insult to the mucosa. Patients present within 6h of ingestion with nausea and vomiting, explosive bloody diarrhea, abdominal pain, and upper GI bleeding. If there are no GI symptoms within 6h, it is probably not a serious ingestion.
2nd stage: a quiescent phase (in which the patient appears to improve and recover) may begin 3-4h after ingestion and last 48h. Metabolic abnormalities may occur at this time.
3rd stage: 12-48h after ingestion, the patient may have a worsening upper GI bleed, lethargy or coma, cardiovascular collapse, severe metabolic acidosis (from impaired oxidative phosphorylation), liver damage, and heart failure.
4th stage: gastric scarring/outlet obstruction and small bowel obstruction.

•Evaluation•
1) Check CBC, electrolytes, glucose, BUN/Cr, ABG, PT/PTT, and LFTs. Check abdominal film for concretions (although 50% of children with large ingestions have a negative film).
2) Check serum iron levels every 2h x 4; a level >500 ug/dl is definitely toxic; levels >300 ug/dl are usually toxic.
3) Total iron binding capacity (TIBC) > serum iron concentration (SIC) is not a valid indicator of toxicity (it had been thought that if TIBC > SIC, then all iron is bound to transferrin and not available to cause toxicity).

•Treatment•
1) Establish IV access. Place patient on monitor. Administer oxygen. Assess and stabilize the airway. If altered mental status, check glucose and consider administering naloxone.

2) Consider gastric lavage and whole bowel irrigation. Activated charcoal is not effective if only iron was ingested. Administer IV fluids.

3) Consider chelation with deferoxamine. If unstable hemodynamics, first hydrate the patient and then administer deferoxamine 15 mg/kg/h IV infusion; it may cause hypotension. If the patient is stable, administer deferoxamine 90 mg/kg (up to 1 gm in children and 2 gm in adults) IM q4-8h. Deferoxamine combines with free iron to form ferrioxamine, which is excreted in the urine and turns the urine orange-red. If the urine does not turn color (which may take 4-6h), it indicates there is no free iron in the serum, and repeat doses of deferoxamine are unnecessary (however, do not stop treatment if the patient is severely ill).

•Disposition•

1) Admit and monitor if significant ingestion, if symptomatic, or if patient becomes symptomatic during a 6h ED observation.

2) If unknown amount of ingestion, and negative abdominal film, serum iron level < 300 ug/dl at 4 hours post-ingestion, no anion gap acidosis, and asymptomatic after a 6h observation, then the patient may be discharged.

XX. ISOPROPYL ALCOHOL

•General•

1) It is found in rubbing alcohol and solvents; it is twice as potent as ethanol.

2) The toxic dose of 70% isopropanol is 1 ml/kg; the lethal dose is 2-4 ml/kg.

•Clinical Presentation•

1) Patients present with abdominal pain, nausea and vomiting, headache, CNS depression, ataxia, and acetone on their breath.

2) The onset of symptoms is 30-60 minutes, with a peak in 2-3h.

•Evaluation•

1) Check glucose, electrolytes, BUN/Cr, isopropanol level, toxicology screen, and serum osmolarity; consider ABG.

2) Isopropyl alcohol is metabolized to acetone, which is a ketone, but not a ketoacid. Therefore, isopropyl alcohol produces an osmolar gap

without metabolic acidosis (or minimal acidosis) and patients will have a normal anion gap and pH. Ketonuria and ketonemia (without elevated glucose or glycosuria) may develop.

•Treatment•

1) Establish IV access. Place patient on monitor. Administer oxygen. Assess and stabilize the airway. If altered mental status, check glucose and consider administering naloxone.

2) Treatment is supportive. Consider gastric lavage if the patient presents <2h after ingestion; activated charcoal is not effective if only isopropyl alcohol was ingested. Consider administering IVNS, thiamine, and glucose.

3) Consider dialysis if signs of hypoperfusion or worsening clinical status.

XXI. LEAD

•General•

1) Lead is the most common cause of chronic heavy metal poisoning; it remains an important environmental illness affecting children. Lead affects virtually all organ systems, and can have serious detrimental affects on the developing brain. Lead interferes with enzymatic activity by combining with sulfhydryl groups in proteins.

2) Lead can be found in lead-based paint or gasoline, soldering materials, lead bullets, and glassmaking materials.

•Clinical Presentation•

Lead toxicity mainly affects children, who may present with irritability, abdominal pain, lethargy, headaches, or encephalopathy. GI symptoms are more common with acute ingestions. Patients may be asymptomatic.

•Evaluation•

1) Check whole blood levels, CBC, electrolytes, BUN/Cr, LFTs, and uric acid.

2) Lead levels > 10 mcg/dL are considered toxic.

3) Patients may have a normocytic or microcytic anemia, and may have evidence of hemolysis. The reticulocyte count may be elevated. The peripheral smear may show basophilic stippling of the RBCs (which

is not universal, and is not specific for lead poisoning).

4) Obtain abdominal x-rays in children (which may demonstrate radiopaque foreign bodies in the GI tract). X-rays of long bones may demonstrate horizontal lead bands. Consider head CT if mental status changes.

5) On exam, the patient may have lead lines on gingival tissue.

•Treatment•

1) If the patient is asymptomatic with blood levels below 60 mcg/dL, and there is no persistent exposure to lead, consider outpatient chelation. Asymptomatic children with lead levels > 45 mcg/dL should receive chelation; levels between 20-44 mcg/dL may require chelation.

2) If the patient is severely symptomatic, establish IV access and administer normal saline. If abdominal films demonstrate radiopaque flecks, perform GI irrigation with polyethylene glycol. Begin chelation. Treat seizures with benzodiazepines and phenobarbital.

3) Chelating agents bind to lead and facilitate its excretion. Parenteral chelating agents include Dimercaprol (BAL) 3-5 mg/kg IM q 4h and EDTA (calcium disodium edetate) 50-75 mg/kg/d IM/IV. Oral chelators include D-penicillamine 25-35 mg/kg po, and succimer (DMSA) 10 mg/kg po q 8h for days 1-5, then 10 mg/kg po q 12h for days 6-14.

XXII. LITHIUM

•General•

1) Lithium toxicity primarily affects the CNS, but may also cause GI, renal, and cardiac dysfunction. There is a higher risk for toxicity if the patient has diabetes, chronic renal failure or hypertension.

2) Peak levels occur 2-4h after ingestion. Lithium clearance is mostly through the kidneys.

•Clinical Presentation•

Initial symptoms include nausea, vomiting, and mild CNS dysfunction; this is followed by confusion, dysarthria, ataxia, extrapyramidal signs, seizure and coma. Clinical assessment (more than serum levels) indicates toxicity.

•Evaluation•

1) Check lithium level, ECG, glucose, electrolytes, toxicology screen, and BUN/Cr.
2) Check repeat lithium levels to document a trend. Toxicity is rare if level <1.5 mEq/L; levels >4 mEq/L are life threatening.

•Treatment•

1) Establish IV access. Place patient on monitor. Administer oxygen. Assess and stabilize the airway. If altered mental status, check glucose and consider administering naloxone.
2) Consider gastric lavage, especially within 1h of ingestion; activated charcoal is indicated only if a coingestion is suspected. Consider whole bowel irrigation, especially if ingestion of sustained-release lithium.
3) Hydrate with normal saline to correct any sodium and fluid deficits (which are common in lithium toxicity). Diuretics have no role in the treatment of lithium toxicity.
4) Dialysis may be indicated if there is preexisting renal insufficiency or failure; level >4.0 mEq/L in chronic ingestion or >6-8 mEq/L in an acute ingestion (even if asymptomatic); or level >2.5 mEq/L and serious CNS or cardiovascular symptoms. Large saline diuresis is almost as effective as dialysis.
5) Admit and monitor if significant ingestion.

XXIII. METHANOL

•General•

1) Methanol is added as a solvent to windshield fluid, antifreeze, and paint removers. The lethal dose is 1-2 cc/kg. The half-life of methanol is 14-20h, which increases to 24-30h with severe toxicity; ethanol prolongs the half-life.
2) Methanol is metabolized (mostly in the liver) to formaldehyde and then to the toxic formic acid. Formic acid is the primary toxin and accounts for most of the metabolic acidosis, anion gap, and ocular toxicity (it causes swelling of axons in the optic disc).

•Clinical Presentation•

1) Unless large amounts are ingested, there is an asymptomatic 18-24h latent period (methanol must first be metabolized to its toxins).
2) Then, patients have symptoms of headache, lethargy, vertigo, nausea

and vomiting, cloudy vision, and abdominal pain. This is followed by a metabolic acidosis and CNS depression.

•Evaluation•

1) Check ABG, ECG, electrolytes, glucose, BUN/Cr, serum osmolarity, toxicology screen, and methanol level.

2) Methanol produces high anion gap and osmolal gaps.

3) Both ethylene glycol and methanol cause a metabolic acidosis and an elevated anion gap. However, the first metabolites are osmotically active but do not cause acidosis; subsequent metabolites cause acidosis. Thus, shortly after ingestion, the patient may have a significantly increased osmolal gap with a normal acid-base status; as the methanol or ethylene glycol is metabolized, the osmolal gap decreases, and the production of toxic acids elevates the anion gap.

•Treatment•

1) Establish IV access. Place patient on monitor. Administer oxygen. Assess and stabilize the airway. If altered mental status, check glucose and consider administering naloxone.

2) Consider gastric lavage if ingestion was within 30-45 minutes of presentation; activated charcoal is not beneficial if only methanol was ingested.

3) If acidotic, give bicarbonate (use caution, as it may cause sodium overload and calcium deposition with resultant hypocalcemia).

4) The antidote is fomepizole (Antizol) 15 mg/kg IV over 30 min, which is a competitive inhibitor of alcohol dehydrogenase and blocks the formation of toxic metabolites. Begin treatment immediately if suspicion of methanol ingestion.

5) If fomepizole is not given, administer ethanol (the loading dose of a 10% solution in dextrose is 7.6 ml/kg, then maintenance dose of 0.83 ml/kg/h if non-alcoholic and 1.96 ml/kg/h if alcoholic; keep ethanol level 100-150 mg/dL); it competes for alcohol dehydrogenase, preventing the conversion of methanol to its toxic metabolites.

6) Folinic acid 1 mg/kg IV every 4h x 24h helps convert formate to H_2O and CO2.

7) Consider hemodialysis if anion gap >30, visual disturbances, level >25-50 mg/dl (the exact level is controversial), severe acidosis, renal insufficiency, or ingestion >40 ml (hemoperfusion is not recommended

as there is rapid saturation of the charcoal).

8) Administer thiamine 100 mg every 6h.

XXIV.   METHEMOGLOBINEMIA

•General•

Methemoglobinemia may be congenital or acquired (from nitrates, lidocaine and other local anesthetics, or shoe dye). Methemoglobin (metHgb) has iron in an oxidized ferric state and is unable to carry oxygen.

•Clinical Presentation•

1) MetHgb causes clinical cyanosis if levels >10-15%; if levels are 25-45%, symptoms include headache and fatigue; if 55-70%, symptoms include seizure and coma; levels >70% are frequently fatal. Blood with metHgb has a chocolate brown color.

2) Consider methemoglobinemia in cyanotic patients without evidence of cardiac or pulmonary disease and no response to supplemental oxygen.

•Evaluation•

1) Check ABG, ECG, pulse oximetry, and electrolytes. Consider CXR.

2) Check metHgb levels with a co-oximeter ABG. A non co-oximeter ABG will usually demonstrate a normal pO2 and saturation, as an ABG measures dissolved oxygen (which may remain normal) and then calculates saturation; it assumes the absence of dyshemoglobins (only a co-oximeter directly measures the oxygen saturation and the concentration of different forms of Hgb).

3) The pulse oximetry reading is usually low (pulse oximetry does not accurately reflect the level of metHgb; as levels reach 30% and higher, pulse oximetry will not go below 85%). If there is a saturation gap (a difference between the calculated saturation and the co-oximeter de-termined saturation), it indicates that a dyshemoglobin is present.

•Treatment•

1) Establish IV access. Place patient on monitor. Administer 100% oxygen. Assess and stabilize the airway. If altered mental status, check glucose and consider administering naloxone.

2) If symptomatic (change in mental status, ischemic chest pain) or ECG

changes and metHgb level >30%, administer methylene blue 1-2 mg/kg (0.1 mg/kg of a 1% solution) over 5 minutes. Methylene blue reduces methemoglobin to hemoglobin. Avoid methylene blue if the patient has G6PD deficiency, as it may cause severe red cell hemolysis.

3) If treatment fails, consider exchange transfusion and hyperbaric oxygen.

XXV. POISONS/ANTIDOTES

Acetaminophen	N-acetylcysteine
Anticholinergics	Physostigmine 1-2 mg IV
Anticoag- heparin	Protamine 1 mg IV
Anticoag- warfarin	Vitamin K 10 mg s.c., FFP
Benzodiazepines	Flumazenil 0.2 mg IV
Beta-blockers	Glucagon 2-10 mg IV
Botulism	Botulism antitoxin
Ca channel blockers	10% Calcium chloride 1-2 g IV
Carbon Monoxide	Oxygen/hyperbaric O_2
Cholinergics	Atropine 0.5-2 mg IV; Pralidoxime 1-2 g IV
Cyanide	Amyl nitrate, sodium nitrite, sodium thiosulfate
Digoxin	Digibind
Ethylene glycol	Antizol 15 mg/kg IV; ethanol; pyridoxine
Iron	Deferoxamine 90 mg/kg IM
Isoniazid	Pyridoxine 5 g IV
Lead	BAL, EDTA
Methanol	Antizol 15 mg/kg IV; ethanol; folinic acid
Methemoglobin	Methylene blue 1-2 mg/kg IV
Opioids	Naloxone 0.4-2 mg IV/IM/ETT
Salicylates	Sodium bicarbonate, dialysis
Tricyclics	Sodium bicarbonate 1-2 mEq/kg IV

| XXVI. SALICYLATES |

•General•

1) Salicylates stimulate the CNS, causing hyperventilation, decreased pCO_2 and respiratory alkalosis; interference with oxidative phosphorylation produces an anion gap metabolic acidosis and hyperthermia.

2) The toxic dose is 200-300 mg/kg; a potentially lethal dose is 500 mg/kg.

•Clinical Presentation•

Mild- symptoms include tachypnea, tinnitus, nausea and vomiting.

Moderate- symptoms include hyperpnea, hyperthermia, anion gap metabolic acidosis, and CNS and coagulation abnormalities.

Severe- above symptoms plus coma, convulsions, and cardiovascular collapse.

•Evaluation•

1) Check salicylate level, glucose, electrolytes, BUN/Cr, ABG, CPK, toxicology screen, and ECG. Perform a rectal exam for occult blood. Consider LP to rule out meningitis.

2) If an acute ingestion, check salicylate levels every 2h until levels fall. Aspirin has a large, changing volume of distribution, so levels may not be accurate; treat the patient, not the level.

3) Check CXR, as the patient may develop ARDS or pulmonary edema (which usually occurs with chronic poisoning).

4) The ferric chloride test (add 3 drops of 10% ferric chloride to 1 ml of urine, which turns purple if salicylic acid is present) is sensitive, but confirm with blood test.

5) The Dome nomogram may indicate the degree of toxicity, but can only be used with a single acute ingestion of non-enteric coated aspirin.

6) Metabolic acidosis predominates in children, as they have a higher metabolic rate.

•Treatment•

1) Establish IV access. Place patient on monitor. Administer oxygen. Assess and stabilize the airway. If altered mental status, check glucose and consider administering naloxone.

2) Administer activated charcoal 1 gm/kg. Consider gastric lavage.
3) Hydrate with D5 normal saline to keep urine output 2-3 ml/kg/h. Avoid overly aggressive hydration, as it may lead to pulmonary edema.
4) If salicylate level is > 35 mg/dL, or if patient is symptomatic with rising salicylate levels or metabolic acidosis, consider urine alkalinization with 1-2 mEq/kg HCO_3 bolus, then start infusion with HCO_3 2 amps and KCl 20-40 mEq in 1 L D5W at 150-250 cc/h. The target urine pH is 7.5-8. Urinary alkalinization promotes excretion of weakly acidic agents. Avoid HCO_3 in the presence of noncardiogenic pulmonary edema, as it may worsen volume overload.
5) Correct potassium, as hypokalemia inhibits urinary alkalinization.
6) Dialyze if coma, pulmonary edema, severe acidosis, chronic renal failure, or salicylate level of 120 mg/dl in an acute ingestion or 60 mg/dl in a chronic ingestion.
7) Consider beta-blockers if markedly increased heart rate.
8) Treat hyperthermia with cooling measures.

•Disposition•
Admit if salicylate level > 50 mg/dl, severe symptoms, or significant electrolyte or acid-base abnormalities.

XXVII. SEROTONIN SYNDROME

•General•
1) Serotonin syndrome occurs because of an increase in central serotonergic neurotransmission, usually occurring after ingestion of serotonin reuptake inhibitors; it may also be caused by MAOIs (Nardil, Eldepryl). Demerol, amphetamines, cocaine, trazodone, and tricyclic antidepressants also have serotonin reuptake inhibitor properties.
2) Symptoms often occur after an increase in the dose of a serotonergic agent, or after the addition of a second serotonergic agent. If a neuroleptic agent has recently been started or increased, consider the diagnosis of neuromalignant syndrome.

•Clinical Presentation•
1) Patients may present with altered mental status, autonomic dysfunction, fever, hypertension, mydriasis, diaphoresis, neuromuscular abnormalities, myoclonus, hyperreflexia, seizure, and ataxia.

2) Rigidity, if limited to the lower extremities, is a sensitive indicator of serotonin syndrome. Lead-pipe rigidity is more consistent with neuromalignant syndrome.

•Evaluation•

Check CBC, electrolytes, glucose, BUN/Cr, ECG, and toxicology screen. Consider head CT, LP, and infectious evaluation.

•Treatment•

1) Establish IV access. Place patient on monitor. Administer oxygen. Assess and stabilize the airway. If altered mental status, check glucose and consider administering naloxone.

2) Discontinue the inciting medication; treatment is mostly supportive.

3) Treat hyperthermia and rigidity aggressively with cool mist, and, if needed, further anti-hyperthermic measures. Antipyretics are generally ineffective.

4) Consider benzodiazepines.

5) Consider serotonin antagonists: cyproheptadine 4-8 mg (max 32 mg; 12 mg in children); methysergide; or propranolol.

6) Dantrolene may be toxic itself.

XXVIII. SULFONYLUREAS

•General•

1) Sulfonylureas stimulate the secretion of insulin by the pancreas and decrease the hepatic insulin clearance; they may also decrease insulin resistance peripherally. All sulfonylureas have a long duration of action (from 6-24h, except for chlorpropamide, which has a 60h duration).

2) Hepatic disease may result in a prolonged duration of action, as all sulfonylureas undergo hepatic metabolism. Chlorpropamide, glyburide, and glimepiride also undergo renal excretion.

Agents

1st generation: Chlorpropamide (Diabinase); Tolbutamide (Orinase); Acetohexamide (Dymelor); Tolazamide (Tolinase).

2nd generation: Glipizide (Glucatrol); Glyburide (Micronase, Diabeta).

3rd generation: Glimepiride (Amaryl).

•Clinical Presentation•

Patients may present with symptoms of hypoglycemia (diaphoresis, tremulousness, and mental status changes).

•Treatment•

1) Establish IV access and administer glucose (1-2 ampules of D50). Monitor glucose frequently, as glucose administration may stimulate additional insulin release and result in a prolonged rebound hypoglycemia.

2) If hypoglycemia is refractory (usually in massive ingestions or hepatic/renal impairment), some suggest administering octreotide, which suppresses the secretion of insulin and may prevent rebound hypoglycemia. Also, consider diazoxide, which raises blood glucose.

•Disposition•

1) Generally, admit and observe patients, as all agents have a long half-life.

2) Some suggest that if hypoglycemia has not developed within 8h, it may be safe to discharge the patient.

3) In asymptomatic pediatric patients, some recommend checking glucose levels every 1-2h, and allowing the child to eat (no IV glucose). If the glucose remains normal for 8h, then it is safe to discharge the patient; if hypoglycemia develops, the patient should be admitted.

XXIX. THEOPHYLLINE

•General•

1) Theophylline stimulates the CNS and has positive inotropic and chronotropic effects on the heart.

2) Peak levels occur 90-120 minutes after oral ingestion. The half-life is 4-8h. Macrolides, ranitidine, and cimetidine decrease theophylline clearance.

•Clinical Presentation•

Toxic symptoms include nausea and vomiting, abdominal pain, tachydysrhythmias, hypotension, tremors, seizure, lethargy, and coma.

•Evaluation•

1) Check ECG, theophylline level, CBC, glucose, BUN/Cr, electrolytes (hypokalemia develops in 25-50% of patients with acute toxicity), Mg, Ca, phosphate, ABG, and toxicology screen. Check theophylline

levels every 2-4h until levels fall.

2) Toxic symptoms usually appear at levels of 20-25 mg/L, with major toxicity at levels >60 mg/L (chronic toxicity occurs at lower levels).

•Treatment•

1) Establish IV access. Place patient on monitor. Administer oxygen. Assess and stabilize the airway. If altered mental status, check glucose and consider administering naloxone.

2) Consider gastric lavage. Administer multiple doses of activated charcoal (1 g/kg q3-4h); give cathartics with the first dose of charcoal.

3) Consider hemoperfusion or dialysis if intractable seizures, coma, significant cardiovascular complications, acute level >90-100 mg/L, or chronic level >60 mg/L. Hemoperfusion is preferred over dialysis.

4) Administer a beta-blocker (esmolol) for tachydysrhythmias.

5) If seizure, administer benzodiazepines or phenobarbital. Phenytoin is contraindicated.

6) Admit if signs of toxicity or if theophylline level > 25 mg/L.

XXX. TRICYCLIC ANTIDEPRESSANTS

•General•

1) Tricyclic antidepressants (TCAs) stimulate catecholamine release and block reuptake. TCAs have anticholinergic and alpha-adrenergic blocking actions. TCAs have a quinidine-like effect on the myocardium, as TCAs block sodium channels, prolonging depolarization.

2) A 10-15 mg/kg ingestion of TCAs may be potentially lethal, but death has occurred in an adult with a 500 mg ingestion.

•Clinical Presentation•

1) Patients may present with mental status changes, tachycardia, anticholinergic symptoms, or seizures.

2) 15-20% of patients develop hypotension. Patients may quickly decompensate.

•Evaluation•

1) Check ECG, electrolytes, glucose, BUN/Cr, ABG, toxicology screen, and TCA serum levels (although serum levels don't always correlate with toxicity).

2) Early ECG signs of toxicity include tachycardia, increased QT inter-

val, and a prominent R in AVR. These changes are followed by a prolonged PR interval, a widened QRS interval, right axis deviation of the terminal 40 ms of the QRS interval in the limb leads, and a high degree A-V block.

•Treatment•

1) Establish IV access. Place patient on monitor. Administer oxygen. Assess and stabilize the airway. If altered mental status, check glucose and consider administering naloxone.

2) Consider gastric lavage. Administer activated charcoal 1 gm/kg (administer activated charcoal up to several hours after ingestion, as the anticholinergic effects of TCAs inhibit peristalsis).

3) If the patient is unstable (ventricular arrhythmias, seizure, hypotension unresponsive to 0.5-1.0 L normal saline, or QRS interval >100 ms), administer HCO3 1 mEq/kg over 1 min (HCO3 decreases free TCA levels and overrides sodium channel blockade). Start infusion of 2 amps HCO3 in D5W at 150-200 ml/h until the QRS interval is <100 ms, arrhythmias have ceased, and the patient has a normal blood pressure. Check ABG to maintain pH 7.45-7.55. Intermittent boluses may be more effective than an infusion.

4) Administer lidocaine for stable ventricular arrhythmias unresponsive to HCO3. Do not use procainamide, as it is similar to TCAs. Avoid beta-blockers, calcium channel blockers, and quinidine.

5) If persistent hypotension, administer dopamine and, if still persistent, administer norepinephrine.

6) Consider administering Mg.

7) If seizure or agitation, administer benzodiazepines (phenytoin use for seizure may increase the risk of ventricular dysrhythmias). A normal QRS interval does not rule out the potential for seizures.

8) Dialysis and hemoperfusion are not effective, as TCAs are highly protein bound.

9) The value of prophylactic HCO3 with a normal QRS interval is unknown.

•Disposition•

If asymptomatic, normal ECG, normal heart rate, and active bowel sounds 6h after lavage/activated charcoal, the patient may be medically cleared. Otherwise, admit to ICU.

XXXI. WARFARIN (COUMADIN)

•General•

1) Warfarin and other coumarin derivatives inhibit the synthesis of the vitamin K dependent coagulation factors (II, VII, IX, and X), and the anticoagulant proteins C and S.

2) Warfarin is used therapeutically as an anticoagulant, while other coumarin derivatives are used as rodenticides. The superwarfarins (used as rodenticides) are extremely potent, and may cause anticoagulation for months.

•Clinical Presentation•

The patient may be asymptomatic, or may present with occult or gross bleeding.

•Evaluation•

1) Check CBC, PT/PTT, INR, electrolytes, and toxicology screen. Consider type and screen.

2) The PT may become elevated 8-12h after ingestion, but typically is delayed 1-2 days. A normal PT 48-72h after ingestion indicates no significant ingestion.

3) Evaluate for any signs of bleeding.

•Treatment•

1) If there is evidence of significant bleeding, establish IV, place patient on monitor, and resuscitate as needed with IVNS, packed RBCs, and FFP.

2) If acute ingestion, administer activated charcoal 1 gm/kg.

3) If acute ingestion and the INR is elevated, administer vitamin K. Do not administer vitamin K prophylactically.

4) If it is a chronic intoxication, treatment depends on the INR and the underlying reason for the patient's anticoagulation. Generally, an INR < 6 only requires temporary cessation of warfarin use. If INR is greater than 6, consider vitamin K. If the effects of warfarin need to be reversed, and the patient's underlying medical condition necessitates continued anticoagulation, heparin can be given while the effects of warfarin are reversed.

5) Admit if any evidence of bleeding.

CHAPTER 26

TRAUMA

I. ABDOMINAL TRAUMA

A. Blunt Abdominal Injury

•Evaluation•

1) Conduct a systematic primary survey (rapid assessment of airway, breathing, circulation, disability, and expose patient), followed by a more detailed secondary survey. Perform rectal and genitourinary exams. Evaluate for other injuries.

2) Perform serial abdominal exams; document any tenderness. Have a high index of suspicion for serious injury if the patient has lap belt bruises or abrasions. Some patients with splenic or hepatic rupture have no tenderness.

3) Consider obtaining CBC, platelets, type and screen, electrolytes, BUN/Cr, LFTs, urinalysis, toxicology screen, and ABG. There is some controversy regarding the utility of initial labs in the otherwise healthy patient. An elevated amylase on arrival is neither sensitive nor specific for pancreatic injury.

4) Hemodynamically unstable patients should be taken to surgery. Clinical predictors of significant abdominal injury include decreased blood pressure, pelvic ring disruption, base deficit <-6, abdominal wall contusion/abrasion, GCS <12, femoral fracture/hip dislocation, or rib fracture below 6th intercostal space. The decision to obtain a diagnostic study depends on the mechanism of injury, physical exam, hemodynamic stability, and the mental status of the patient. Options include:

a) <u>Bedside ultrasound</u>- It has been shown to be accurate for the rapid identification of free intraperitoneal fluid. Rapid bedside ultrasound has a moderate sensitivity for solid organ injury, and poor sensitivity for hollow viscus injury; it does not evaluate the retroperitoneum or diaphragm.

b) <u>Abdominal CT</u>- CT is the preferred imaging method for stable patients. It is sensitive and specific for retroperitoneal and solid organ injury, but not as sensitive as DPL for small intestine injury; it may miss diaphragmatic injuries. The patient must be hemodynamically stable for transfer to radiology. Generally, oral and IV contrast improve the quality of an abdominal CT (however, some advocate withholding oral contrast because of the time delay and risk of aspiration). Do not delay CT for oral contrast; if the contrast is given as soon as decision for CT is made, enough time usually elapses for gastric emptying (the goal is to opacify the duodenum and jejunum, which are the most often injured parts of the intestines).

c) <u>Diagnostic peritoneal lavage (DPL)</u>. The best indications for DPL include patients who go to surgery for other injuries and cannot have their abdomen evaluated; unstable patients with multisystem injuries and an unreliable abdominal exam; in stab wounds where the superficial fascia has been violated; if there is a suspicion of bowel or diaphragmatic injury and the patient is not going to surgery; and gunshot wounds where peritoneal penetration is highly unlikely. CT better evaluates the retroperitoneum and solid organs. DPL is positive if there is >10 cc aspiration of blood, grossly bloody lavage, >100,000 RBCs, or >500 WBCs. Elevated amylase and alkaline phosphatase in DPL fluid may indicate small bowel injury. All gun shot wound DPLs are positive if >5000-10,000 RBCs. Perform DPL after insertion of a urinary catheter and NG tube. Do an open supraumbilical DPL if there is a previous scar, or pelvic fracture, or the patient is gravid.

5) Obtain necessary radiographs (cervical spine, chest, and pelvis).

•Treatment/Disposition•

1) For all significant trauma, establish at least 2 large bore IVs, monitor the patient, and administer oxygen. Maintain cervical spine precautions. Assess and stabilize the airway. Consult surgery.

2) If hypotension is unresponsive to 2L normal saline (or two boluses of 20 cc/kg), consider blood transfusion.

3) Hemodynamically unstable patients should be taken to surgery. Otherwise, the treatment and disposition depend on the hemodynamic status, the results of the imaging studies, and clinical presentation.

4) Unless contraindicated, an NG tube and urinary catheter should be inserted in all seriously injured patients.

5) Administer tetanus prophylaxis as necessary.

B. Penetrating Abdominal Injury

•Evaluation•

1) Conduct a systematic primary survey (rapid assessment of airway, breathing, circulation, disability, and expose patient), followed by a more detailed secondary survey. Perform rectal and genitourinary exams. Evaluate for other injuries. Obtain necessary radiographs (cervical spine, chest, pelvis).

2) Indications for immediate laparotomy in penetrating abdominal injury include hypotension, gun shot wound through the peritoneal cavity, peritoneal signs, evisceration, free air, or if there is gross blood per NG tube, DPL or rectal. Otherwise, the location of the injury determines the optimal diagnostic evaluation:

   a) Thoracoabdominal injury (defined as below the nipples/scapulae and above the costal margin). Consider DPL (which is positive if >5000-10,000 RBCs), CXR, CT, echocardiogram, and prophylactic chest tube (CT is a poor test for diaphragmatic injury, and is not as sensitive as DPL for GI tract injury).

   b) Back and flank injury (defined as between the tips of the scapulae and iliac crest, posterior to the mid-axillary line). Consider DPL (which is positive if >10,000 RBCs); consider triple-contrast CT.

   c) Anterior abdominal stab wound (defined as from the costal margin to the inguinal ligament, anterior to the mid-axillary line). Consider DPL, which is positive if >100,000 RBCs. In a stab wound, if the patient is stable with no signs of peritoneal violation, then explore for fascial penetration; if there is no fascial penetration, consider observation or discharge with close follow-up. If penetration is documented, consider CT or DPL.

•Treatment/Disposition•

1) For all significant trauma, establish at least 2 large bore IVs, monitor the patient, and administer oxygen. Maintain cervical spine precautions. Assess and stabilize the airway. Consult surgery.

2) If hypotension is unresponsive to 2L normal saline (or two boluses of 20 cc/kg), consider blood transfusion.

3) Hemodynamically unstable patients should be taken to surgery. Otherwise, the treatment and disposition depend on the hemodynamic status, the results of the imaging studies, and clinical presentation.

4) Unless contraindicated, an NG tube and urinary catheter should be inserted in all seriously injured patients.

5) Administer tetanus prophylaxis as necessary.

II. GLASGOW COMA SCALE (GCS)

•General•

GCS is a point system that attempts to quantify the level of consciousness. Patients are assigned points based on their responses in 3 categories: eye opening, best verbal response, and best motor response. The points from each category are then added for the patient's GCS; the lowest possible point total is 3.

Eyes

4- Eyes open spontaneously

3- Eyes open to command

2- Eyes open to pain

1- No response

Best Verbal Response

5- Normal speech

4- Confused speech

3- Inappropriate speech

2- Incomprehensible speech

1- Nothing

Best Motor Response

6- Obeys commands

5- Localizes pain

4- Withdraws from pain

3- Flexure posturing

2- Extensor posturing

1- Nothing

III. HEAD TRAUMA

A. General Head Injury

•Clinical Presentation•

1) A patient with a basilar skull fracture may present with hemotympanum, otorrhea, raccoon's eyes, and Battle's sign (ecchymosis of mastoid).

2) The Cushing response is hypertension and bradycardia secondary to increased intracranial pressure.

3) Cheyne-Stokes breathing is alternating apnea and hyperpnea, and may indicate impending tentorial herniation.

4) Increased intracranial pressure may result in cerebral herniation, compressing cranial nerve III, resulting in a dilated ipsilateral pupil. Bilateral pupillary dilation is more consistent with brainstem injury.

5) If there is an intracranial hematoma, it is ipsilateral to a fixed, dilated pupil in 80-90% of patients, contralateral to hemiparesis in 71%, and under a scalp hematoma in 97%. (5% of the population has anisocoria.)

•Evaluation•

1) Conduct a systematic primary survey (rapid assessment of airway, breathing, circulation, disability, and expose patient), followed by a more detailed secondary survey.

2) Perform a complete neurologic exam, including pupillary response. Determine the patient's Glasgow Coma Scale (GCS). Assess for other injuries (especially cervical spine).

3) Obtain head CT and urgent neurosurgical consult if the patient has a depressed level of consciousness, focal CNS signs, or a palpable depressed skull fracture.

4) Consider head CT if GCS <15, if patient is on anticoagulants, > 60 years old, <2 years old, any loss of consciousness, progressive headache, use of alcohol or drugs, vomiting, seizure, or signs of basilar skull fracture.

5) Consider observation only if patient is asymptomatic or has only mild headache, dizziness, or scalp laceration/contusion.

6) In general, skull films are not recommended. Obtain necessary radiographs (cervical spine, chest, pelvis). Consider checking blood alcohol level.

7) In infants, clinical signs are poor indicators of intracranial injury. Consider imaging all infants with blunt head trauma, especially those

with loss of consciousness, vomiting, drowsiness, abnormal CNS exam, or local scalp findings; one strategy suggests obtaining a head CT on patients with symptoms suggestive of brain injury, and that asymptomatic infants with scalp findings should have skull films, followed by head CT if there is a skull fracture.

•**Treatment**• (if severe head injury)

1) For all significant trauma, establish at least 2 large bore IVs, monitor the patient, and administer oxygen. Maintain cervical spine precautions. Check glucose level; consider administering naloxone and thiamine.

2) If necessary, perform a rapid sequence intubation using etomidate 0.2-0.4 mg/kg IV (which decreases ICP while maintaining mean arterial pressure), midazolam or a decreased dose of thiopental (avoid hypotension) as induction agents. Consider lidocaine 1.5-2.0 mg/kg IV to decrease the gag response; consider fentanyl (50-100 mcg IV) to blunt the sympathetic response to intubation. If paralysis is necessary, consider rocuronium 0.9-1.2 mg/kg IV, which is a nondepolarizing agent with an onset similar to succinylcholine and does not increase ICP; if succinylcholine 1-2 mg/kg IV is administered, first use a defasciculating dose of 0.01 mg/kg IV or a nondepolarizing agent to prevent fasciculations. Keep pCO2 35-40 mm Hg. (In several studies, hyperventilation resulted in increased ischemia and brain injury and worsened outcomes; however, limited hyperventilation is appropriate if there is an acute significant increase in intracranial pressure.)

3) CT scan may dictate the need for emergent surgical intervention (e.g., subdural or epidural hematoma).

4) Consider mannitol 0.25-1.0 gm/kg over 15-30 min, which has a maximal effect within 30-60 min and lasts 90 min-6h. Consider empiric administration of mannitol if there are signs of transtentorial herniation (focal CNS signs, unilateral dilated pupil, or progressive neurologic deterioration). If the patient is stable, mannitol should not be administered without CT scan and neurosurgical consultation. Avoid hypovolemia.

5) Steroids are not indicated.

6) Avoid hypotension and hypoxia; keep patient euvolemic. Keep pa-

tient euglycemic.

7) Elevate the head of the bed to 30 degrees; keep the patient sedated with benzodiazepines.

8) If patient is hypertensive, consider labetalol if SBP >200 mm Hg (avoid nitroprusside and vasodilators, as they will increase cerebral blood flow).

9) If a focal brain lesion is present, load with phenytoin 18 mg/kg.

10) Unless contraindicated, an NG tube and urinary catheter should be inserted in all seriously injured patients.

11) Administer tetanus prophylaxis as necessary.

12) Consult neurosurgery.

B. Concussion

1) Concussion is defined as altered mental status induced by head trauma ± loss of consciousness (grade 1 concussion is confusion lasting <15 minutes without loss of consciousness; grade 2 is confusion lasting >15 minutes without loss of consciousness; grade 3 is loss of consciousness).

2) The post-concussive syndrome may present with headache, dizziness, memory impairment, or nausea and vomiting; it occurs following minor head injury. Perform a complete physical and neurologic exam. It usually resolves spontaneously over hours to days.

C. Epidural Hematoma (EDH)

1) An EDH is a collection of blood in the epidural space, between the dura and the inner table of the skull. It is usually secondary to a skull fracture that tears an artery (most commonly the middle meningeal artery in the temporoparietal region).

2) There is usually no significant underlying brain injury.

3) Patients may be conscious or comatose. Patients may have a palpable bony step-off, a dilated pupil ipsilateral to the hematoma, and contralateral hemiplegia. The patient may have a "lucid interval" between the initial injury and a subsequent decreasing level of consciousness.

4) Head CT may demonstrate a hyperdense extraaxial biconvex or lenticular shaped hemorrhage; it usually does not cross suture lines.

5) Treatment involves surgical evacuation. Consider emergent burr hole if neurosurgery is unavailable and the patient is herniating. In gen-

eral, the burr hole is placed in the area of hemorrhage located by the CT. If a CT has not been obtained, consider placing a burr hole on the side of the dilated pupil 3 cm anterior and 4 cm superior to the tragus of the ear.

D. Subdural Hematoma (SDH)

1) A SDH is a hemorrhage that occurs in the subdural space, between the arachnoid and dura. There may be underlying brain injury. A SDH usually arises from a torn bridging vein; patients with brain atrophy (from alcoholism or age) are at greater risk for SDH, because the bridging veins traverse greater distances and are more easily torn.

2) A SDH may be classified by its age. Acute SDHs are less than 24 hours old and usually secondary to trauma; subacute SDHs are between 24h and 2 weeks old. Chronic SDHs are older than 2 weeks.

3) On exam, patients may have evidence of a skull fracture, an altered level of consciousness, a dilated pupil ipsilateral to the hematoma, or contralateral hemiparesis.

4) Head CT may demonstrate an acute hyperdense crescent shaped hematoma exterior to the brain parenchyma but inside the skull with possible signs of mass effect; as the hematoma ages, it becomes isodense or hypodense. Check CBC, PT/PTT, electrolytes, and glucose.

5) Surgical intervention is indicated in patients with acute SDHs larger than 5 mm, and producing any neurological symptoms. Chronic SDHs may require surgical decompression if there is evidence of mass effect.

IV. MAXILLOFACIAL TRAUMA

•General•

1) Assess and stabilize the airway, and maintain cervical spine precautions; assume cervical spine injury/associated injuries until proven otherwise.

2) Midline maxillary or frontal bone fractures require significant force, while nasal bone or zygomatic fractures are relatively low impact injuries.

•Fractures/Treatment•

1) Mandible

   a) On physical exam, malocclusion (one indication of malocclusion is that the patient is unable to hold a tongue blade between the molars against resistance) may indicate a fracture; pain and abnormal mobility and crepitus may also indicate a fracture.

   b) A panoramic dental x-ray or PA and lateral views may demonstrate a fracture. Consider CT for diagnosis.

   c) Ensure patient has no airway compromise. Stable fractures require ice, soft or liquid diet, and evaluation by an oral surgeon.

2) Midface

   a) Midface fractures are described by the Le Fort classification. A Le Fort I fracture is from the lateral nasal apertures through the maxilla, separating the palate from the midface. A Le Fort II is a pyramidal fracture through the nasal bones and maxillary sinuses, separating them from the frontal bone and zygoma. A Le Fort III (craniofacial disjunction) is a fracture line through the glabella, orbits, and frontozygomatic suture lines.

   b) Instability of the midface can be assessed by gently pulling on the midface on the alveolar ridge. There are often associated injuries, as a significant force is required for a midface fracture. Also, CSF leakage may occur.

   c) Management includes protecting the airway. Blind nasotracheal intubation is contraindicated in patients with midfacial trauma; a cricothyroidotomy may be necessary. Antibiotics are recommended. Admit patient for airway management and operative repair.

3) Nasal Bone

   a) Physical exam may reveal deviation of the nose, edema, tenderness, epistaxis, and septal hematoma or deviation.

   b) X- rays (lateral and Waters view) may or may not demonstrate a fracture.

   c) Septal hematomas (blue swelling over the septum) should be incised and drained to avoid long-term morbidity. If the patient has persistent bleeding, insert a nasal packing. Patients with septal deviation should be referred to an ENT specialist for elective reduction; or, consider immediate reduction under local anesthesia (with the handle of a scalpel), followed by nasal packing and external splinting. Consider antibiotics, as a nasal fracture may communicate with paranasal sinuses.

4) Orbit

See Ophthalmology: Trauma

V. NECK TRAUMA

A. Blunt Neck Injury

•General•

1) Impact to the anterior neck may result in damage to the trachea or larynx, and may compress the esophagus against the spinal column.
2) Blunt neck trauma may cause cervical spine injury or vascular injury.

•Evaluation•

1) Conduct a systematic primary survey (rapid assessment of airway, breathing, circulation, disability, and expose patient), followed by a more detailed secondary survey.
2) Examine the airway. Examine vascular structures and the oropharynx. Evaluate for associated chest or cervical spine injuries. Perform a neurologic exam.
3) Any expanding hematoma requires emergent investigation and possible airway control.
4) Dysphonia, dysphagia, hemoptysis, or loss of anatomic landmarks may indicate a laryngeal fracture or esophageal injury.
5) Consider cervical spine x-rays, CXR, and soft tissue neck x-rays. Consider CT. Consider esophagoscopy and laryngoscopy. Consider angiography to evaluate for possible vascular injuries.

•Treatment•

1) For all significant trauma, establish at least 2 large bore IVs, monitor the patient, and administer oxygen. Maintain cervical spine precautions. Assess and stabilize the airway.
2) If hypotension is unresponsive to 2L normal saline (or two boluses of 20 cc/kg), consider blood transfusion.
3) Control bleeding with direct pressure.
4) Obtain a surgical evaluation.
5) Unless contraindicated, a urinary catheter should be inserted in all

seriously injured patients.

6) Administer tetanus prophylaxis as necessary.

B. Penetrating Neck Injury

•Evaluation•

1) Conduct a systematic primary survey (rapid assessment of airway, breathing, circulation, disability, and expose patient), followed by a more detailed secondary survey.

2) Perform a complete vascular and neurologic exam. Examine the oropharynx. Evaluate for associated chest injuries. Obtain CXR. Consider plain neck films to evaluate for fracture or air.

3) Any expanding hematoma requires emergent investigation and possible airway control.

4) Anterior neck injury is defined as through the platysma and anterior to the posterior border of the sternocleidomastoid. The evaluation is usually determined by which region (zone) of the neck is involved:

Zone I (thoracic outlet to cricoid cartilage)- Consider obtaining an angiogram of the aortic arch and great vessels; consider imaging the esophagus and trachea. Obtain CXR. Consider echocardiogram.

Zone II (cricoid to angle of mandible)- Consider surgical exploration (not mandatory) or angiogram of the carotid/vertebral arteries; ultrasound may be an alternative.

Zone III (above angle of mandible)- Consider obtaining a carotid angiogram and perform an oropharynx exam.

Posterior neck- Consider an angiogram of the vertebral arteries.

•Treatment•

1) For all significant trauma, establish at least 2 large bore IVs, monitor the patient, and administer oxygen. Maintain cervical spine precautions. Assess and stabilize the airway.

2) If hypotension is unresponsive to 2L normal saline (or two boluses of 20 cc/kg), consider blood transfusion.

3) Control bleeding with direct pressure.

4) Obtain a surgical evaluation.

5) Unless contraindicated, a urinary catheter should be inserted in all seriously injured patients.

6) Administer tetanus prophylaxis as necessary.

VI. PEDIATRIC TRAUMA (Blunt)

•**Evaluation**•

1) Conduct a systematic primary survey (rapid assessment of airway, breathing, circulation, disability, and expose patient), followed by a more detailed secondary survey.

2) Obtain necessary radiographs (cervical spine, chest, and pelvis).

3) If the patient is unstable with a possible abdominal injury, consider diagnostic peritoneal lavage (DPL) or immediate surgery.

4) If the patient is stable with a possible abdominal or chest injury, consider CT and serial exams. Check CBC, LFTs, urinalysis, CXR, and pelvic films.

•**Diagnosis**•

1) **Abdominal CT**- Peritoneal fluid, bowel wall thickening, and bowel dilation are sensitive and specific indicators of bowel wall rupture; extraluminal air is usually not seen.

2) **Cervical Spine X-rays**- Cervical spine injuries in children most often occur in the high cervical vertebra. Normal soft tissue dimensions: the prevertebral space should be 7 mm at C2 and 14 mm at C6; the pre-dens space should be <5 mm. In children <8 years old, pseudosubluxation of C2-C3 and C3-C4 are seen in 24% and 14%, respectively. The anterior aspect of spinous process of C2 should fall within 2 mm of a line drawn through the anterior aspects of the spinous processes of C1-C3. In 20% of children, more than 2/3 of anterior arch of atlas is above tip of the dens. In the very young, C3-C4 vertebral bodies often appear wedged.

3) **CXR**- The pediatric chest wall is extremely compliant; assume underlying organ injury if the CXR demonstrates a rib fracture.

4) **DPL**- DPL may be too sensitive and lead to unnecessary laparotomy; consider abdominal/pelvic CT if intra-abdominal injury is suspected by exam or mechanism, especially if the patient has a depressed level of consciousness.

5) **LFTs**- In hemodynamically stable children, elevated LFTs are associated with hepatic contusion or laceration.

6) **Physical Exam**- Serial abdominal exams are sensitive for small bowel injury. A linear ecchymosis from a lap belt may indicate a vertebral

fracture or intestinal injury. In restrained motor vehicle accident patients with abdominal wall contusions and a vertebral column fracture, there is a high incidence of intestinal injury.

7) **Urinalysis**- Hematuria is a reliable, nonspecific indicator of intra-abdominal injury; consider abdominal CT in all pediatric patients with blunt trauma and any degree of hematuria (adult criteria do not apply).

•Treatment•

1) For all significant trauma, establish 2 large bore IVs (in children, the preferred IV sites are antecubital and femoral, or, if necessary, intraosseous), monitor the patient, and administer oxygen. Maintain cervical spine precautions. Assess and stabilize the airway. Check temperature and glucose. Consult surgery.

2) The lowest acceptable blood pressure in children is 70 + (2 x age in years). If hypotension is unresponsive to two boluses of 20 cc/kg, administer packed RBCs in a 10 cc/kg bolus mixed with normal saline or whole blood 20 cc/kg; consider immediate surgery. Vasopressors are generally not indicated.

3) Unless contraindicated, an NG tube and urinary catheter should be inserted in all seriously injured patients (generally, NG tubes are not placed unless the airway has been secured, especially in infants, who are obligate nose breathers).

4) If the patient has abdominal tenderness or there is a suspicion of intra-abdominal injury, consider observation and serial exams; or, depending on the results of the abdominal CT and surgical consult, consider laparotomy. 80-90% of children with blunt splenic or liver injury can be treated without laparotomy.

VII. PELVIS/GENITOURINARY TRAUMA

A. Blunt Pelvic Injury

•Evaluation•

1) Conduct a systematic primary survey (rapid assessment of airway, breathing, circulation, disability, and expose patient), followed by a more detailed secondary survey.

2) Perform a rectal and genitourinary exam. Examine patient for associ-

ated cervical spine, abdominal, chest, or genitourinary injuries. There is an association between pelvic fractures and injury to the thoracic aorta.

3) Tenderness with gentle compression of the ileac wings may indicate a fracture; do not rock the pelvis, as this may increase hemorrhage. An acetabular fracture causes pain when the sole of the foot is percussed; it is associated with a hip dislocation (obtain Judet x-ray views).

4) Destot's sign (a hematoma above the inguinal ligament or perineum) may indicate a pelvic fracture.

5) Check pelvis x-ray; consider CBC, BUN/Cr, type and screen, and urinalysis.

6) 10% of patients with blunt pelvic trauma have a urethral injury; consider performing a retrograde urethrogram before insertion of a urinary catheter (especially if there is blood at the meatus, a scrotal hematoma, or a high prostate), and then perform a cystogram.

7) Indications for abdomen/pelvis CT include gross hematuria, microscopic hematuria in hemodynamically unstable patients, penetrating abdominal or flank injuries, or significant flank tenderness. To evaluate the kidneys, an abdomen/pelvis CT is generally the preferred imaging method (over IVP), as CT provides better anatomic detail, and also provides information on associated abdominal injuries; an IVP may be performed as a screening evaluation if CT is unavailable. In hemodynamically stable adult patients with blunt trauma and only microscopic hematuria, no acute evaluation of the kidneys is required; however consider CT to evaluate for associated injuries.

X-Ray

1) Obtain an A-P view of the pelvis. Closely examine the sacro-ileac joint for widening, and examine the inferior pubic borders for asymmetry. If the symphysis pubis is >10 mm in child or >8 mm in adult, consider dislocation.

2) Inlet views demonstrate A-P displacement of fracture; outlet views show sacral fracture or superior/inferior displacement.

3) Obtain Judet views if there is a suspicion of an acetabular fracture.

Classification of Traumatic Pelvic Fractures

I: Fracture of individual bones without a break in the ring (e.g., avulsions, horizontal sacral fracture, ileal wing fracture, single pubis or ischial ramus fracture).

II: Single break in the ring (nondisplaced ipsilateral rami fractures, nondisplaced ilium body fracture near sacroiliac joint, or vertical sacral fracture).

III: Double break in the ring; class III fractures are unstable (bilateral double rami fracture, fracture dislocation of pubis, double vertical fractures, open book pelvis, or multiple displaced fractures).

IV: Acetabular fractures.

•Treatment•

1) For all significant trauma, establish at least 2 large bore IVs, monitor the patient, and administer oxygen. Maintain cervical spine precautions. Assess and stabilize the airway. Consult surgery.

2) If hypotension is unresponsive to 2L normal saline (or two boluses of 20 cc/kg), consider blood transfusion.

3) Stabilize the fracture (isolated rami fractures are stable; ipsilateral superior and inferior rami fractures are usually stable; double breaks are unstable); stable fractures with continued bleeding will not benefit from an external fixator. Consult orthopedics.

4) Displacement >0.5 cm of any ring fracture is unstable and may require blood replacement. Open- book fractures may result in significant hemorrhage. Consider embolization of pelvic arteries if patient is hemodynamically unstable (although most bleeding is venous).

5) Administer tetanus prophylaxis as necessary.

B. Penetrating Pelvic Injury

•Evaluation•

1) Conduct a systematic primary survey (rapid assessment of airway, breathing, circulation, disability, and expose patient), followed by a more detailed secondary survey.

2) Perform a rectal and genitourinary exam.

3) Check CBC, BUN/Cr, type and screen, and urinalysis. Obtain x-ray.

4) Evaluate the outlet tracts; consider cystogram, proctoscopy, and vaginal speculum exam. Consider diagnostic peritoneal lavage, which is positive if >10,000 RBCs.

5) Penetrating trauma with any hematuria requires imaging (abdominal CT) to evaluate for possible injury to the urinary tract.

•Treatment•

1) For all significant trauma, establish at least 2 large bore IVs, monitor the patient, and administer oxygen. Maintain cervical spine precautions. Assess and stabilize the airway. Consult surgery.

2) If hypotension is unresponsive to 2L normal saline (or two boluses of 20 cc/kg), consider blood transfusion.

3) Treatment depends on the specific underlying injury.

4) Administer tetanus prophylaxis as necessary.

VIII. PREGNANCY AND TRAUMA

•Clinical Presentation•

1) Patients with abdominal injury may be asymptomatic, or may present with abdominal pain and vaginal bleeding. Only 50% of patients who abrupt have the classic abdominal pain, vaginal bleeding, and uterine irritability. Some pregnant women with massive hemoperitoneum have no peritoneal signs.

2) Suspect uterine rupture if hemodynamic instability is associated with abdominal pain, absent fetal heart tones, vaginal bleeding, and an indistinct fundal exam; treatment includes immediate laparotomy.

3) Normal physiologic changes in pregnancy include increased HR and decreased BP.

•Evaluation•

1) Conduct a systematic primary survey (rapid assessment of airway, breathing, circulation, disability, and expose patient), followed by a more detailed secondary survey. The evaluation attempts to exclude maternal or fetal injury, including placental abruption.

2) Check CBC, urinalysis, and type and screen; consider the Kleihauer-Betke test to identify fetomaternal hemorrhage.

3) Document the presence or absence of fetal heart tones, fetal movement, contractions, fundal tenderness or vaginal bleeding.

4) The indications for imaging studies in the evaluation of head, neck, thoracic, abdominal, pelvic, or extremity trauma are generally similar to non-pregnant patients. Obtain all necessary radiographic studies, but shield the uterus when possible.

5) Ultrasound is only 50% diagnostic for placental abruption; fetal monitoring is most sensitive.

6) If vaginal bleeding is present in the third trimester, consider placenta previa; perform a speculum exam in the operating room.

•Treatment•

1) For all significant trauma, establish at least 2 large bore IVs, monitor the patient, and administer oxygen. Maintain cervical spine precautions. Assess and stabilize the airway.

2) If hypotension is unresponsive to 2L IV fluid (or two boluses of 20 cc/kg), consider blood transfusion. Use lactated Ringer's, as normal saline may cause hyperchloremic acidosis. If vasopressors are required, consider ephedrine.

3) Hemodynamically unstable patients should be taken to surgery. Otherwise, the treatment and disposition depend on the hemodynamic status, the results of the imaging studies, and clinical presentation.

4) Position the patient on a left lateral tilt to avoid compression of the inferior vena cava by the gravid uterus.

5) If the patient is over 20 weeks estimated gestational age, arrange fetal monitoring for 4h with minor trauma and 24h with major trauma. 2-4% of patients with minor trauma abrupt.

6) Administer Rhogam (50 mcg if ≤12 weeks gestational age and 300 mcg if >12 weeks gestational age) if fetomaternal hemorrhage is suspected.

7) If necessary, a peri-mortem c-section should be done with a generous vertical incision; perform within 4 minutes of cardiac arrest.

8) Unless contraindicated, an NG tube and urinary catheter should be inserted in all seriously injured patients.

9) Administer tetanus prophylaxis as necessary (it is safe in pregnancy).

10) Consult OB/Gyn.

IX. SPINAL TRAUMA

A. Cervical Spine Trauma

•Evaluation•

1) Conduct a systematic primary survey (rapid assessment of airway, breathing, circulation, disability, and expose patient), followed by a more detailed secondary survey.

2) Maintain cervical spine precautions and do a complete neurological

exam.

3) Cervical spine x-rays may be deferred if there is no midline cervical tenderness, no intoxication, normal mental status, no focal neurological deficits, and no distracting injury.

4) If the patient cannot be clinically cleared, obtain cervical spine films.

5) If there is a fracture on plain films, if the patient has any neurological deficits, or if the patient has persistent pain despite negative x-rays, consider CT or MRI.

6) Children and the elderly usually sustain upper cervical injuries, while other adults usually sustain lower cervical injuries. There is an increased incidence of odontoid fractures in the elderly; if the patient has persistent neck pain and negative plain films (especially if there is underlying arthritis), consider CT.

7) Evaluate for associated injuries.

<u>Normal X-Ray Patterns in Adults</u>

Normal soft tissue dimensions- The soft tissue is best evaluated on the lateral view. At C1-C4, the prevertebral space should be 7 mm or 1/3 the width of the vertebral body. At C5-T1, it should be 22 mm or the width of the vertebral body. The normal pre-dens space is <3 mm.

Lateral view- Alignment is evaluated by ensuring a smooth continuous curve in the anterior vertebral line (a line connecting the anterior margins of the vertebral bodies), the posterior vertebral line (a line connecting the posterior margins of the vertebral bodies), the spinolaminal line (a line connecting the bases of the spinous processes), and a line connecting the tips of the spinous processes. The lateral x-ray shows the transverse process superimposed on the vertebral body; the pedicles are not seen. The posterior cortex of the articular masses connects the superior and inferior facets and should be superimposed to form the posterior cortical line; the posterior laminal line is the posterior extent of the spinal canal. Inferior to C3, the interspinous process spaces should be equal. Evaluate the cortex of each vertebral body, the disc spaces, and the soft tissues.

A-P view- The articular masses are superimposed. Therefore, the lateral cortical margins should appear continuous and undulating. The spinous processes should form a straight line, and the spaces between spinous processes should be equal.

Open mouth/Odontoid view- The lateral atlantoaxial joint spaces should be open and the contiguous surfaces should be parallel. The lateral margins should be on the same plane. The space on each side of the dens should be symmetrical. Evaluate the odontoid.

Oblique views- The oblique view shows the pedicles, foramina, articular masses, and laminae (which should appear to be shingled in a vertical direction).

Normal X-Ray Patterns in Pediatrics

Normal soft tissue dimensions- The prevertebral space should be 7 mm at C2 and 14 mm at C6; the pre-dens space should be <5 mm.

Normal variants- In children <8 years old, pseudosubluxation of C2-C3 and C3-C4 is seen in 24% and 14% of patients, respectively. The anterior aspect of the spinous process of C2 should fall within 2 mm of a line drawn through the anterior aspects of the spinous processes of C1-C3. In 20% of children, more than 2/3 of the anterior arch of the atlas is above the tip of the dens. In the very young, the C3-C4 vertebral bodies often appear wedged. Cervical spine injuries in children most often occur in the high cervical vertebra.

Innervation

C3-C4- Innervates trapezius. Test by shoulder elevation; it is sensory to shoulder.
C4- Innervates diaphragm.
C5-C6- Innervates biceps. Test by forearm flexion; it is sensory to thumb.
C7- Innervates triceps. Test by forearm extension; it is sensory to index.
C8- Innervates flexor digitorum. Test by finger flexion; it is sensory to small finger.
T1- Innervates interossei. Test by finger abduction.

•Specific Injuries•

Type of Injury by Mechanism

Extension rotation- causes *Pillar fracture*.

Flexion- These injuries result in compression of the anterior column and distraction of the posterior column. Examples include: *Flexion Teardrop* (a triangular fragment is displaced from the anteroinferior part of the vertebra; extensive anterior and posterior disruption and cord injury result); *Anterior Subluxation*; *Bilateral Interfacetal Dislocation* (this injury is unstable with complete ligamentous disruption; the lateral shows anterior displacement of ≥50% of one vertebra over the lower one); *Wedge Compression Fracture*; *Clay Shoveler Fracture* (a spinous process fracture of C6-T1).

Flexion rotation- causes *Unilateral Interfacetal Dislocation* (on lateral, there is anterior dislocation of <50% of one vertebra over the lower one, and above the injury the vertebrae appear to be in an oblique projection; the oblique view shows a disruption of the normal "shingles" appearance; this injury is generally considered stable).

Hyperextension- dislocation- These injuries result in compression of the posterior column and distraction of the anterior column. Examples include: *Avulsion of Anterior Arch*; *Laminar Fracture*; *Hangman's fracture* (bilateral C2 pedicle fracture; it is unstable); *Extension Teardrop* (triangular anterior, inferior fragment is avulsed off the vertebra, but the posterior ligaments are intact; this injury is unstable in extension); *Posterior Neural Arch Fracture (posterior arch of C1 fracture)*.

Vertical compression- These injuries result in axial loading of both the anterior and posterior columns. Examples include: *Jefferson Fracture* (burst of ring of C1; the odontoid view shows lateral displacement of the articular masses of C1 and the lateral view shows a widened pre-dental space); *Vertebral Burst Fracture* (pieces of the vertebral body may be forced into the spinal canal).

Other Cervical Spine Injuries

Odontoid Fracture- Type I is an avulsion of the tip of the dens; Type II is a fracture of the base of the dens; Type III is a fracture of the dens which extends into the body of the axis. Odontoid fractures are more common in the elderly.

SCIWORA (spinal cord injury without radiographic abnormality)- It results from spinal cord trauma from a displacement of the vertebral elements (e.g., subluxation, ligamentous impingement, or disc herniation), which has reduced spontaneously. SCIWORA accounts for up to 25-50% of pediatric cervical spine injuries. Consider MRI.

•Treatment•
1) Immobilize the patient. For all significant trauma, establish at least 2 large bore IVs, monitor the patient, and administer oxygen. Assess

and stabilize the airway.

2) Consider methylprednisolone 30 mg/kg loading dose over 15 min, then 5.4 mg/kg/h infusion. Methylprednisolone is indicated for an acute spinal cord injury within 8h of the injury, and is contraindicated in the presence of the cauda equina syndrome, gun shot wound, pregnancy, or other life-threatening illness; it is controversial in children younger than 13 years old.

3) Consult neurosurgery.

4) Unless contraindicated, an NG tube and urinary catheter should be inserted in all seriously injured patients.

5) Administer tetanus prophylaxis as necessary.

B. Spinal Cord Injury Syndromes

1) **Anterior Cord Syndrome**- It is secondary to compression of the anterior spinal cord form forced hyperflexion. It results in motor paralysis and loss of pain and temperature sensation distal to the lesion; the posterior columns are spared.

2) **Brown-Sequard Syndrome**- It is an injury to one side of the spinal cord. It results in paralysis and loss of proprioception on the ipsilateral side of the lesion and loss of pain and temperature sensation on the contralateral side; it is usually from penetrating wounds.

3) **Central Cord Syndrome**- It is secondary to forced hyperextension in which the ligamentum flavum contuses the medial aspects of the cord. It results in motor and sensory loss that is greater in the arms than the legs.

4) **Neurogenic Shock**- It results in vasomotor instability from loss of sympathetic tone. The SBP is usually 80-100 mm Hg, but the patient has warm skin, adequate urine output, and paradoxical bradycardia; often other autonomic symptoms are present. Neurogenic shock only occurs in acute spinal cord injuries above the T6 level; hypotension in association with spinal cord injury below the T6 level is likely due to hemorrhage. If blood loss has been excluded, treat with judicious normal saline and consider dopamine.

5) **Spinal Shock**- It results in distal areflexia, loss of sphincter tone, priapism, and flaccid quadriplegia; it may be transient.

C. Thoracolumbar Trauma

•Evaluation•

1) Conduct a systematic primary survey (rapid assessment of airway, breathing, circulation, disability, and expose patient), followed by a more detailed secondary survey.

2) Maintain cervical spine precautions and do a complete neurological exam. Document any point tenderness or neurovascular deficits.

3) Obtain thoracolumbar x-rays if there is point tenderness or neurologic deficits on exam. The rib cage stabilizes the thoracic spine, and therefore a significant force is required to cause a thoracic fracture dislocation.

4) If there is a fracture on plain films or if the patient has any neurological deficits, consider CT or MRI.

5) Evaluate for associated injuries.

X-Ray

1) On the lateral film, check the anterior and posterior height of the vertebral bodies, the alignment of the vertebral bodies, and the interspinous distance.

2) On the A-P view, check the height of the vertebral bodies and the width between the pedicles.

Innervation

L1-L2- Innervates iliopsoas. Test by hip flexion; it is sensory to medial thigh.

L3-L4- Innervates quadriceps. Test by knee extension.

L5- Innervates extensor hallucis; it is sensory to lateral calf.

S1- Innervates biceps. Test by knee flexion; it is sensory to lateral foot.

S1-S2- Innervates gastrocs. Test by foot plantar flexion.

S2-S4- Innervates sphincter; it is sensory to perianal area.

•Specific Injuries•

Wedge/compression fracture- It occurs from axial loading. It is usually stable, but may become unstable if the vertebral body has lost >50% of its height. Treatment is symptomatic.

Burst fracture- It occurs from axial loading. The vertebral end plates fracture, exploding the body; the posterior portion may protrude into the canal. Obtain urgent neurosurgical consult and CT/MRI.

•Treatment•- If spinal cord injury or unstable fracture:

1) Immobilize the patient. For all significant trauma, establish at least 2 large bore IVs, monitor the patient, and administer oxygen. Assess and stabilize the airway.

2) Consider methylprednisolone 30 mg/kg loading dose over 15 min, then 5.4 mg/kg/h infusion. Methylprednisolone is indicated for an acute spinal cord injury within 8h of the injury, and is contraindicated in the presence of the cauda equina syndrome, gun shot wound, pregnancy, or other life-threatening illness; it is controversial in children younger than 13 years old.

3) Consult neurosurgery.

4) Unless contraindicated, an NG tube and urinary catheter should be inserted in all seriously injured patients.

5) Administer tetanus prophylaxis as necessary.

X. THORACIC TRAUMA

A. Blunt Thoracic Injury

•Evaluation•

1) Conduct a systematic primary survey (rapid assessment of airway, breathing, circulation, disability, and expose patient), followed by a more detailed secondary survey.

2) Perform pulmonary, abdominal, and cardiac exams; auscultate for cardiac murmur. Evaluate for chest wall deformity or rib fracture. Tracheal deviation, decreased breath sounds, and hypotension may indicate tension pneumothorax, which requires an emergent thoracostomy. Patients with blunt traumatic aortic injuries may have no physical findings suggestive of injury.

3) Obtain CXR to evaluate for pneumothorax, hemothorax, rib fracture, or pulmonary contusion. Indications of aortic rupture on CXR include a wide mediastinum (the most sensitive sign), no aortic knob, deviation of the trachea to the right, the presence of a pleural cap, elevation of the right mainstem bronchus, depression of the left mainstem bronchus, and the NG tube pushed to the right (which may be the most accurate sign). Up to 1/3 of patients with an aortic rupture may have a normal initial CXR.

4) Consider spiral chest CT/arch angiogram to evaluate the aorta if there

is a significant mechanism of injury (deceleration from >30 mph, fall >30 feet), abnormal CXR or abnormal physical exam. Consider transesophageal echocardiography.

5) Consider ECG, CBC and type and screen. Evaluate for other injuries. Obtain necessary radiographs (cervical spine, pelvis).

•Treatment•

1) For all significant trauma, establish at least 2 large bore IVs, monitor the patient, and administer oxygen. Maintain cervical spine precautions. Assess and stabilize the airway. Consult surgery.

2) If hypotension is unresponsive to 2L normal saline (or two boluses of 20 cc/kg), consider blood transfusion. Hemodynamically unstable patients require an immediate surgical evaluation.

3) If there is a traumatic aortic injury, consider maintaining blood pressure between 100 and 120 mmHg with beta-blockers and nitroprusside (as in aortic dissection); this will decrease shear forces on the aorta.

4) If a chest tube is placed for a pneumothorax, insert the tube in the 4th or 5th intercostal space at the anterior or midaxillary line, and direct the tube toward the anterior apex; for a hemothorax, direct the tube posteriorly and laterally. Consider a thoracotomy if unstable vital signs, initial output from chest tube > 20 ml/kg, 1500 ml of blood from chest tube in the first 12h or >300 ml/h x 3-4h, or if there is a 50% hemothorax; blunting of the costophrenic angles on an upright CXR is seen with 200 cc of fluid. If massive hemothorax, consider autotransfusion of the chest tube output back into the patient.

5) If a subclavian line is placed, insert the line on the side of the injury to avoid collapse of the uninvolved lung.

6) A resuscitative thoracotomy may be beneficial if the patient is in profound shock unresponsive to fluids or there were signs of life within 5 minutes of arrival to the ED, and the patient has penetrating wounds of the chest or neck. Blunt trauma victims will not benefit.

7) If the ECG is abnormal (especially if the patient has comorbid disease and is unstable), admit to rule out MI and obtain an echocardiogram (emergently if the patient is unstable).

8) Unless contraindicated, an NG tube and urinary catheter should be inserted in all seriously injured patients.

9) Administer tetanus prophylaxis as necessary.

•Specific Injuries•

1) Aortic Rupture

a) Most aortic tears occur in the descending aorta at the isthmus; they usually occur from rapid deceleration.

b) Patients most often present with chest or intrascapular pain. Patients may have lower extremity pulse deficits. The physical exam is insensitive for diagnosis.

c) CXR may demonstrate a wide mediastinum (the most sensitive sign), no aortic knob, deviation of the trachea to the right, the presence of a pleural cap, elevation of the right mainstem bronchus, depression of the left mainstem bronchus, widened paratracheal stripe, and the NG tube pushed to the right (which may be the most accurate sign). Consider CT, transesophageal echocardiography (which can be performed at the bedside), or aortography.

d) Management is surgical. If patient is hypertensive, consider esmolol and nitroprusside.

2) Flail Chest

a) Flail chest is a mobile segment of the chest wall that results from a fracture of 3 or more adjacent ribs in 2 places.

b) Flail chest is usually diagnosed by physical exam; during inspiration, the flail segment paradoxically moves inward, and then outward with expiration. It is associated with pulmonary contusion; check ABG.

c) Treatment includes oxygen, cardiac monitoring, and stabilizing the flail segment with a sandbag (or positioning the patient with the injured side down). Isolated flail chest does not mandate intubation.

3) Myocardial Contusion

a) Suspect a contusion in any patient who presents with chest signs or symptoms following a motor vehicle accident > 35 mph. Most patients have external signs of thoracic trauma.

b) A contusion may result in dysrhythmias or reduced cardiac output. Tachycardia, new atrial fibrillation or multiple PVCs may be demonstrated on the ECG. CK-MB does not appear to correlate with injury. Consider obtaining an echocardiogram.

c) If a contusion is suspected, consider admission to telemetry (although most patients with contusions do well, so some recommend only admitting those with coronary disease, hemodynamic instability or ECG evidence of ischemia or arrhythmias); if no dysrhythmias develop within 12h and CK-MB determinations are normal, then cardiac injury is unlikely. A normal ECG with normal hemodynamics signifies no clinically significant cardiac contusion.

4) Pneumothorax/Hemothorax

a) Accumulation of air in the pleural space may be classified as a simple pneumothorax (no communication with the atmosphere), a communicating pneumothorax, or a tension pneumothorax. A hemothorax is an accumulation of blood in the pleural space; the bleeding is usually from injured lung parenchyma.

b) Patients typically present with dyspnea and chest pain, and may or may not be hemodynamically stable. Physical exam may reveal decreased breath sounds and hyperresonance. A tension pneumothorax results when the injury allows air to enter on inspiration, but does not allow air to escape in exhalation; eventually, there is a mediastinal shift to the uninvolved hemithorax and compression of the great vessels with subsequent hypotension, jugular venous distention, and tachycardia.

c) Check CXR (consider expiration films); consider CT.

d) Treat tension pneumothoraces immediately with needle decompression in the second intercostal space in the midclavicular line. Communicating pneumothoraces should be covered with the dressing taped down on 3 sides. The treatment of simple pneumothoraces depends on their size and the patient's hemodynamic status; chest tubes are generally placed in the fifth intercostal space, anterior to the midaxillary line. A hemothorax is treated with large-bore (38 French) tube thoracostomy in the anterior axillary line, at the level of the nipple; the amount of hemorrhage is monitored.

5) Pulmonary Contusion

a) A pulmonary contusion may result from blunt trauma or high velocity missile wounds. Patients may present with tachypnea, dyspnea, hypotension, or tachycardia. There may be associated rib fractures.

b) A pulmonary contusion may manifest on CXR within minutes of the injury (always within 4-6h), and may show patchy infiltrates or consolidation. Consider CT. Usually, ABG demonstrates a low pO2.

c) Treatment involves maintaining oxygenation (consider CPAP) and aggressive supportive care. Pneumonia is a common complication, but prophylactic antibiotics are not indicated.

B. Penetrating Thoracic Injury

•Evaluation•

1) Conduct a systematic primary survey (rapid assessment of airway, breathing, circulation, disability, and expose patient), followed by a more detailed secondary survey.

2) Perform pulmonary, abdominal, and cardiac exams; auscultate for cardiac murmur. Evaluate for chest wall deformity or rib fracture. Tracheal deviation, decreased breath sounds, and hypotension may indicate tension pneumothorax, which requires an emergent thoracostomy.

3) Obtain CXR to evaluate for pneumothorax, hemothorax, pulmonary parenchymal injury, and aortic injury. Indications of aortic rupture on CXR include a wide mediastinum (the most sensitive sign), no aortic knob, deviation of the trachea to the right, the presence of a pleural cap, elevation of the right mainstem bronchus, depression of the left mainstem bronchus, and the NG tube pushed to the right (which may be the most accurate sign). Up to 1/3 of patients with an aortic rupture may have a normal initial CXR.

4) Consider ECG, CBC and type and screen. Evaluate for other injuries. Obtain necessary radiographs (cervical spine, pelvis).

5) **Anterior cardiac box injury** (defined as the sternal notch to the costal margin, between the nipples; or consider using the boundaries of the sternal notch to the costal margin, and the mid-clavicular line on the right and anterior axillary line on the left): consider obtaining an echocardiogram or chest CT.

6) **Posterior cardiac box injury** (defined as between the scapulae): if gun shot wound, consider a chest CT/arch angiogram, esophagram and endoscopy. If stab wound, obtain CXR and consider chest CT/angiogram, esophagram, and endoscopy (especially if the mediastinum is abnormal on the CXR).

7) If the patient has a stab wound that is not in the anterior or posterior box, obtain a CXR. If the initial CXR is negative, repeat an inspiratory/expiratory A-P and lateral CXR in 6h; if still negative for pneumothorax/hemothorax, then it is safe to discharge the patient.

•Treatment•

1) For all significant trauma, establish at least 2 large bore IVs, monitor the patient, and administer oxygen. Maintain cervical spine precautions. Assess and stabilize the airway. Consult surgery.

2) If hypotension is unresponsive to 2L normal saline (or two boluses of 20 cc/kg), consider blood transfusion. Hemodynamically unstable patients require an immediate surgical evaluation.

3) If a chest tube is placed for a pneumothorax, insert the tube in the 4th or 5th intercostal space at the anterior or midaxillary line, and direct the tube toward the anterior apex; for a hemothorax, direct the tube posteriorly and laterally. Consider a thoracotomy if unstable vital signs, 1500 ml of blood from chest tube in the first 12h or >300 ml/h x 3-4h, or if there is a 50% hemothorax; blunting of the costophrenic angles on an upright CXR is seen with 200 cc of fluid.

4) If a subclavian line is placed, insert the line on the side of the injury to avoid collapse of the uninvolved lung.

5) A resuscitative thoracotomy may be beneficial if there were signs of life within 5 min of arrival to the ED, and the patient has penetrating wounds of the chest or neck. Blunt trauma victims will not benefit.

6) Unless contraindicated, an NG tube and urinary catheter should be inserted in all seriously injured patients.

7) Administer tetanus prophylaxis as necessary.

XI. VASCULAR TRAUMA (Penetrating)

•Evaluation•

1) Conduct a systematic primary survey (rapid assessment of airway, breathing, circulation, disability, and expose patient), followed by a more detailed secondary survey.

2) Document the location of the injury, the color of the skin, and the presence and character of the pulse. Document a neurologic exam. 25% of arterial injuries have no pulse deficits. Evaluate for other injuries.

3) Using a Doppler device, measure the arterial pressure index (the systolic pressure measured at a site distal to the injury in the affected extremity divided by the same measurement in the normal extremity); a value <0.9 is abnormal.

4) Indications for immediate operative intervention or an emergent angiogram include signs of arterial occlusion, active hemorrhage, signs of ischemia, expanding or pulsatile hematoma, bruit, thrill, or involvement of a central vessel (e.g. subclavian, axillary, or femoral).

5) A proximity angiogram (i.e., obtaining an angiogram if the injury is in close proximity to a vessel) is not indicated, except for high-risk injuries.

6) Doppler ultrasound may be another option for the evaluation of vessels.

7) Consider x-ray of the involved extremity.

•Treatment•

1) For all significant trauma, establish at least 2 large bore IVs, monitor the patient, and administer oxygen. Maintain cervical spine precautions. Assess and stabilize the airway. Avoid placing IV lines in the injured extremity.

2) If hypotension is unresponsive to 2L normal saline (or two boluses of 20 cc/kg), consider blood transfusion.

3) Control bleeding with direct pressure; stabilize the extremity. Do not apply clamps blindly to vessels, as this may permanently damage vessels and injure other neurovascular structures. Avoid tourniquets.

4) Consult vascular surgery. Unstable patients with obvious vascular injuries require immediate surgical intervention.

5) Administer IV antibiotics for skeletal injury (bullets are not sterile).

6) Unless contraindicated, an NG tube and urinary catheter should be inserted in all seriously injured patients.

7) Administer tetanus prophylaxis as necessary.

APPENDICES

(Adapted from American Heart Association Guidelines)

I. A: BASIC LIFE SUPPORT: <u>CPR/RESCUE BREATHING</u>

A. Airway: Open airway with head tilt-chin lift method or jaw thrust (if trauma is present).

B. Breathing: Look, listen, and feel. If breathing resumes, place patient in recovery position.

BREATHING

Maneuver	Adult (>8yrs)	Child (1-8yrs)	Infant (<1yr)
Initial	2 breaths @ 2 sec/breath	2 breaths @ 1-1.5 sec/breath	2 breaths @ 1-1.5 sec/breath
Subsequent	10-12 breaths/min	20 breaths/min	20 breaths/min
Airway Obstruction	Heimlich maneuver	Heimlich maneuver	Back blows/chest thrusts

CIRCULATION

Maneuver	Adult (>8 yrs)	Child (1-8 yrs)	Infant (<1 yr)
Pulse Check	Carotid	Carotid	Brachial or femoral
Compression Landmarks	Lower half of sternum	Lower half of sternum	1 finger width below nipples
Compression Method	Heel of one hand, other hand on top	Heel of one hand	2 thumbs-encircled hands, or 2 or 3 fingers
Compression Depth	1.5-2 inches	1-1.5 inches	0.5-1 inch
Compression Rate	100/min	100/min	100-120/min
Compression: ventilation ratio	15:2	5:1	5:1

I. B. BASIC LIFE SUPPORT: <u>FOREIGN BODY/AIRWAY OBSTRUCTION</u>

	Adult	Child (1-8 yrs)	Infant (<1 yr)
1	Ask: Are you choking? Can you speak?	Ask: Are you choking? Can you speak?	Confirm airway obstruction
2	Perform abdominal thrusts/Heimlich maneuver; or chest thrusts for pregnant or obese patients	Perform abdominal thrusts/Heimlich maneuver	Perform up to 5 back blows and 5 chest thrusts
3	Repeat thrusts until effective or patient becomes unresponsive	Repeat thrusts until effective or patient becomes unresponsive	Repeat step 2 until effective or patient becomes unresponsive
	Patient becomes unresponsive	Patient becomes unresponsive	Patient becomes unresponsive
4	Activate EMS	If 2nd rescuer is available, have him activate EMS	If 2nd rescuer is available, have him activate EMS
5	Perform tongue-jaw lift, then finger sweep to remove object	Perform tongue-jaw lift; if object is seen, remove it with finger sweep	Perform tongue-jaw lift; if object is seen, remove it with finger sweep
6	Open airway and attempt ventilation; if still obstructed, reposition head and attempt ventilation again	Open airway and attempt ventilation; if still obstructed, reposition head and attempt ventilation again	Open airway and attempt ventilation; if still obstructed, reposition head and attempt ventilation again
7	Perform up to 5 abdominal thrusts	Perform up to 5 abdominal thrusts	Perform up to 5 back blows and 5 chest thrusts
8	Repeat steps 5-7 until effective	Repeat steps 5-7 until effective	Repeat steps 5-7 until effective
9		Activate EMS if obstruction is not relieved after 1 min	Activate EMS if obstruction is not relieved after 1 min

II. A. *ACLS PROTOCOLS*: <u>VENTRICULAR FIBRILLATION/PULSELESS VENTRICULAR TACHYCARDIA</u>

•<u>VFIB/PULSELESS VTACH</u>•

Perform CPR.

⇩

Defibrillate up to 3 times; start at 200 J, then 300 J, then 360 J.

⇩

If persistent VF/VT, continue CPR and intubate.

⇩

• **Epinephrine** 1 mg IVP every 3-5 min.
• <u>Or</u>, **Vasopressin** 40 U IV, single dose, 1 time only.

⇩

Defibrillate with 360 J within 30-60 sec.

⇩

• Consider **Amiodarone** 300 mg IVP (may repeat with 150 mg IVP); **Lidocaine** 1.0-1.5 mg/kg IV (may repeat with 0.5-0.75 mg/kg IV in 5 minutes for total of 3 mg/kg); **Magnesium** 1-2 g IV (if hypomagnesemic); **Procainamide** 20 mg/min (max 17 mg/kg) or 100 mg IVP every 5 minutes for intermittent/recurrent VF/VT.
• Defibrillate at 360 J 30-60 seconds after each medication.
• Consider **sodium bicarbonate** 1 mEq/kg IV bolus if prolonged resuscitation with effective ventilation or upon return of spontaneous circulation after a prolonged arrest.

412

II. B. *ACLS PROTOCOLS*: <u>PEA</u>

•<u>PULSELESS ELECTRICAL ACTIVITY</u>•

Perform CPR; Intubate.

⇩

Consider etiology of PEA: hypoxia; hypovolemia; tension pneumothorax; hypothermia; cardiac tamponade; MI; pulmonary embolism; overdose; hyperkalemia; acidosis.

⇩

- **Epinephrine** 1 mg IVP every 3-5 minutes.
- If bradycardic, **Atropine** 1 mg IV every 3-5 minutes as needed (max total dose 0.04 mg/kg).

- Perform primary and secondary ABCD surveys.
- Place and secure the airway and establish IV as soon as possible.
- Assess for occult blood flow (pseudo-EMT").
- Search for and treat reversible causes.

* Pulseless Electrical Activity (PEA) is a rhythm on a monitor without a detectable pulse.

II. C. *ACLS PROTOCOLS*: <u>ASYSTOLE</u>

•<u>ASYSTOLE</u>•

Perform CPR; Intubate; Consider pacing.

Consider etiology of asystole: hypoxia; hypovolemia; tension pneumothorax; hypothermia; cardiac tamponade; MI: pulmonary embolism; overdose; hyperkalemia; acidosis.

- **Epinephrine** 1 mg IV every 3-5 minutes.
- **Atropine** 1 mg IV every 3-5 minutes (max total dose 0.04 mg/kg).

- Perform primary and secondary ABCD surveys.
- Place and secure the airway and establish IV as soon as possible.
- Search for and treat reversible causes.
- If asystole persists, consider withholding resuscitation efforts.

II. D. *ACLS PROTOCOLS*: __ATRIAL FIBRILLATION__

If unstable, perform cardioversion (usually only if the ventricular rate is >150 beats/min).

Otherwise, if stable hemodynamics, the goal is to control the heart rate. Consider converting rhythm and anticoagulation.

⇩

IF PRESERVED HEART FUNCTION

For rate control ⇨ Use 1 of the following: Diltiazem, Verapamil, or Beta Blockers.

To convert rhythm:
If duration < 48h ⇨ Consider DC cardioversion, amiodarone, ibutilide, flecainide, propafenone or procainamide.

If duration > 48h ⇨ Avoid non-emergent cardioversion unless clot precautions are taken (IV heparin and TEE); use antiarrhythmics with extreme caution. Consider delayed cardioversion after 3 weeks of anticoagulation, followed by 4 more weeks of anticoagulation.

IF IMPAIRED HEART FUNCTION

For rate control ⇨ Digoxin, Diltiazem, or Amiodarone.

To convert rhythm:
If duration < 48h ⇨ Consider DC cardioversion or amiodarone.
If duration > 48h ⇨Anticoagulate for 3 weeks, then cardioversion.

IF ATRIAL FIBRILLATION AND WPW ⇨ DC cardioversion or amiodarone. If preserved heart function, also consider flecainide or procainamide or propafenone or sotalol. Consider anticoagulation, especially if duration > 48h.

II. E. *ACLS PROTOCOLS*: <u>NARROW COMPLEX TACHYCARDIA</u>

•<u>NARROW COMPLEX SVT (stable)</u>•

Vagal maneuvers (which include Valsalva and carotid sinus massage; ocular pressure is contraindicated).

⇩

Adenosine 6 mg IV rapid push.

⇩

Adenosine 12 mg rapid push.

If persistent narrow complex SVT:

<u>Junctional Tachycardia, preserved heart function</u> ⇨ NO DC CARDIOVERSION. Consider amiodarone; beta-blocker; calcium channel blocker.

<u>Junctional Tachycardia, impaired heart function</u> ⇨ NO DC CARDIOVERSION. Consider amiodarone.

<u>PSVT, preserved heart function</u> ⇨ Priority order: DC cardioversion; calcium channel blocker; beta blocker; digoxin. Consider procainamide; amiodarone; sotalol.

<u>PSVT, impaired heart function</u> ⇨ Priority order: digoxin, amiodarone, diltiazem. Consider DC cardioversion.

<u>Ectopic Atrial Tachycardia, preserved heart function</u> ⇨ NO DC CARDIOVERSION. Consider calcium channel blocker, beta-blocker, amiodarone.

<u>Ectopic Atrial Tachycardia, impaired heart function</u> ⇨ NO DC CARDIOVERSION. Consider amiodarone, diltiazem.

II. F. *ACLS PROTOCOLS*: <u>STABLE VENTRICULAR TACHYCARDIA</u>

•<u>STABLE VENTRICULAR TACHYCARDIA (VT)</u>•

*Note: may go directly to cardioversion.

<u>**Monomorphic VT, normal heart function**</u> ⇨ Procainamide (20 mg/min; max 17 mg/kg); or sotalol; or amiodarone (150 mg bolus over 10 minutes; may repeat every 10 minutes; or give as infusion 360 mg over 6h); or lidocaine (1-1.5 mg/kg IVP; repeat 0.5-0.75 mg/ kg every 5-10 minutes, max total dose 3 mg/kg).

<u>**Monomorphic VT, impaired heart function**</u> ⇨ Amiodarone 150 mg IV bolus over 10 minutes; or lidocaine 0.5-0.75 mg/kg IVP; then, synchronized cardioversion.

<u>**Polymorphic VT, normal baseline QT interval**</u> ⇨ Treat ischemia and correct electrolytes. Consider beta-blockers or lidocaine or amiodarone or procainamide or sotalol. If impaired heart function, use amiodarone 150 mg IV bolus over 10 minutes; or lidocaine 0.5-0.75 mg/kg IVP; then, synchronized cardioversion.

<u>**Polymorphic VT, prolonged baseline QT interval**</u> ⇨ Correct electrolytes. Consider magnesium (1-2 g) or overdrive pacing or isoproterenol (2-10 mcg/min) or phenytoin or lidocaine (1-1.5 mg/kg IVP; repeat 0.5-0.75 mg/kg every 5-10 minutes, max total dose 3 mg/kg).

II. G. *ACLS PROTOCOLS*: <u>BRADYCARDIA</u>

•<u>BRADYCARDIA</u>•
If serious signs or symptoms due to bradycardia:
(Patient not in cardiac arrest)

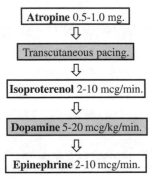

Atropine 0.5-1.0 mg.
⇩
Transcutaneous pacing.
⇩
Isoproterenol 2-10 mcg/min.
⇩
Dopamine 5-20 mcg/kg/min.
⇩
Epinephrine 2-10 mcg/min.

If no serious signs or symptoms **AND** patient is in Type II second degree AV block or third degree AV block.		• Prepare for transvenous pacer. • If symptoms develop, use a transcutaneous pacemaker until a transvenous pacer is placed.
If no serious signs or symptoms and patient is **NOT** in Type II second degree AV block or third degree AV block.		Observe.

II. H. *ACLS PROTOCOLS*: <u>PULMONARY EDEMA</u>

•<u>PULMONARY EDEMA</u>•

| 1st Line | ⇨ | • Furosemide IV 0.5-1.0 mg/kg.
 • Morphine IV 2-4 mg.
 • Nitroglycerin SL.
 • Oxygen/intubation/CPAP as needed. |

| 2nd Line |

⇩

| If systolic BP <70 mm Hg (signs of shock) | ⇨ | Consider **norepinephrine** (0.5-30 mcg/min IV). |

| If systolic BP 70-100 mm Hg (signs of shock) | ⇨ | Consider **dopamine** (5-15 mcg/kg/min IV). |

| If systolic BP 70-100 mmHg (no signs of shock) | ⇨ | Consider **dobutamine** (2-20 mcg/kg/min IV). |

| If systolic BP >100 mm Hg | ⇨ | Consider **nitroglycerin** (10-20 mcg/min IV) or **nitroprusside** (0.1-5.0 mcg/min IV). |

Consider other options:
• Pulmonary artery catheter.
• Intra-aortic balloon pump.
• Angiography for ischemia/AMI.

II. I. *ACLS PROTOCOLS*: <u>HYPOTHERMIA</u>

> **IF PULSE OR BREATHING ARE ABSENT:**

⇩

Perform CPR; Defibrillate if VF or pulseless VT (200 J, 300 J, 360 J); Intubate and establish IV access.

⇩

| **If temp <30°C** | ⇨ | Continue CPR. Do not administer IV medications. Limit shocks to 3. Provide active internal rewarming (options include warm IV fluids, warm humidified O2, lavage of peritoneum, stomach, bladder, or pleural cavity, and extracorporeal bypass). |

| **If temp >30°C** | ⇨ | Continue CPR. Administer meds at longer intervals. Provide active internal rewarming (options include warm IV fluids, warm humidified O2, lavage of peritoneum, stomach, bladder, or pleural cavity, and extracorporeal bypass). |

> **IF PULSE AND BREATHING ARE PRESENT:**

⇩

| **If Temp 34-36°C (Mild)** | ⇨ | Passive rewarming (remove wet clothes; give blankets); active external rewarming (heated blankets). |

| **If Temp 30-34°C (Moderate)** | ⇨ | Passive rewarming; actively rewarm truncal areas only. |

| **If Temp <30°C (Severe)** | ⇨ | Active internal rewarming (options include warm IV fluids, warm humidified O2, lavage of peritoneum, stomach, bladder, or pleural cavity, and extracorporeal bypass). |

III. A: *PEDIATRIC ALS*: <u>BRADYCARDIA</u>

•<u>BRADYCARDIA</u>•

Assess and stabilize the airway. Administer oxygen.

⇩

If bradycardia is causing poor perfusion, hypotension, respiratory difficulty, or altered mental status:

⇩

Ventilate with 100% O2.

⇩

Start chest compressions if heart rate <60 beats/min and poor perfusion despite oxygenation and ventilation.

⇩

Epinephrine 0.01 mg/kg (1:10,000, 0.1 ml/kg) IV/IO; or 0.1 mg/kg (1:1000, 0.1 ml/kg) endotracheal. Repeat same dose every 3-5 min.

⇩

Atropine 0.02 mg/kg (minimum dose 0.1 mg; max 0.5 mg for child, 1 mg for adolescent). May repeat once.

⇩

Consider pacing.

• Consider epinephrine or dopamine infusions.
• Identify and treat possible causes: hypoxemia; hypothermia; head injury; heart block; toxins.

III. B: *PEDIATRIC ALS*: <u>ASYSTOLE/PEA</u>

•<u>ASYSTOLE/PULSELESS ELECTRICAL ACTIVITY</u>•

Perform CPR. Establish IV access and administer oxygen. Secure the airway and hyperventilate.

⇩

Consider possible etiologies: hypoxia; acidosis; hypovolemia; hyperkalemia; pulmonary embolism; cardiac tamponade; hypothermia; tension pneumothorax; overdose.

⇩

Epinephrine, first dose: 0.01 mg/kg (1:10,000, 0.1 ml/kg) IV/IO; or 0.1 mg/kg (1:1000, 0.1 ml/kg) endotracheal.

⇩

Epinephrine, second and subsequent doses: Dose as above, or consider 0.1 mg/kg (1:1000, 0.1 ml/kg) IV/IO/ET. May repeat every 3-5 minutes.

III. C. *PEDIATRIC ALS*: <u>TACHYCARDIA</u>

Provide oxygen and ventilation as needed. Assess circulation.

⇩

Evaluate QRS duration.

⇩

If narrow QRS (<0.08 sec)

⇩

If probable SVT:

⇩

Consider vagal maneuvers.

⇩

If **poor perfusion**, perform immediate cardioversion with 0.5-2.0 J/kg or immediate **Adenosine** 0.1 mg/kg IV/IO (max 6 mg); may double and repeat dose.

If **adequate perfusion**, consider **Adenosine** 0.1 mg/kg IV/IO (max 6 mg); may double and repeat dose. Consider cardioversion with 0.5-1.0 J/kg.

If wide QRS (>0.08 sec)

⇩

If probable ventricular tachycardia and **poor perfusion**, perform immediate cardioversion with 0.5-1.0 J/kg.

⇩

Consider **Amiodarone** 5 mg/kg IV over 20-60 min; or **Procainamide** 15 mg/kg IV over 30-60 min; or **Lidocaine** 1 mg/kg IV bolus.

If **adequate perfusion**, consider **Amiodarone** 5 mg/kg IV over 20-60 min; or **Procainamide** 15 mg/kg IV over 30-60 min; or **Lidocaine** 1 mg/kg IV bolus. Consider cardioversion with 0.5-1.0 J/kg.

Identify and treat possible causes, including hypoxia; acidosis; hypovolemia; hyperkalemia; pulmonary embolism; cardiac tamponade; hypothermia; tension pneumothorax; overdose.

III. D. *PEDIATRIC ALS*: <u>VF/PULSELESS VT</u>

•<u>VENTRICULAR FIBRILLATION/ PULSELESS VENTRICULAR TACHYCARDIA</u>•

Perform CPR. Establish IV access and administer oxygen. Secure the airway and hyperventilate.

⇩

Defibrillate up to 3 times with 2 J/kg, then 4 J/kg, then 4 J/kg.

⇩

Epinephrine, first dose: 0.01 mg/kg (1:10,000, 0.1 ml/kg) IV/IO; or 0.1 mg/kg (1:1000, 0.1 ml/kg) endotracheal.

⇩

Defibrillate with 4 J/kg 30-60 seconds after each medication.

⇩

Amiodarone 5 mg/kg bolus IV/IO or **Lidocaine** 1 mg/kg IV/IO/PT. **Magnesium** 25-50 mg/kg IV/IO (max 2 g) for Torsades de pointes or hypomagnesemia.

⇩

Epinephrine, second and subsequent doses: Dose as above, or consider 0.1 mg/kg (1:1000, 0.1 ml/kg) IV/IO/ET; may repeat every 3-5 minutes.

III. E. *PEDIATRIC* VITAL SIGNS

•<u>PEDIATRIC VITAL SIGNS</u>•

BLOOD PRESSURE (children 1-10 years of age):

<u>**Average Systolic Blood Pressure**</u>:
   90 mm Hg + (age of child in years x 2)

<u>**Lower Limits of Systolic Blood Pressure**</u>:
   70 mm Hg + (age of child in years x 2).

NORMAL HEART RATE (beats/min)

Newborn – 3 mon	85-205
3 mon – 2 years	100-190
2 years to 10 years	60-140
>10 years	60-100

NORMAL RESPIRATORY RATE (breaths/min)

Infant	30-60
Toddler	24-40
Preschooler	22-34
School age	18-30
Adolescent	12-16

III. F. *PEDIATRIC* RESUSCITATION SUPPLIES

Equipment	Newborn 3-5 kg	Infant 6-9 kg	Toddler 10-11 kg	Sm child 12-14 kg	Child 15-18 kg	Child 19-22 kg	Lg child 24-30 kg
Laryngo-scope	0-1 straight	1 straight	1 straight	2 straight	2 str. or curved	2 str. or curved	2-3 str. or curved
ET tube	3.0-3.5 uncuffed	3.5 uncuffed	4.0 uncuffed	4.5 uncuffed	5.0 uncuffed	5.5 uncuffed	6.0 cuffed
ETT length (cm at lip)	10-10.5	10-10.5	11-12	12.5-13.5	14-15	15.5-16.5	17-18
NG tube (F)	5-8	5-8	8-10	10	10-12	12-14	14-18
Urinary catheter (F)	5-8	5-8	8-10	10	10-12	10-12	12
Chest tube (F)	10-12	10-12	16-20	20-24	20-24	24-32	28-32

IV. A. *NEONATAL* RESUSCITATION

Assess infant for respirations, heart rate, and color. Assess for amniotic fluid. Provide warm environment and suction mouth and nose. If meconium is present and infant is depressed, use laryngoscope and suction hypopharynx and then intubate and suction trachea.

⇩

Stimulate infant with slaps to soles of feet and rubbing back.

⇩

If inadequate respirations or if heart rate < 100 beats/min, deliver positive pressure ventilation with 100% O2 for 15-30 seconds.

⇩

If heart rate <60 bpm: Continue ventilations; start chest compressions. **If heart rate >60 bpm:** Continue ventilations. If infant is pink, and heart rate > 100 bpm, assess for spontaneous respirations.

⇩

If heart rate < 60 bpm after 30 seconds of positive pressure ventilation and chest compressions (or if the initial heart rate is zero):

⇩

Epinephrine 0.01-0.03 mg/kg (0.1-0.3 ml/kg of a 1:10,000 solution) IV/IO or endotracheal. May repeat every 3-5 minutes.

⇩

Consider 10 ml/kg NS, RL, or O-negative blood if there is suspected acute blood loss (pallor, or faint pulses with heart rate > 100 bpm).

⇩

If documented hypoglycemia, administer **Glucose** 200 mg/kg (2 ml/kg of 10% dextrose) slow IV push. Consider **Sodium bicarbonate** 1-2 mEq/kg if prolonged arrest.

⇩

If continued depression, consider pneumothorax or diaphragmatic hernia. Consider **Dopamine**. Consider **Naloxone** 0.1 mg/kg IV/IO/ET.

IV. B. *NEONATAL* RESUSCITATION (cont.)
APGAR SCORING

Sign	0	1	2
Heart Rate	Absent	< 100 bpm	> 100 bpm
Respirations	Absent	Slow, irregular	Good, crying
Muscle Tone	Limp	Some flexion	Active motion
Reflex Irritability	No response	Grimace	Cough, cry
Color	Blue or pale	Pink body, blue ext.	Completely pink

ENDOTRACHEAL TUBE AND LARYNGOSCOPE

Gestational Age (weeks)	Weight (g)	ETT (mm)	Insertion depth (cm from lip)	Laryngoscope
< 28	< 1000	2.5	6.5-7	Miller 0
28-34	1000-2000	3.0	7-8	Miller 0
34-38	2000-3000	3.5	8-9	Miller 0
> 38	> 3000	3.5-4.0	> 9	Miller 1

TERM NEWBORN VITAL SIGNS

Heart Rate (awake):	100-180 bpm
Respiratory Rate:	30-60 breaths/min
Systolic Blood Pressure:	39-59 mm Hg
Diastolic Blood Pressure:	16-36 mm Hg

V. METRIC CONVERSIONS

I. Volume
1 teaspoon = 5 ml
1 tablespoon = 15 ml
1 fluid ounce = 30 ml
1 cup = 240 ml
1 pint = 473 ml
1 quart = 946 ml

II. Length
1 inch = 2.54 cm
1 cm = 0.394 inch

III. Weight
1 grain = 64.8 mg
1 ounce = 28.4 gm
1 pound = 0.454 kg
1 kilogram = 2.2 lb

IV. Temperature
$T(F) = (9/5) * T(C) + 32$
$T(C) = (5/9) * (T(F) - 32)$

TEMP

C	F
40.6	105.1
40.4	104.7
40.2	104.3
40.0	104.0
39.8	103.7
39.6	103.3
39.4	102.9
39.2	102.6
39.0	102.2
38.8	101.8
38.6	101.5
38.4	101.2
38.2	100.8
38.0	100.4
37.8	100.1
37.6	99.7
37.4	99.3
37.2	99.0
37.0	98.6
36.0	96.8
35.0	95.0
34.0	93.2
33.0	91.4
32.0	89.6
31.0	87.8
30.0	86.0
29.0	85.2
28.0	82.4
27.0	80.6

WEIGHT

Kg	lbs
125	275
120	264
115	253
110	242
105	231
100	220
95	209
90	198
85	187
80	176
75	165
70	154
65	143
60	132
55	121
50	110
45	99
40	88
35	77
30	66
25	55
20	44
15	33
10	22
7	15
5	11
3	6.6
2	4.4
1	2.2

VI. NORMAL LAB VALUES

<u>Hematology</u>		<u>Coagulation</u>
WBC	4.5-11x10⁹/L	
RBC	4.5-6.3x10¹²/L	
Hemoglobin	14-17 g/dL	
Hematocrit	42-52%	
MCV	83-97	
MCH	27-31 pg/cell	
MCHC	32-36 g/dL	
Neutrophils	54-75%	
Bands	3-8%	
Lymphocytes	20-40%	
Monocytes	2-8%	
Eosinophils	1-4%	
Basophils	0.5-1%	
Platelets	130K-400K	

	<u>Coagulation</u>	
PT (prothrombin time)	10-30 s
aPTT	22-34 s
Fibrinogen	200-400 mg/dL
Fibrin split products	<10 mg/L
Plasminogen	65-125%

<u>Chemistry</u>		<u>Cardiac Enzymes</u>	
Sodium	136-145 mEq/L	CPK	18-209 U/L
Potassium	3.5-5.5 mEq/L	CK-M	0-4.1 ng/ml
Chloride	95-107 mEq/L	CK-MB	0-1.9
CO2	20-28 mEq/L	(relative index)	
BUN	7-21 mg/dL	Troponin	<1.5 ng/ml
Creatine	0.7-1.2 mg/dL	Myoglobin	<110 ng/ml
Glucose	65-110 mg/dL		
Calcium	8.5-10.6 mg/dL		
Magnesium	1.3-2.1 mEq/L		
Amylase	50-150 U/L		
Bilirubin total	0.2-1.3 mg/dL		
Bilirubin direct	0.1-0.3 mg/dL		
Bilirubin indirect	0.2-0.7 mg/dL		
ALT	<48 U/L		
AST	<42 U/L		

A

Abdominal aortic aneurysm 10–11

Abdominal pain
Differential diagnosis 106

Abdominal trauma 380–383
Blunt injury 380–382
Penetrating injury 382–383

Abortion, spontaneous 227–230

Abruption, placental 224–225

Abscess
Anorectal 107

Acetaminophen, toxicity 338–339

Achilles tendon rupture 244
Treatment 246

Acid ingestions 347–348

Acid-base disorders 183–184

Acidosis, metabolic 183

ACLS protocols
Asystole 414
Atrial fibrillation 415
Bradycardia 418
Hypothermia 420
Narrow complex tachycardia 416
PEA 413
Pulmonary edema 419
Pulseless electrical activity 413
Ventricular fibrillation 412
Ventricular tachycardia, pulseless 412
Ventricular tachycardia, stable 417

Activated charcoal
in poisoning 334–335

Acute chest syndrome 148
Treatment 149

Acute coronary syndromes 37–47

Acute mountain sickness 88

Acute myocardial infarction 37–47

Acute renal failure 322

Adrenal insufficiency 61–62

Airway obstruction 411

Alcohol
Complications 358
Hepatitis 358
Ketoacidosis 358
Wernicke's 359
Intoxication 356
Seizures 357–358
Withdrawal 356–357

Alkali ingestions 347–348

Alkalosis, metabolic 183

Allergic contact dermatitis 57

Allergic reactions 1–4

Altered mental status
In the elderly 190–191

Alternative airway
Options 8–9

Amphetamines, toxicity 340–341

Amputations, hand 250–251

Anal fissure 107

Analgesia
in pediatrics 275

Anaphylaxis 1–2

Aneurysm

Abdominal aortic 10–11
Angina, unstable 46–47
Angioedema 3–4
Animal bites 71
Anion gap
    Definition 183
    Etiology 183
Ankle injuries 244–246
Anorectal abscess 107
Anterior cord syndrome 400
Anterior subluxation, cervical 398
Anthrax 95–96
Anticholinergics, toxicity 341–342
Aortic aneurysm, abdominal 10–13
Aortic dissection 11–13
Aortic rupture 404
Apgar scoring 428
Aplastic crisis 148
Appendicitis 108–110
Arrhythmias
    Atrial fibrillation 13
    Multifocal atrial tachycardia 15–16
    Paroxysmal atrial tachycardia 16
    PSVT 16–17
    Ventricular bigeminy 17–18
    Ventricular tachycardia 18
        Distinguishing from SVT 18
Arthritis
    Septic 264
Arthritis, acute 331–332
    Reactive 331
    Reiter's 331

Septic 332
Aspiration pneumonia 166
Asthma 323–324
Asystole
    ACLS protocols 414
    Pediatric ALS protocols 422
Atrial fibrillation 13–15
    ACLS protocols 415

B

Back pain 259–262
Bacterial vaginosis 171
Barotrauma of ascent 81
Barotrauma of descent 80
Barton fracture 249
Basic life support
    Airway obstruction 411
    CPR 410
    Foreign body 411
    Rescue breathing 410
Bell's palsy 191–192
Benign positional vertigo 215–216
Bennet's fracture 252
Benzodiazepines, toxicity 342–343
Beta blockers, toxicity 343–344
Bezold-Jarisch reflex 213
Bilateral interfacetal dislocation 398
Biological warfare agents 94–99
    Anthrax 95–96
    Botulinium toxin 96
    Plague 96–97
    Ricin 97
    Smallpox 97–98
    Tularemia 98–99
    Viral hemorrhagic fevers 99

Bites
  Animal 71
  Human 72–73
Blepharitis 237
Blood products 142
  Cryoprecipitate 142
  Fresh frozen plasma 142
  Packed RBCs 142
  Platelets 142
Botulinim toxin 96
BPV 215–216
Bradycardia
  ACLS protocols 418
  Pediatric ALS protocols 421
Breath holding in children 285
Breech delivery 219
Bronchiolitis 293–294
Bronchitis, in COPD 328
Brown-Sequard syndrome 400
Brugada rules 19
Bullous myringitis 304
Bundle branch blocks 31–32
Burns 74–76
Burst fracture 401

C

Calcaneal fracture 247
Calcium channel blockers,
    toxicity 344–345
Calcium disorders 184–185
  Hypercalcemia 184–185
  Hypocalcemia 185
Candida diaper dermatitis 285
Carbon monoxide, toxicity 345–
    347
Cardiac tamponade 50
Cardiomyopathy 21–22

Dilated 21
  Hypertrophic 21–22
  Restrictive 22
Cat scratch disease 72
Cathartics
  in poisoning 334
Cauda equina syndrome 261
Caustic ingestions 347–348
Cellulitis 151–152
  Orbital 231–232
  Periorbital 231
Central cord syndrome 400
Central vertigo 216
Cerebral edema, high altitude 88
Cerebrovascular accident. See
    Stroke
Cervical spine trauma 396–400
  Injuries 398–399
  X-ray 397
Chalazion 237
CHAMP toxins 364
Chancroid 171
Chemical warfare agents 99–
    101
  Mustards 100
  Nerve agents 100–101
Chicken pox 310–314
Childbirth. See Delivery
Chlamydia
  in PID 169–171
  pneumonia in children 306
  Pneumoniae 168
Chloral hydrate
  in pediatric sedation 275
Cholangitis 117–118
Cholecystitis 118–119
Cholelithiasis 119–120
Cholinergics, toxicity 348–349

Ciguatera 114
Clay shoveler's fracture 399
Cluster headache 193
   Treatment 195
CMV 155
COBRA 181–182
Cocaine, toxicity 349–351
Cold illness
   Frostbite 77–78
   Hypothermia 78–80
Colles fracture 249
Concussion 386
Condylar fracture 255
Congenital heart disease
   in children 280–282
Congestive heart failure 22–25
   in children 282–283
Conjunctivitis 232–233
   in newborn 294
Constipation 110
   in children 284–285
Constrictive pericarditis 50
COPD 328–330
Corneal abrasion 233–234
Coumadin, toxicity 379
CPR 410
Cricothyroidotomy 8
Crohn's disease 124–125
Croup 294–296
Cryoprecipitate 142
Cryptococcus 155
CVA. *See* Stroke
Cyanide, toxicity 351–353
Cyanosis
   in children 285

D

Decompression sickness 81–82
Decreased vision 234
Deep venous thrombosis 26–29
   of upper extremity 28
Delirium 190
Delivery procedure 218
   Breech 219
   Shoulder dystocia 218–219
Dementia 190
Dental conditions
   Fractures 55
   Infection 55
   Post-extraction 55
   Subluxation/avulsion 56
DeQuervain's tenosynovitis 273
Dermatitis, allergic contact 57
Diabetic ketoacidosis 62–64
Diaper dermatitis 285
Diarrhea 111–114
   Invasive infections 112–113
   Toxigenic infections 113–114
Digital method (intubation) 8
Digoxin, toxicity 353–354
Diplopia 235
Dislocation
   Acromioclavicular 269
   Anterior shoulder 269–270
   Bilateral interfacetal 398
   Elbow 255
   Hand 251
   Hip 267
   Inferior shoulder 270
   Knee 258
   Lunate 273
   Perilunate 273
   Posterior shoulder 269

Unilateral interfacetal 399
Diverticulitis 114–115
Diverticulosis 116
DKA. *See* Diabetic ketoacidosis
Drowning 89–90
Duodenal ulcer. *See* Peptic ulcer disease
DVT. *See* Deep venous thrombosis
Dysbarism 80–82
    Barotrauma of ascent 81
    Barotrauma of descent 80
    Decompression sickness 81–82
Dysfunctional uterine bleeding 220
Dysphagia 116–117

E

ECG diagnosis
    AV-Block 30–31
    Bundle branch blocks 31–32
    Evidence of ischemia 34
    Hypertrophy 32–33
    Normal Values 30
Eclampsia 226–227
Ecstasy, toxicity 355–356
Ectopic pregnancy 222–224
Effusion, pericardial 50–51
Elbow injuries 254–256
    Dislocation 255
Electrical injury 82–84
Electrocution. *See* Electrical injury
Emphysema 328
EMTALA 181–182
Encephalitis, viral 158
Endocarditis 152–153

Epididymitis 135–136
Epidural hematoma 386–387
Epiglottitis 296–297
Episcleritis 240
Epistaxis 68–69
Epley maneuver 216–217
Erysipelas 151–152
Erythema infectiosum 297
Erythema multiforme 57–59
Ethanol, toxicity 356–359
Ethylene glycol, toxicity 359–361
Extension teardrop fracture 399
External otitis. *See* Otitis externa
Eye disorders. *See* Ophthalmologic disorders

F

Febrile child 290–293
Febrile seizures 318–319
Felon 252
Fibrinolytic therapy
    in myocardial infarction 43
    in stroke 207
Fifth disease 297
Fishhooks (removal) 102
Fitz-Hugh-Curtis syndrome 170
Flail chest 404
Flexion teardrop fracture 398
Flexor tendon injuries 254
Food poisoning 111–114
Foot injuries 246–248
Forearm injuries 248–250
Foreign body removal 102–105
    Cutaneous 102–103
    Ear 103
    Gastrointestinal 103–104

Nasal 104–105
Respiratory 105
Fractures
Ankle 245
Barton 249
Bennet's 252
Bimalleolar 245
Burst 401
Calcaneal 247
Clay shoveler's 399
Colles 249
Condylar 255
Extension teardrop 399
Fibular shaft 245
Fifth metatarsal 246
Flexion teardrop 398
Galeazi 249
Greenstick 262
Hangman's 399
Hill-Sachs 270
Hip 267
Humerus 256
Hutchinson 249
Jefferson 399
Jones 247
Knee 258
Lateral malleolus 245
Lisfranc's 247
Maisoneuve 245
Mandible 388
Metacarpal 252
Metatarsal 247
Midface 388
Monteggia 249
Nasal bone 388
Nightstick 249
Odontoid 399
Olecranon 256

Pelvis 266
Phalanx 251
Pilon 245
Radial head 256
Rolando 252
Scaphoid 274
Smith 249
Supracondylar 255
Talus 247
Tibial shaft 245
Toddler 263
Torus 263
Vertebral burst 399
Wedge compression
Cervical 399
Thoracolumbar 401
Fresh frozen plasma 142
Frostbite 77–78
Fulminant colitis 126

G

Galeazi fracture 249
Gallbladder disease 117–120
Cholangitis 117–118
Cholecystitis 118–119
Cholelithiasis 119–120
Gamekeeper's thumb 253
Gamma-hydroxy butyrate,
toxicity 361–362
Gastric lavage
in poisoning 335
Gastric ulcer. See Peptic ulcer
disease
Gastritis 129–130
Gastroenteritis
in children 287–288
Gastroesophageal reflux 120

Gastrointestinal bleed 120–122
Genitourinary trauma 392–395
GHB, toxicity 361–362
GI bleed 120–122
Glasgow coma scale 383
Glaucoma 236–237
Globe rupture 241
Gout 332–333
Greenstick fracture 262
Group B strep pneumonia 306
Guillain-Barre syndrome 192–
    193

H

H. pylori 130
Hallpike test 215
Hand, foot and mouth disease
    297
Hand injuries 250–254
Hangman's fracture 399
Head trauma 383–387
    Concussion 386
    Epidural hematoma 386–387
    Subdural hematoma 387
Headache 193–196
    Cluster 193
        Treatment 195
    Migraine 193–194
        Treatment 195
    Temporal arteritis 194
        Treatment 196
    Tension-type 194
        Treatment 196
Heat illness 85–88
    Heat cramps 85
    Heat exhaustion 85–86
    Heat stroke 86–88

HELLP syndrome 226
Hematoma, epidural 386–387
Hematoma, subdural 387
Hemolytic-uremic syndrome
    288–289
Hemophilia 142–144
Hemorrhagic fevers 99
Hemorrhagic stroke 205
    Treatment 206
Hemorrhoids 107–108
Hemothorax 405
Henoch-Schonlein purpura 289–
    290
Hepatitis 122–123
Herniated disk 260–261
Herpes zoster 153–154
HIINK 64–65
High altitude medicine 88–89
    Acute mountain sickness 88
    High altitude cerebral edema
        88
    High altitude pulmonary
        edema 89
Hill-Sachs fracture 270
Hip injuries 265–268
HIV
    CNS disease 154–155
        Cryptococcus 155
        Toxoplasmosis 155
    Drug reactions 156
    Ophthalmologic disease 155
        CMV 155
    Pulmonary disease 155–156
        PCP 156
Hordeolum (stye) 237
Human bites 72–73
Human papilloma virus 171
Humerus injuries 254–256

Hunt and Hess classification 210
Hutchinson fracture 249
Hypercalcemia 184–185
Hyperglycemic hyperosmolar non-ketotic coma 64–65
Hyperkalemia 185–187
Hypernatremia 188
Hypertensive crisis 36–37
Hyperthyroidism 65–66
Hypocalcemia 185
Hypokalemia 187–188
Hyponatremia 188–189
Hypothermia 78–80
    ACLS protocols 420
Hypothyroidism 66–67

I

Impetigo 297–298
Infectious disease
    Cellulitis 151–152
    Diarrhea 111–114
    Endocarditis 152–153
    Epididymitis 135–136
    Herpes zoster 153–154
    HIV illnesses 154–156
    Influenza 156–158
    Lyme disease 175–176
    Meningitis 158–160
    Otitis externa 160–161
    Pediatrics 290–311
    Pharyngitis 161
    Pneumonia 162–168
    Pyelonephritis 179–180
    Rheumatic fever 168–169
    Rocky mountain spotted fever 176–177
    Sexually transmitted diseases 169–173
    Sinusitis 173–174
    Tetanus 174–175
    Urinary tract infection 177–179
    Zoster 153–154
Inflammatory bowel disease 124–126
    Complications 126
    Crohn's disease 124–125
    Ulcerative colitis 125–126
Influenza 156–158
Inhalants, toxicity 362–364
Inhalation injury 76–77
Intubation
    Nasotracheal 9
    Procedure in adults 5–8
    Procedure in children 277–280
    Retrograde 9
Intussusception 311–312
Ipecac
    in poisoning 335
Iritis 242–243
Iron, toxicity 364
Ischemia
    Mesenteric 126–128
    Myocardial 37–47
Ischemic stroke 204
    treatment 206
Isopropyl alcohol, toxicity 366–367

J

Janeway lesions 153
Jaundice 124

in children 312–313
Jefferson fracture 399
Jones criteria 169
Jones fracture 247

K

Kawasaki disease 298
Ketamine
  in adult intubation 6
  in pediatric intubation 279
  in pediatric sedation 275
Kidney stones. *See* Nephrolithiasis
Knee injuries 256–259

L

Lab values, normal 430
Lachman test 257
Laryngotracheobronchitis 294–296
Lead, toxicity 367–368
Legal issues 181–182
  COBRA 181–182
  EMTALA 181–182
Legg-Calve-Perthes disease 263
Legionnaire's disease 168
Lice 59–60
Lid disorders 237–238
Ligament injuries
  Hand 253
  Knee 258
Lightning 84–85
Lisfranc's fracture 247
Lithium, toxicity 368–369
Low back pain 259–262
Lunate dislocation 273
Luxatio erecta 270

Lyme disease 175–176
Lymphadenitis 298–299
Lymphogranuloma venereum 172

M

Maisoneuve fracture 245
Mallet finger 253
Mandible fracture 388
Maxillofacial trauma 387–389
McMurray test 257
Measles 299
Meniere's disease 216
Meningitis
  in adults 158–160
  in children 299–302
Meniscal injuries 258
Mesenteric ischemia 126–128
Metabolic acidosis 183
Metabolic alkalosis 183
Metacarpal fractures 252
Metatarsal fractures 247
Methanol, toxicity 369–371
Methemoglobinemia 371–372
Metric conversions 429
Midface fracture 388
Migraine 193–194
  Treatment 195
Mononucleosis 302
Monteggia fracture 249
Multifocal atrial tachycardia 15–16
Multiple sclerosis 196–197
Mustards 100
Myasthenia gravis 197–198
Mycoplasma
  Pneumonia in children 307

Mycoplasma pneumoniae 168
Myocardial contusion 404
Myocardial infarction 37–47
    and LBBB 45
    ECG correlation 39
    Fibrinolytic therapy 43–44
    PCI 43
    Posterior infarction 46
    Right ventricle infarction 46
Myocarditis 47
Myxedema coma 67

N

Nail injuries 253
Nasal fracture 388
Nasotracheal intubation 9
Near drowning 89–90
Neck trauma 389–390
    Blunt injury 389–390
    Penetrating injury 390
Neonatal resuscitation 427
Nephrolithiasis 137–140
Nerve agents (warfare) 100–101
Neurocardiogenic syncope 212–
    213
Neurogenic shock 400
Neutropenic fever 144–145
Newborn vital signs 428
Nightstick fracture 249
Nursemaid's elbow 264
Nylen-Barany test 215

O

Occult bacteremia
    in children 290
Odontoid fracture 399
Olecranon fracture 256

Omphalitis 303
Oncologic emergencies 144–146
    Neutropenic fever 144–145
    Spinal cord compression
        145–146
    Superior vena cava syndrome
        146
Open globe. *See* Globe rupture
Ophthalmologic disorders
    Blepharitis 237
    Cellulitis
        Orbital 231–232
        Periorbital (preseptal) 231
    Chalazion 237
    Conjunctivitis 232–233
    Corneal abrasion 233–234
    Decreased vision 234
    Diplopia 235
    Glaucoma 236–237
    Hordeolum 237
    Iritis 242–243
    Lid disorders
        Blepharitis 237
        Chalazion 237
        Hordeolum (stye) 237
    Medications 235–236
    Painful eye 235
    Retinal artery occlusion 238–
        239
    Retinal detachment 239–240
    Scleritis 240
    Trauma
        Globe rupture 241
        Lid lacerations 241–242
        Orbital fractures 242
    Uveitis 242–243
Orbital cellulitis 231–234
Orbital fractures 242

Orthopedic injuries
  Achilles tendon 244
  Ankle injuries 244–246
  Elbow injuries 254–256
  Foot injuries 246–248
  Forearm injuries 248–250
  Hand injuries 250–254
  Hip injuries 265–268
  Humerus injuries 254–256
  Knee injuries 256–259
  Low back pain 259–262
  Patellar 259
  Pediatrics 262
  Pelvis injuries 265–268
  Shoulder injuries 268–272
  Wrist injuries 272–274
Orthostatic hypotension 213
Osgood-Schlatter disease 263
Osler nodes 153
Osmol gap
  Definition 183
  Etiology 183
Osteomyelitis 303
Otitis externa 160–161
Otitis media 303–305
  with effusion 304
Ottowa rules
  for ankle 244
  for foot 246
  for knee 257

P

Packed RBCs 142
Painful eye 235
PALS. *See* Pediatric ALS
Pancreatitis 128–129
Panic disorder 320–321

Paroxysmal atrial tachycardia 16
Patellar injuries 259
PCP 156
PEA
  ACLS protocols 413
  Pediatric ALS protocols 422
Pediatric ALS
  Asystole 422
  Bradycardia 421
  PEA 422
  Pulseless ventricular tachycardia 424
  Tachycardia 423
  Ventricular fibrillation 424
Pediatric resuscitation supplies 426
Pediatric trauma 391–392
Pediatric Vital Signs 425
Pediatrics
  Analgesia/sedation 275
  Asthma 323–324
  Cardiovascular 280–284
    Congenital heart disease 280–282
    Congestive heart failure 282–283
    SVT 283–284
  Constipation 284–285
  Cyanosis 285
  Dermatology 285–287
    Diaper dermatitis 285
    Seborrheic dermatitis 286
    Tinea capitis 286–287
    Tinea corporis 287
  Gastroenteritis 287–288
  Hemolytic-uremic syndrome 288–289

Henoch-Schonlein purpura 289–290
Infectious disease 290–311
Intussusception 311–312
Jaundice 312–313
Metabolic requirements 313
Reye's syndrome 313–314
Seizures 314–319
Febrile seizures 318–319
Sickle cell disease 146–149
Stridor 319
Pediculosis 59
Pelvic inflammatory disease 169–171
Pelvis injuries 265–268
Pelvis trauma 392–395
Blunt injury 392–394
Penetrating injury 394–395
Peptic ulcer disease 129–130
Pericardial effusion 50–51
Pericarditis 49–50
Constrictive 50
Perilunate dislocation 273
Periorbital cellulitis 231
Peripheral vertigo 215–216
Peritonsillar abscess 69–70
in children 307–308
Pertussis 164, 307
Pharyngitis 161–162
Phlegmasia alba dolens 29
Phlegmasia cerulea dolens 29
Photophobia 235
PID 169–171
Pilon fracture 245
Pityriasis rosea 305
Placenta previa 225–226
Placental abruption 224–225
Plague 96–97

Platelets 142
Pneumonia 162–168
Aspiration 166
Chlamydia 168
H. flu 166
in children 305–307
Chlamydia 306
Group B strep 306
Mycoplasma 307
Pertussis 307
Klebsiella 166
Legionnaire's disease 168
M. catarrhalis 167
Mycoplasma 168
Pseudomonas 167
S. aureus 167
S. pneumoniae 167
Tuberculosis 167
Pneumothorax 405
Poison ivy 57
Poisons/antidotes 372
Post-partum hemorrhage 219–220
Posterior myocardial infarction 46
Potassium disorders 185–188
Hyperkalemia 185–187
Hypokalemia 187–188
Preeclampsia 226–227
Pregnancy
and trauma 395–396
Delivery 218
Ectopic 222–224
Post-partum hemorrhage 219–220
Pseudoseizures 203
PSVT 16–17
Psychiatry

Panic disorder 320–321
Psychosis 320–321
Psychosis 320–321
Pulmonary contusion 405–406
Pulmonary edema
    ACLS protocols 419
    High altitude 89
Pulmonary embolus 51–54
Pulseless electrical activity
    ACLS protocols 413
    Pediatric ALS protocols 422
Puncture wounds 102
Pyelonephritis 179–180
    in children 309–310

R

Rabies 73–74
Radial head fracture 256
Radial head subluxation 264
Radiation injuries 90–92
Ramsey-Hunt 191
Rapid sequence intubation. *See*
    Intubation
Reactive arthritis 331
Reflux, gastroesophageal 120
Reiter's syndrome 331
Renal failure 322
Respiratory
    Asthma 323–324
    COPD 328–330
Retention, urinary 140
Retinal artery occlusion 238–239
Retinal detachment 239–240
Retrograde intubation 9
Retropharyngeal abscess 307–308

Reye's syndrome 313–314
RH sensitization 229
Rheumatic fever 168–169
Rheumatology
    Acute arthritis 331–332
    Gout 332–333
Ricin 97
Right ventricle infarction 46
Rings (removal) 102
Ringworm. *See* Tinea corporis
Rocky mountain spotted fever
    176–177
Rolando fracture 252
Roseola 308–309
Rubeola 299

S

Salicylates, toxicity 373–374
Salter-Harris classification 262
Scabies 59–60
Scaphoid fracture 274
Scapholunate dissociation 274
SCIWORA 399
Scleritis 240
Scombroid 114
Seborrheic dermatitis
    in children 286
Sedation
    in pediatrics 275
Seizures 198–203
    Alcohol 357–358
    Febrile 318–319
    Generalized 198–199
    in children 314–319
    Partial (focal) 199
    Pseudoseizures 203
Septic arthritis 264, 332

Serotonin syndrome 374–375
Sexual assault, prophylaxis after
172–173
Sexually transmitted diseases
169–173
    Bacterial vaginosis 171
    Chancroid 171
    Chlamydia 169–171
    Human papilloma virus 171
    Lymphogranuloma venereum
        172
    N. gonorrhea 169–171
    Syphilis 172
    Trichomonas 172
    Vaginal candidiasis 172
Shellfish poisoning
    Neurotoxic 114
    Paralytic 114
Shoulder dystocia- delivery
    218–219
Shoulder injuries 268–272
Sickle cell disease 146–149
Sinusitis 173–174
Slipped capital femoral epiphysis
    264–265
Small bowel obstruction 131–
    132
Smallpox 97–98
Smith fracture 249
Snakebites 92–94
Sodium disorders 188–189
    Hypernatremia 188
    Hyponatremia 188–189
Spinal cord compression 145–
    146
Spinal cord injury syndromes
    400
    Anterior cord 400

Brown-Sequard 400
Central cord 400
Neurogenic shock 400
Spinal shock 400
Spinal shock 400
Spinal trauma 396–402
    Cervical spine 396–400
    Cord injury syndromes 400
    Thoracolumbar 400–402
Splenic sequestration crisis 148
Splinters (removal) 103
Spontaneous abortion 227–230
    RH sensitization 229
Status epilepticus
    in adults 201–202
    treatment in children 316
STDs 169–173
Stevens-Johnson Syndrome 57–
    59
Stingers (removal) 103
Stokes-Adams attacks 212
Strep throat. See Pharyngitis
Stridor 319
Stroke 203–208
    Fibrinolytic therapy 207–208
    Hemorrhagic stroke
        syndromes 205
    Ischemic stroke syndromes
        204
Stye 237
Subarachnoid hemorrhage 209–
    212
Subdural hematoma 387
Sulfonylureas, toxicity 375–376
Sunburn 60
Superior vena cava syndrome
    146
Supracondylar fracture 255

Supraglottitis. *See* Epiglottitis
SVT, in children 283–284
Syncope 212–215
Synovitis, transient 265
Syphilis 172

T

Tachycardia
    Multifocal atrial 15–16
    Paroxysmal atrial 16
    Paroxysmal supraventricular
      16–17
    Pediatric ALS protocols 423
    Ventricular 18
Talus fracture 247
Tamponade, cardiac 50
Temporal arteritis 194
    Treatment 196
Tendon injuries 253
Tenosynovitis 253
    DeQuervain's 273
Tension-type headache 194
    Treatment 196
Testicular torsion 136–137
Tet spells 282
Tetanus 174–175
    Wound management 175
Theophylline, toxicity 376–377
Thompson test 244
Thoracic trauma 402–407
    Blunt injury 402–406
      Aortic rupture 404
      Flail chest 404
      Hemothorax 405
      Myocardial contusion 404
      Pneumothorax 405
      Pulmonary contusion
        405–406

    Penetrating injury 406–407
Thoracolumbar trauma 400–402
    Injuries 401
Thrombophlebitis, superficial 28
Thrombotic thrombocytopenic
      purpura 149–150
Thyroid storm 66
TIA 208–209
Tick-borne illnesses 175–177
    Lyme disease 175–176
    Rocky mountain spotted fever
      176–177
Tinea capitis
    in children 286–287
Tinea corporis
    in children 287
Toddler fracture 263
Torsades de Pointes 19
Torsion
    Appendix testes 137
    Testicular 136–137
Torus fracture 263
Toxic megacolon 126
Toxicology
    Acetaminophen 338–339
    Amphetamines 340–341
    Anticholinergics 341–342
    Benzodiazepines 342–343
    Beta blockers 343–344
    Calcium channel blockers
      344–345
    Carbon monoxide 345–347
    Caustic ingestions 347–348
    Cholinergics 348–349
    Cocaine 349–351
    Coumadin 379
    Cyanide 351–353
    Differential diagnosis 336–

338
  Digoxin 353–354
  Ecstasy 355–356
  Ethanol 356–359
  Ethylene glycol 359–361
  General approach 334
  GHB 361–362
  Hemodialyzable toxins 335–
    338
  Hemoperfusable toxins 335
  Inhalants 362–364
  Interventions 334–335
  Iron 364–366
  Isopropyl alcohol 366–367
  Lead 367–368
  Lithium 368–369
  Methanol 369–371
  Methemoglobinemia 371–
    372
  Poisons/antidotes 372
  Salicylates 373–374
  Serotonin syndrome 374–375
  Sulfonylureas 375–376
  Theophylline 376–377
  Toxidromes 335–336, 335–
    338
  Tricyclics 377–378
  Warfarin 379
Toxidromes 335–338
Toxoplasmosis 155
Transient ischemic attack 208–
  209
Transient synovitis 265
Trauma
  Abdominal 380–383
    Blunt injury 380–382
    Penetrating injury 382–
      383

Genitourinary 392–395
Glasgow coma scale 383
Head 383–387
  Concussion 386
  Epidural hematoma 386–
    387
  Subdural hematoma 387
in pregnancy 395–396
Maxillofacial 387–389
Neck 389–390
  Blunt injury 389–390
  Penetrating injury 390
Pediatric 391–392
Pelvis 392–395
  Blunt injury 392–394
  Penetrating injury 394–
    395
Spinal 396–402
  Cervical 396–400
  Cord injury syndromes
    400
  Thoracolumbar 400–402
Thoracic 402–407
  Blunt injury 402–406
  Penetrating injury 406–
    407
Vascular 407–408
Trichomonas 172
Tricyclic antidepressants, toxicity
  377–378
Trigger finger 254
TTP 149–150
Tuberculosis 167
Tularemia 98–99

U

Ulcer, peptic 129–130

Ulcerative colitis 125–126
Unilateral interfacetal dislocation 399
Unstable angina 46–47
Urinary retention 140
Urinary tract infection 177–179
    in children 309–310
Urticaria 3–4
UTI 177–179
Uveitis 242–243

V

Vaginal candidiasis 172
Varicella 310–314
Vascular trauma 407–408
Vasovagal syncope 212–213
Ventricular bigeminy 17–18
Ventricular fibrillation
    ACLS protocols 412
    Pediatric ALS protocols 424
Ventricular tachycardia 18
Ventricular tachycardia, pulseless
    ACLS protocols 412
    Pediatric ALS protocols 424
Ventricular tachycardia, stable
    ACLS protocols 417
Vertebral burst fracture 399
Vertigo 215–217
    Benign positional 215–216
    Central 216
    Epley maneuver 216–217
    Peripheral 215–216
Viral encephalitis 158
Viral hemorrhagic fevers 99
Vital signs
    in children 425
    in newborns 428

Volvulus
    Cecal 132
    Sigmoid 132–133
Vomiting 133–134
Von Willebrand disease. *See*
    Hemophilia

W

Warfare
    Biological agents 94–99
        Anthrax 95–96
        Botulinim toxin 96
        Plague 96–97
        Ricin 97
        Smallpox 97–98
        Tularemia 98–99
        Viral hemorrhagic fevers 99
    Chemical agents 99–101
        Mustards 100
        Nerve agents 100–101
Warfarin, toxicity 379
Washed out syndrome 350
Wedge compression fracture
    Cervical 399
    Thoracolumbar 401
Wellen's syndrome 40
Wernicke's encephalopathy 359
Whole bowel irrigation
    in poisoning 335
Withdrawal, alcohol 356–357
WPW 20–21
Wrist injuries 272–274

Z

Zippers (removal) 103
Zoster 153–154

References

References include:

Tintanelli J. Emergency Medicine. McGraw-Hill; 1996.

Rosen P. Emergency Medicine. Mosby; 1998.

Stine, R, Chudnofsky, C. A Practical Approach to Emergency Medicine. Little, Brown, and Co; 1994.

Simon, R, Koenigknecht, S. Emergency Orthopedics. Appleton and Lange; 1995.

ACLS Guidelines

ATLS Guidelines

Emergency Medicine Reports

Annals of Emergency Medicine

Emergency Medicine for the Primary Care Physician

Emedicine.com